MW00513713

CONTENTS

INTRODUCTION

The Keto diet is the solution you've always been waiting for.

Here's to shedding weight effortlessly; optimizing your health; and unleashing your inner athlete. The Keto diet will transform your life!

Yes, I know...

These sound like outlandish claims. I'd be the first to agree that I start to sound like some crazy infomercial when I start talking about the Keto diet. But it's not my fault; Keto made me do it!

Jokes aside though, I have real reasons to be this excited; I reaped a ton of benefits.

Bear with me as I take you down a few years of memory lane.

I was in my senior year at college, juggling multiple jobs to keep myself financially afloat; and I was sick. Not sick with a terrible virus but sick not to be as bouncy as I ought to be.

Sick to the bone! Exhausted, overweight, sluggish, depressed, still struggling with acne, and extremely worried about my ever-increasing waistline.

You see, I wasn't your stereotypical college kid. I didn't have terrible eating habits, at least I didn't think I did; I'd always been careful with my diet. Despite my crazy sweet tooth, and my passionate love for cream (mmmm), I'd listened to the health authorities.

I'd stuck to zero-fat foods. Opted for the "diet" versions of foods when available. Tried to live on low-fat pasta dishes, 'slimming' menus of limp boiled fish, boiled potatoes and mushy boiled vegetables. I'd forgone my favorite foods because I was told that healthy people didn't eat those. I was stuck to the foods I hated just because that's what I was told was healthy.

...But, the weight just kept piling on.

So, I slashed my portion sizes. I started to skip meals. I went utterly zero fat. I tried to ignore the fact that my food tasted bland, unappetizing and, at times, even horrible. In my head, it was worth it, so I kept encouraging myself, but my body kept ballooning. Up another clothing size. And another and another.

Would it ever end?...

WHAT IS THE KETO DIET?

Let me cut straight to the chase.

Simply, the Keto diet termed a "low-carb" diet burns fuel from fat in the body instead of carbohydrates. It allows you to shed weight efficiently, enjoy an endless source of energy and carves the body into the best state of health both physically and mentally.

Unlike many other low carb diets, you don't stuff yourself with processed foods, unhealthy fried foods (hello Atkins) and all the junk your body craves, which you know are bad for you.

It is about eating whole foods, which are, as close to their pure state as possible, just like nature intended. It is going back to the basics and enjoying real food. ...Real Good Food! The kind that makes you sigh with pleasure feel completely satisfied and causes you to make it repeatedly.

The Keto diet is NOT a hunger strike; you don't need to deprive yourself or limit your food intake in any way. It's about healing your destructive relationship with food, i.e., eating only healthy fun stuff that boosts your self-image and makes you fall in love with exciting food all over again just as you were made to be.

How does the Keto diet work?

While I don't plan to get too deep into the science of the Keto diet, there are a few core principles you should know about.

- Firstly, Dr. Russel Wilder, MD of the Mayo Clinic invented the Keto diet in 1921 as a way to treat epilepsy in kids. It worked! While not recognizing the other benefits it came with at the time; this diet has currently taken the world by storm.
- On a diet, you strictly reduce your carb intake to allow the body to enter into a state called 'Ketosis.' At this point, the body switches from using carbs but fats to produce energy, and that is where the weight loss magic happens. The lipids are shed!
- So, to keep the body pumped with ketones, you ought to ensure a good intake of healthy fats to keep yourself adequately fuelled and healthy.
- Expect to eat around 70%-80% fat, 25% protein, and 5% carbs. For best results, keep your net carbs under 20g per day (although a more conservative aim would be around 50g)

Why no carbs?

I don't hate carbs. They're one of nature's way of fueling our bodies and brains. However, we eat far too much of this stuff by the way we live lately. Mostly, in the form of processed sugars, refined carbs, and other high carb foods.

They spell disaster for your body, and you start piling on weight in those places you hate the most. In your stomach, your hips, your legs, your butt, your arms, your neck. Everywhere that's wrong! It leaves you more vulnerable to health problems such as type 2 diabetes, metabolic syndrome, depression and anxiety, certain cancers and just many more.

Foods that are high in carbs

Before you read this list, prepare not to panic. Seeing what's off the menu, may make you wonder what on earth you'll eat. Take a chill pill; this is normal and shows how addicted to carbs you are!

I'll walk you through the foods you can eat shortly after this list, and you will feel more excited.

Deep breath

Sugar
Sugar is about as high carb as it gets. Avoid it in all forms, including the following foods.

- Soft drinks
- Fruit yogurt
- Premade cereal bars
- Smoothies
- Candy
- Boxed Juice
- Sports drinks
- Chocolate
- Cake
- Buns
- Pastries
- Ice cream
- Donuts
- Cookies
- Breakfast cereals

Grains
Grains are also extremely high in carbs. You'll need to skip the following:

- Wheat
- Barley
- Oats
- Rice
- Rye
- Corn
- Quinoa
- Millet
- Bulgur
- Amaranth
- Sprouted Grains
- Buckwheat

Remember that it's not just about the grains themselves but also the foods made from them, which include:

- Bread
- Pasta
- Rice
- Potatoes
- French fries
- Potato chips
- Porridge
- Muesli

Beans & Lentils
Beans and lentils are another carb offender. Get the following off the menu.

- Red, green, brown and black lentils
- Red Kidney beans
- Black-Eye beans
- Chickpeas
- Black beans
- Green peas
- Lima beans
- Pinto beans
- White beans
- Fava beans

How was it for you? Not as bad as you thought, right?

If I can't eat carbs, what can I eat?
Let's look at the other side of the coin. You're about to be pumped!

Meat, poultry, fish, and seafood
Eat as much as you like. Stick to organic, and grass-fed options if you can afford it. Keep the fat on!
- Beef
- Pork
- Lamb
- Game
- Chicken
- Turkey
- Organ meats
- Salmon
- Mackerel
- Sardines
- Herring
- Cod
- Seafood

Eggs
Eggs are excellent on Keto since they are versatile and rich in nutrients. Enjoy them however you like, and choose free-range, farm-raised types if possible.

Dairy Products
Wave goodbye to those tasteless zero fat products - we're about the whole dairy here! They taste better, they're much more satisfying, and they're exactly what your body needs. This includes:
- Butter
- Cream
- Sour Cream
- Soft/Hard Cheese
- Greek/Bulgarian Yogurt
- Regular Yogurt (sugar-free)

Just a quick word - avoid drinking milk. It's surprisingly high in carbs. Instead, go for nut milk like almond milk and coconut milk.

Fats, oils, and sauces
Awesome! We can include as many fatty foods as we like. Such as:
- Butter
- Cream
- Coconut oil
- Olive oil
- Ghee
- Chicken fat
- Avocados
- Mayonnaise
- High-fat sauces

Please stick to wholefood, healthy fats and avoid those refined polyunsaturated fats and trans fats. They're just not good for you man!

Vegetables
Many veggies are high carb, so you'll need to avoid them. However, there are still much more you can enjoy. They'll bring extra flavor, nutrition and excitement to your meals and help your digestive system to keep working optimally. Enjoy these:
- Green leafy veggies
- Broccoli/Cabbage
- Brussels sprouts
- Asparagus
- Zucchini
- Eggplant
- Olives
- Mushrooms
- Cucumber
- Lettuce
- Avocado
- Onions & Garlic

Herbs and spices

You can eat as much of these as you like, but please do check the ingredients list on pre-prepared spice blends- they often have some sugar sneaked in.

Sauces and condiments

Certain go-to condiments may be off the menu with Keto, but you can still enjoy the sugar-free versions of the following:

- Soy Sauce
- Lemon and lime juice
- Sriracha Sauce
- Homemade mayo
- Dijon mustard
- Wholegrain mustard (check the label)
- Hot sauces (check the label)
- Salad dressings (homemade only)

Sweeteners

Some Keto purists don't agree that sweeteners should be allowed. For me, a little touch of sweetness can be a welcome treat.

- Erythritol
- Stevia
- Splenda
- Brand-name sugar replacements
- Monk Fruit Sugar & Syrup

Alcoholic and Non-Alcoholic Drinks

There are plenty of great drinks options on the Keto diet.

Start with the basics - tea, coffee, and water. These quench your thirst brilliantly and have zero-carb, provided you avoid non- keto syrups, sugars, and excessive milk. If you like this idea, I'd advise you check out bulletproof coffee. You might have a pleasant surprise!

You'll be happy to know that you can also drink alcohol on the Keto diet, provided you stick with a few safe options, like:

- Champagne (sugar-free)
- Red or white wine
- Whiskey/Brandy
- Tequila
- Vodka Soda
- Dry Martini

Be careful to avoid liquors and alcopops as these are quite high in sugar.

ASK ME ALL YOU WANT

Whenever I tell someone that the Keto diet is the life hack responsible for the impressive changes in me, I usually get bombarded with questions, and that's fine by me.

I'm happy when people are curious, I want them to give it a go themselves, and the more information I can provide the more fulfilled I feel. So, why not you too?

I've gathered some of my most asked questions, and I provide honest answers based on my experience. Let's delve in.

Q: Will I go through detox?

A: Yes, most people experience symptoms when they start the Keto diet, because of your body's transition from using carbs to using fats for fuel. It includes anything from minor headaches and perhaps not feeling like yourself, to more flu-like symptoms. Your experience is very personal and depends on how addicted to carbs you were.

Q: How should I cope with detox symptoms?

A: If you do experience detox symptoms, make sure to slow down, drink plenty of water and sleep as much as you can. Even if you feel rotten for a day or two, remember that it's all for a terrific cause. Today is the first day of a stronger, slimmer and unstoppable you.

Q: Can anyone follow the Keto diet?

A: Yes! Anyone can follow the Keto diet and notice incredible results because it's a healthy and transformative diet and lifestyle. Remember, it was first created for kids with epilepsy, so it's naturally safe. Nevertheless, if you're pregnant, breastfeeding, under 18 years old, diabetic, or have high blood pressure, please consult your doctor first.

Q: I'm morbidly obese. Can I still do the diet?

A: Absolutely! Keto is probably the answer you've been looking for. I'm not going to lie; it will challenge you. You might suffer from regular cravings at the beginning of your journey as you transition to using fats for energy, but it will be worth it. Read the next chapter Obese to Fit: Weight Loss Tips with Keto for more useful tips.

Q: What benefits can I expect from going Keto?

A: There are tons of benefits to reap. I've already shared some of them with you when I spoke about my journey with Keto. But there are many more that I might not have covered. Some are:

- **Weight loss** — No more nibbling lettuce leaves to shed weight. Keep eating the tasty fatty stuff precisely as you want and your body will burn the fats for energy. There'll be no more reserved fats for a bulging stomach.
- **Increased brainpower** — An increase in healthy fat consumption will feed your brain and encourage you to become more productive than ever before, learn new things quickly and get on top of your game.
- **Increased stamina and endurance** — Want to run a marathon? Keto is your diet. Whereas stored sugars will run out on a regular run, this doesn't happen with Keto. Instead, you'll use stored fats, which is fantastic.
- **Healthier hormones** — Whether you're male or female, switching to Keto will help regulate your hormones, help you sleep better and help you feel better 24/7.
- **No more binge eating** — Keto enables you to feel satisfied so you don't find yourself snacking or binge eating all the time.
- **Reduced cholesterol levels** — The Keto diet reduces bad cholesterol and increases the good ones.
- **Eased symptoms of epilepsy** — This diet was designed for you, remember?
- **No more migraines** — Keto works brilliantly for people who suffer from crippling migraines and headaches.
- **Reduced risk of cancer** — Carbs feed cancerous cells in your body, so getting rid of them instantly helps protect you against one of our greatest fears.

Again, I've kept this nice and simple so you can quickly understand Keto and get started righ away!

8 NO-FAIL TIPS TO HELP YOU LIVE A HAPPIER KETO LIFESTYLE

Don't you wish that someone would just hand you a list of Keto lifestyle hacks that would help you get to grips and lose weight, gain energy and feel terrific faster?
Well, today's your lucky day because that's what I've just done for you.

Make Yours!

I feel like a full flute of champagne with an attitude saying this; you've got to make yours!
When you start a Keto diet, it often seems like an easy thing to get the carbs of the menu. Just skip the bread, pasta, potatoes, and rice, and you're done! It isn't that simple; I'm afraid to say. Carbs and more specifically, sugars are in almost every processed food you buy from yogurts, to condiments, to sauces and much more in between.
The best way to beat these carbs is to merely avoid these foods entirely and make your versions. Not only can you control the carbs like this, but you can also tweak the recipe, so it's exactly how you love your food to be. If you absolutely must eat processed food, check your labels!

Counting your macros is essential!

I'm a laid-back kind of a person, and I like to think that once I've understood a concept, I can go ahead without worrying about the details. However, you can't do this when it comes to Keto. As unusual as it might seem, you absolutely must count your macros - your net carb, protein, and fat intake.

Ditch those carb-rich foods before you start

There's nothing worse than feeling like you're comfortable on the Keto diet and super-happy with your progress, only to find a packet of potato chips or long-forgotten cheese fries lurking at the back of the pantry. Bang! There goes your willpower! Even if you have firm resolve, it's quite likely you'll succumb to temptation.
Avoid this problem by thoroughly cleaning your pantry before you get started with Keto.
I understand that if you have a partner or family members around who aren't following the Keto diet, this can be a hard task. In this case, I suggest you grab a large box, place their high-carb foods inside and keep it out of sight! If you're the one doing the family cooking, a lot of discipline is needed not to have a bite of those pasta dishes when you make them. Let the others do the taste checks when you cook.

Treat yourself!

Just because you're going Keto, doesn't mean you should start eating horrible stodgy foods. Don't follow such boring websites that show these; Keto can be fun-loving. This isn't about eating trash. It's about nourishing your body with exactly what it needs, and that includes your taste buds too.

You absolutely can continue eating like a foodie and enjoy those tender gnocchi in marinara sauce, or fragrant Nasi goreng, or fantastically spiced Indian Lamb Curry. That's exactly why I've written this book; there's a way to go about it.

Greens! Greens! Greens!

It's vital that you eat plenty of green leafy veggies while you're on Keto. They are one of the planet's best sources of minerals and add more fiber, antioxidants and even protein to your healthy diet. I love kale, spring greens, and spinach, but any will do.

Don't be afraid to include plenty of other low carb veggies too. Provided you keep your eye on your macros, they make a very nourishing, healthy addition to your diet that will keep your heart healthy, help prevent cancer and boost your digestive system too.

Get organized

The Organization is key to simplifying your Keto lifestyle, which helps you to stick to the diet. Plan your meals at the start of the week, organize a grocery list and go shopping ideally once to save you some time and energy.

It's also a good idea to cook extra portions of food at once while cooking. Most of the recipes in this book work excellently (and often taste better!) when made in advance. Use your fridge and freezer to store the leftovers, and you'll only have to reheat.

Drink plenty of water & Exercise

As well as eating the right foods, it's also important to stay hydrated. Get a refillable water bottle, fill it up and carry it with you. Aim for a minimum of 2 liters of water per day. Staying active with stressless exercises helps your body get into Ketosis and burns more fat while being excellent for your entire body, mind, and spirit.

Nevertheless, remember, it will take a couple of weeks for your body to adjust to the Keto lifestyle to start seeing the weight loss results you hope for, so don't go too hard on yourself. Slow and steady exercises do the trick.

Make sense of eating out

There's nothing worse than being 'that person' who can't eat a thing on the menu at a restaurant. So, do your homework!

Before you go anywhere, check out your local restaurants and find out if there's anything on the menu that will suit you. Check out the restaurants' online menus or pick up the phone and give them a call.

It is fantastic to find your perfect restaurant; once you do, visit them often for your comfort.

Got it? Awesome! There's just one last topic I'd like to cover before we move forward to the recipes, and that's weight loss. Yes, I know I've talked about it plenty of times already, but it does deserve some space. Because, dare I say it, changing your eating habits isn't enough by itself. You need to do some work on yourself too. Keep reading to learn my Keto weight loss tips.

So, the Keto diet was what helped me to lose weight after a crazy number of times trying. Nothing else ever seemed to work. It didn't matter how determined I felt, or how religiously I stuck to the diet. Nothing worked. Until Keto!

But, it would be a lie to say that it was Keto alone that helped me to shift the weight.

Because of course, I had a big part to play! It was hard, I needed to be smart, and I knew there'd be a long road ahead of me.

Here's how it happened.

I faced my issues

My weight problem wasn't just because I overate, ate the wrong foods or didn't get enough exercise. It was about what was going on in my head. I started to ask myself why I made the food choices I did, how my weight was benefiting me (really, it was), and how to move through those issues.

So, whatever is the motivation behind the weight gain, even if it's for beauty purposes, you will have to address that issue at mind and make a change because you can still look jaw-dropping gorgeous with weight loss.

I didn't quit

Even with the most amazing diet in the world, you will experience hard times. I bet you, hard times are signs that you are making progress.

You might struggle with food cravings, battle those early detox symptoms and feel desperate when you think of avoiding sugar long-term. I certainly fought along the way.

But I never gave up. I pushed through the difficulties, I held my head high and pushed on through for myself and for everyone that admires me...wink! Looking at myself right now, it paid off!

I retrained my eating habits

I always had a huge appetite. Even in my thinner days, I'd polish off at least twice the amount that everyone else did. When I felt hungry, I ate.

All the diets I'd ever tried before were hard because I was continually feeling either deprived or hungry. But with Keto, I felt satisfied for longer.

I planned my meals

The worst time to decide what to eat is right before your meals when you're feeling hungry. Do this, and you're very likely to make poor food choices and opt for those high-carb, high-sugar, instant 'hit' foods.

That's why, when I got started, I carefully planned my meals throughout the day, compiled my grocery list and made sure I had everything that I needed to be healthy at home and stuck to my Keto lifestyle.

I kept a food diary

It's far too easy to forget what you've eaten and end up overeating in the course of a day. Forgetting to keep track of your macros (your fat, protein, and carbs) and making poor food choices may become inherent in your habits. So, track your food intake and macros by writing them down to give you control over what goes through your lips.

After a while, you'll be disciplined with the routine and will not need to write your intakes down.

I stayed flexible

OK, so this might sound strange for me to say, considering that I'm writing this book. Nevertheless, the truth is, Keto isn't a strict prescription that you need to stick to 100%. We're all different and have varying lifestyles and needs. A specific maximum number of carbs might be best for one person but be crazily high for you. Listen to your own body and give it what it needs.

I failed. But I kept going

I'm only human. I failed.

One day, I went on a date (my first in years, might I add!) and found myself munching on the free bread they provided while the conversation flowed. Eek! I stopped as soon as I realized my fall, but I still felt painfully guilty. Then, the ultimate question came, should I quit eating now and save the progress, I'd made so far or do I ignore my previous Keto efforts and keep on with my bread? Guess, which option I chose?

I focused on me

About the same time when I went Keto, one of my mother's friends took action to lose weight too. He chose the Keto diet and shifted weight quickly. It was amazing watching him shed those excess pounds and emerge leaner, healthier, more confident, and like a brand-new man.

How about me?

What was happening to my weight loss efforts – so slow? Was I doing something wrong? Should I give up before I make a fool of myself? NO! He had had a different body structure than mine hence the noticeable quick results.

A word of caution: in this age of Instagram, it's easy to forget that we aren't all supposed to be poster boys.

Being different is OK. Instead of thinking about other people and continually comparing my weight loss to theirs, I decided to be bold. I focused on myself instead.

Remember, weight loss isn't always linear. It can be, but more often than not, you might lose four pounds in one week and then gain another the next. Don't panic! It's all part of the journey.

The tips I've shared in this chapter should help you to keep pushing forward and making this shift to a brand new you.

Now that we've got all that out of the way let's talk about food. Sounds good? C'mon then!

TOP 10 KETO RECIPES

Raspberry Almond Pancake with Blackberry Sauce

Ready in about: 40 minutes | Serves: 6
Per serving: Kcal 425, Fat 34.1g, Net Carbs 4.8g, Protein 9.8g

Ingredients

Pancakes

2 cups almond flour
½ tsp salt
2 tsp swerve
1 tsp baking soda
1 tsp baking powder
1 ½ cups almond milk
1 tsp almond extract
2 large eggs
¼ cup olive oil
1 tsp raspberry extract
Whole raspberries to garnish

Blackberry Sauce

3 cups fresh blackberries
½ cup swerve
½ cup water + 1 tbsp water
½ tsp arrowroot starch
A pinch of salt
A squirt of lemon juice

Directions

In a bowl, mix almond flour, salt, swerve, baking soda, and baking powder with a whisk; set aside.
In another bowl, whisk almond milk, almond extract, eggs, olive oil, and raspberry extract together. Then, pour the egg mixture into the almond flour mixture and continue whisking until smooth.
Put the mixture in the fridge to set for 5 minutes while you preheat the griddle pan over medium heat on a stovetop.
Once heated, remove the batter from the refrigerator and pour 1 soup spoonful of batter into the griddle pan. Cook on one side for 2 minutes, flip the pancake, and cook the other side for 2 minutes.
Transfer the pancake to a plate and repeat the cooking process until the batter is exhausted.

The blackberry sauce:

Pour the blackberries and half cup of water into a saucepan, and bring the berries to boil over medium heat, for about 8 minutes.
Then, lower the heat and simmer the berries for 5 minutes so that they are soft and exuding juice.
Stir in the swerve at this point and cook for 5 more minutes. Next, stir in salt and lemon juice, and while they cook, mix arrowroot starch with the remaining water. Pour the mixture into the berries.
Stir and continue cooking the sauce to thicken to your desire. Turn off the heat and let it cool.
Finally, plate the pancakes one on another and generously drizzle the blackberry sauce over them, garnish with the whole raspberries, and serve for breakfast.

Brie and Caramelized Onion Beef Burgers

Ready in about: 35 minutes | Serves: 4
Per serving: Kcal 487, Fat 32g, Net Carbs 7.8g, Protein 38g

Ingredients

1 medium white onion, sliced
1 tbsp olive oil
2 tbsp balsamic vinegar
2 tsp erythritol
A pinch of salt

Burgers

1 lb ground beef
2 tbsp olive oil
Salt and black pepper to season
4 slices French brie cheese
4 low carb hamburger buns, halved
Mayonnaise to serve

Directions

Make the caramelized onions first:

Heat the olive oil in a skillet over medium heat, once it just starts to smoke, reduce the heat to low and add the onions. Sauté for 15 minutes until golden brown and add the erythritol, balsamic vinegar, and salt. Cook for 3 more minutes, turn the heat off and set aside.
Make 4 patties out of the ground beef and season with salt and pepper.
Then, heat a large cast-iron skillet over high heat. When it starts smoking, add the olive oil.Swirl the pan, coat it with the oil, and cook the patties for 4 minutes on each side.
Place a brie slice on each patty and top with the caramelized onions. Put the patties with cheese and onions into two halves of the buns. Serve with mayonnaise as a snack or for lunch.

Zucchini Parmesan Chips with Greek Yogurt Dip

Ready in about: 52 minutes | Serves: 4
Per serving: Kcal 253, Fat 19.4g, Net Carbs 3.8g, Protein 14.5g

Ingredients

½ cup Greek yogurt
½ cup sour cream
1 ½ cups crumbled feta cheese
¼ cup chopped mint
1 tbsp minced garlic
2 zucchinis, thinly sliced
⅓ cup coconut flour
½ cup grated Parmesan cheese
Salt and black pepper to taste
Cooking spray

Directions

To make the yogurt dip: In the food processor, add the Greek yogurt, sour cream, feta cheese, mint, and garlic. Blend the ingredients on medium speed for 2 minutes. Pour into a bowl and season with salt and pepper. Place the bowl in the refrigerator to chill while you make the chips.

Preheat the oven to 450ºF. Grease a baking sheet with cooking spray and set aside.

Mix the coconut flour, Parmesan cheese, salt, and black pepper in a bowl. Then dip and press each zucchini slice in the flour mixture on both sides, coating generously. Place on the baking sheet and cook in the oven for 25 to 30 minutes. Remove when ready and serve with the Greek yogurt dip.

Spicy Ahi Tuna Keto Sushi

Ready in about: 15 minutes | Serves: 4
Per serving: Kcal 120, Fat 1.5g, Net Carbs 1.8g, Protein 27g

Ingredients

½ lb ahi tuna, sushi grade
1 ¼ cups cauli rice
1 ½ tsp sugar-free sriracha sauce
1 ½ tbsp mayonnaise
1 nori sheet
Salt to taste

Directions

First, slice the tuna with a knife into a long tube of a ¼ -inch thickness and set aside.

Microwave the cauli rice for 1 minute, pour into a clean kitchen towel and squeeze as much moisture from it. Then pour into a bowl and stir in the sriracha and mayonnaise.

Lay the nori sheet on a flat surface, spoon the cauli rice on it ¾ way up, and flatten the cauli evenly with the back of the spoon. Lay the tuna strip and sprinkle with salt.

Roll the nori sheet with the rice side up and over the tuna, making sure to tuck in as you move; quite firmly too.

Once you've reached the empty part of the nori sheet, wet your fingers with water and run along the layer to make it moist. After, seal the roll.

Use a sharp knife to cut the sushi into rolls and serve with a sugar-free soy sauce and grated ginger.

Chocolate, Yogurt & Egg Muffins

Ready in about: 45 minutes | Serves: 6
Per serving: Kcal 187, Fat 11.5g, Net Carbs 2.6g, Protein 3.6g

Ingredients

2 cups almond flour
⅓ cup erythritol
¼ cup unsweetened cocoa powder
2 tsp baking powder
½ tsp salt
1 large egg
1 cup plain yogurt
¼ cup olive oil
¾ cup unsweetened dark chocolate chips

Directions

Preheat the oven to 350ºF and line the muffin cups with parchment paper and set aside.

In a medium bowl, whisk almond flour, erythritol, cocoa powder, baking powder, and salt together.

Then, in a separate bowl, whisk the egg, yogurt, and olive oil, and pour the mixture gradually into the flour mixture while mixing with a spatula just until well incorporated. Try not to over-mix.

Fold in some chocolate chips and fill the muffin cups with the batter - three-quarter (¾) way up. Top with the remaining chocolate chips, place on a baking tray, and bake for 20 to 25 minutes.

Once they are ready, turn the oven off and let the muffins sit in there to cool for 15 minutes. Remove onto a flat surface to cool completely. Sift a little erythritol over them and serve for breakfast.

Pesto Chicken Pizza

Ready in about: 35 minutes | Serves: 6
Per serving: Kcal 497, Fat 32.8g, Net Carbs 3.4g, Protein 25.5g

Ingredients

Pizza Bread

3 cups almond flour
3 tbsp butter, melted
⅓ tsp salt
3 large eggs

Pesto Chicken Topping

2 chicken breasts
Salt and black pepper to taste
1 ½ tbsp olive oil
1 green bell pepper, seeded and sliced
1 ½ cups olive oil pesto
1 cup grated mozzarella cheese
1 ½ tbsp grated Parmesan cheese
1 ½ tbsp fresh basil leaves
2 tbsp pine nuts
A pinch of red pepper flakes

Directions

Preheat the oven to 350ºF. In a bowl, mix almond flour, butter, salt, and eggs until a dough forms. Mold the dough into a ball and place it in between two full parchment papers on a flat surface.

Then, use the rolling pin to roll it out into a circle of a ¼ -inch thickness. Slide the pizza dough into the pizza pan and remove the parchment paper. Place the pizza pan in the oven and bake for 20 minutes.

While the dough bakes, bring a pot of water to simmer on a stovetop, season the chicken with salt and pepper, wrap it in plastic wraps and poach it in the simmering water for 15 minutes.

Remove and unwrap the chicken, let rest, then chop it into bite size pieces.

Once the pizza bread is ready, remove it from the oven, fold and seal the extra inch of dough at its edges to make a crust around it.

Apply 2/3 of the pesto on it using a spoon and sprinkle half of the mozzarella cheese on it too. Toss the chopped chicken in the remaining pesto and spread it on top of the pizza. Sprinkle with the remaining mozzarella, bell peppers, and pine nuts and put the pizza back in the oven to bake for 9 minutes.

When it is ready, remove from the oven to cool slightly, garnish with the basil leaves and sprinkle with Parmesan and red pepper flakes. Slice and serve with green salad.

Meatballs and Squash Pasta

Ready in about: 65 minutes | Serves: 6
Per serving: Kcal 470, Fat 28g, Net Carbs 2g, Protein 14g

1 (2 lb) butternut squash
2 lb ground chicken
Salt and black pepper to taste
1 cup pork rinds, crushed
4 cloves garlic
1 onion, chopped
2 stalks celery, chopped
1 cup parsley leaves
3 tbsp olive oil + extra for brushing
2 eggs, cracked into a small bowl
2 cups sugar-free tomato sauce
10 leaves basil, chopped
1 tsp dried oregano
1 cup + 2 tbsp grated Parmesan cheese
Grated Parmesan cheese for garnishing

Directions

Preheat the oven to 450ºF. Cut the squash in half and scoop the seeds out with a spoon. Sprinkle with salt and brush with olive oil.

Place in a baking dish and cover with foil. Roast for 20 minutes, then remove the aluminum foil and continue cooking for 35 minutes. When ready, scrape the pulp into strands. Remove the spaghetti strands to a bowl and toss with 2 tbsp of Parmesan cheese. Season with salt, and plate.

Add garlic, onion, celery, and parsley to the food processor, and blend into a smooth paste for about 2 minutes.

Put the ground chicken in a bowl; pour in half of the celery puree, pork rinds, eggs, and a cup of Parmesan cheese; mix well. Mold out meatballs from the mixture and place them on a baking sheet. Bake the meatballs for just 10 minutes, but not done.

Place a pot over medium heat and warm 3 tbsp of olive oil. Stir-fry the remaining vegetable paste for 5 minutes. Stir in the tomato sauce, oregano, basil, and salt to taste. Let the sauce cook on low-medium heat for 5 minutes, remove, and add in the meatballs. Continue cooking for 15 minutes. Spoon the meatballs with sauce over the spaghetti, sprinkle with extra Parmesan cheese and serve.

Mocha Mug Cake

Ready in about: 10 minutes | Serves: 2
Per serving: Kcal 375, Fat 38g, Net Carbs 2.7g, Protein 12g

Ingredients

6 tbsp almond flour
8 tbsp swerve
4 tbsp unsweetened cocoa powder
4 tsp espresso powder
2 eggs
6 tbsp coconut milk
4 tbsp olive oil
½ tsp baking powder
Whipped cream for topping
Unsweetened chocolate syrup to garnish

Directions

Mix almond flour, swerve, cocoa powder, espresso powder, eggs, coconut milk, olive oil, and baking powder in a bowl. Pour the mix into two mugs ¾ way up and cook in a microwave for 70 seconds.

Remove and swirl a generous amount of whipping cream on the cakes and some chocolate syrup.

To make more cups, repeat the cooking process. I did 2 cups at a time in the microwave.

Spinach Frittata with Chorizo & Tomato Salad

Ready in about: 56 minutes | Serves: 4
Per serving: Kcal 366, Fat 31.5g, Net Carbs 5.2g, Protein 13g

Ingredients

8 eggs
2 tbsp almond milk
Salt and black pepper to taste
10 oz sliced white mushrooms
1 garlic clove, minced
2 tbsp olive oil
6 oz baby spinach, rinsed
¼ cup grated cheddar cheese
Chorizo and Tomato Salad
4 plum tomatoes, cut into wedges
1 small red onion, thinly sliced
4 oz chorizo, thinly sliced
1 tbsp plain vinegar
2 sprigs thyme, leaves picked
2 tbsp olive oil

Directions

Preheat an oven to 350ºF and grease a baking dish with cooking spray; set aside.

Heat 1 tbsp of olive oil in a skillet over medium heat and stir-fry the mushrooms to sweat for about 4 minutes. Add garlic, salt and pepper. Sauté for 30 seconds to make the garlic fragrant. Stir in spinach and cook until wilted, about 5 minutes. Increase the heat and let the excess liquid evaporate.

Beat the eggs in a large bowl and stir in almond milk, salt, pepper, the mushroom/spinach mixture, and cheddar cheese. Pour the mixture into the baking dish and bake in the oven for 25 minutes.

In a salad bowl, add the tomatoes, onion, and thyme. Drizzle the vinegar and a little oil over them, and toss the ingredients with a spoon. Heat a skillet over medium heat and fry the chorizo until browned, about 6 minutes. Add the chorizo to the salad, and drizzle a little oil from the pan atop. Slice the frittata into wedges. Serve warm with the chorizo and tomato salad.

Peanut Butter Pecan Ice Cream

Ready in about: 36 minutes + chilling time | Serves: 4
Per serving: Kcal 302, Fat 32g, Net Carbs 2g, Protein 5g

Ingredients

2 cups heavy cream
1 tbsp erythritol
½ cup smooth peanut butter
1 tbsp olive oil
½ tsp salt
2 eggs yolks
½ cup swerve sweetener confectioners
½ cup chopped pecans

Directions

Melt the heavy cream with peanut butter, olive oil, erythritol, and salt in a small pan over low heat without boiling about 3 minutes. Remove from the heat. In a bowl, beat the egg yolks until creamy in color. Stir the eggs into the cream mixture.

Continue stirring until a thick batter has formed; about 3 minutes. Pour the cream mixture into a bowl. Refrigerate for 30 minutes, and stir in swerve sweetener confectioners.

Pour the mixture into ice cream machine and churn it according to the manufacturer's instructions. Stir in the pecans after and spoon the mixture into loaf pan. Freeze for 2 hours before serving.

SMOOTHIES & BREAKFASTS

Morning Berry-Green Smoothie

Ready in about: 5 minutes | Serves: 4
Per serving: Kcal 360, Fat 33.3g, Net Carbs 6g, Protein 6g

Ingredients

1 avocado, pitted and sliced
3 cups mixed blueberries and strawberries
2 cups unsweetened almond milk
6 tbsp heavy cream
2 tsp erythritol
1 cup ice cubes
⅓ cup nuts and seeds mix

Directions

Combine the avocado slices, blueberries, strawberries, almond milk, heavy cream, erythritol, ice cubes, nuts and seeds in a smoothie maker; blend in high-speed until smooth and uniform.

Pour the smoothie into drinking glasses, and serve immediately.

Breakfast Nut Granola & Smoothie Bowl

Ready in about: 5 minutes | Serves: 4
Per serving: Kcal 361, Fat 31.2g, Net Carbs 2g, Protein 13g

Ingredients

6 cups Greek yogurt
4 tbsp almond butter
A handful toasted walnuts
3 tbsp unsweetened cocoa powder
4 tsp swerve brown sugar
2 cups nut granola for topping

Directions

Combine the Greek yogurt, almond butter, walnuts, cocoa powder, and swerve brown sugar in a smoothie maker; puree in high-speed until smooth and well mixed.

Share the smoothie into four breakfast bowls, top with a half cup of granola each, and serve.

Bacon and Egg Quesadillas

Ready in about: 30 minutes | Serves: 4
Per serving: Kcal 449, Fat 48.7g, Net Carbs 6.8g, Protein 29.1g

Ingredients

8 low carb tortilla shells
6 eggs
1 cup water
3 tbsp butter
1 ½ cups grated cheddar cheese
1 ½ cups grated Swiss cheese
5 bacon slices
1 medium onion, thinly sliced
1 tbsp chopped parsley

Directions

Bring the eggs to a boil in water over medium heat for 10 minutes. Transfer the eggs to an ice water bath, peel the shells, and chop them; set aside.

Meanwhile, as the eggs cook, fry the bacon in a skillet over medium heat for 4 minutes until crispy. Remove and chop. Plate and set aside too.

Fetch out 2/3 of the bacon fat and sauté the onions in the remaining grease over medium heat for 2 minutes; set aside. Melt 1 tablespoon of butter in a skillet over medium heat.

Lay one tortilla in a skillet; sprinkle with some Swiss cheese. Add some chopped eggs and bacon over the cheese, top with onion, and sprinkle with some cheddar cheese. Cover with another tortilla shell. Cook for 45 seconds, then carefully flip the quesadilla, and cook the other side too for 45 seconds. Remove to a plate and repeat the cooking process using the remaining tortilla shells.

Garnish with parsley and serve warm.

Avocado and Kale Eggs

Ready in about: 20 minutes | Serves: 4
Per serving: Kcal 274, Fat 23g, Net Carbs 4g, Protein 13g

Ingredients

1 tsp ghee
1 red onion, sliced
4 oz chorizo, sliced into thin rounds
1 cup chopped kale
1 ripe avocado, pitted, peeled, chopped
4 eggs
Salt and black pepper to season

Directions

Preheat oven to 370ºF.

Melt ghee in a cast iron pan over medium heat and sauté the onion for 2 minutes. Add the chorizo and cook for 2 minutes more, flipping once.

Introduce the kale in batches with a splash of water to wilt, season lightly with salt, stir and cook for 3 minutes. Mix in the avocado and turn the heat off.

Create four holes in the mixture, crack the eggs into each hole, sprinkle with salt and black pepper, and slide the pan into the preheated oven to bake for 6 minutes until the egg whites are set or firm and yolks still runny. Season to taste with salt and pepper, and serve right away with low carb toasts.

Bacon and Cheese Frittata

Ready in about: 25 minutes | Serves: 4
Per serving: Kcal 325, Fat 28g, Net Carbs 2g, Protein 15g

Ingredients

10 slices bacon
10 fresh eggs
3 tbsp butter, melted
½ cup almond milk
Salt and black pepper to taste
1 ½ cups cheddar cheese, shredded
¼ cup chopped green onions

Directions

Preheat the oven to 400ºF and grease a baking dish with cooking spray. Cook the bacon in a skillet over medium heat for 6 minutes. Once crispy, remove from the skillet to paper towels and discard grease. Chop into small pieces. Whisk the eggs, butter, milk, salt, and black pepper. Mix in the bacon and pour the mixture into the baking dish.

Sprinkle with cheddar cheese and green onions, and bake in the oven for 10 minutes or until the eggs are thoroughly cooked. Remove and cool the frittata for 3 minutes, slice into wedges, and serve warm with a dollop of Greek yogurt.

Spicy Egg Muffins with Bacon & Cheese

Ready in about: 30 minutes | Serves: 6
Per serving: Kcal 302, Fat 23.7g, Net Carbs 3.2g, Protein 20g

Ingredients

12 eggs
¼ cup coconut milk
Salt and black pepper to taste
1 cup grated cheddar cheese
12 slices bacon
4 jalapeño peppers, seeded and minced

Directions

Preheat oven to 370ºF.

Crack the eggs into a bowl and whisk with coconut milk until combined. Season with salt and pepper, and evenly stir in the cheddar cheese.

Line each hole of a muffin tin with a slice of bacon and fill each with the egg mixture two-thirds way up. Top with the jalapeno peppers and bake in the oven for 18 to 20 minutes or until puffed and golden. Remove, allow cooling for a few minutes, and serve with arugula salad.

Ham & Egg Broccoli Bake

Ready in about: 25 minutes | Serves: 4
Per serving: Kcal 344, Fat 28g, Net Carbs 4.2g, Protein 11g

Ingredients

2 heads broccoli, cut into small florets
2 red bell peppers, seeded and chopped
¼ cup chopped ham
2 tsp ghee
1 tsp dried oregano + extra to garnish
Salt and black pepper to taste
8 fresh eggs

Directions

Preheat oven to 425ºF.

Melt the ghee in a frying pan over medium heat; brown the ham, stirring frequently, about 3 minutes. Arrange the broccoli, bell peppers, and ham on a foil-lined baking sheet in a single layer, toss to combine; season with salt, oregano, and black pepper. Bake for 10 minutes until the vegetables have softened.

Remove, create eight indentations with a spoon, and crack an egg into each. Return to the oven and continue to bake for an additional 5 to 7 minutes until the egg whites are firm.

Season with salt, black pepper, and extra oregano, share the bake into four plates and serve with strawberry lemonade (optional).

Italian Sausage Stacks

Ready in about: 20 minutes | Serves: 6
Per serving: Kcal 378, Fat 23g, Net Carbs 5g, Protein 16g

Ingredients

6 Italian sausage patties
4 tbsp olive oil
2 ripe avocados, pitted
2 tsp fresh lime juice
Salt and black pepper to taste
6 fresh eggs
Red pepper flakes to garnish

Directions

In a skillet, warm the oil over medium heat and fry the sausage patties about 8 minutes until lightly browned and firm. Remove the patties to a plate.

Spoon the avocado into a bowl, mash with the lime juice, and season with salt and black pepper. Spread the mash on the sausages.

Boil 3 cups of water in a wide pan over high heat, and reduce to simmer (don't boil).

Crack each egg into a small bowl and gently put the egg into the simmering water; poach for 2 to 3 minutes. Use a perforated spoon to remove from the water on a paper towel to dry. Repeat with the other 5 eggs. Top each stack with a poached egg, sprinkle with chili flakes, salt, black pepper, and chives. Serve with turnip wedges.

Dark Chocolate Smoothie

Ready in about: 10 minutes | Serves: 2
Per serving: Kcal 335; Fat: 31.7g Net Carbs: 12.7g, Protein: 7g

Ingredients

8 pecans
¾ cup coconut milk
¼ cup water
1 ½ cups watercress
2 tsp vegan protein powder
1 tbsp chia seeds
1 tbsp unsweetened cocoa powder
4 fresh dates, pitted

Directions

In a blender, add all ingredients and process until creamy and uniform. Place into two glasses and chill before serving.

Five Greens Smoothie

Ready in about: 5 minutes | Serves: 4
Per serving: Kcal 124, Fat 7.8g, Net Carbs 2.9g, Protein 3.2g

Ingredients

6 kale leaves, chopped
3 stalks celery, chopped
1 ripe avocado, skinned, pitted, sliced
1 cup ice cubes
2 cups spinach, chopped
1 large cucumber, peeled and chopped
Chia seeds to garnish

Directions

In a blender, add the kale, celery, avocado, and ice cubes, and blend for 45 seconds. Add the spinach and cucumber, and process for another 45 seconds until smooth.

Pour the smoothie into glasses, garnish with chia seeds and serve the drink immediately.

Almond Waffles with Cinnamon Cream

Ready in about: 25 minutes | Serves: 6
Per serving: Kcal 307, Fat 24g, Net Carbs 8g, Protein 12g

Ingredients

For the Spread

8 oz cream cheese, at room temperature
1 tsp cinnamon powder
3 tbsp swerve brown sugar
Cinnamon powder for garnishing

For the Waffles

5 tbsp melted butter
1 ½ cups unsweetened almond milk
7 large eggs
¼ tsp liquid stevia
½ tsp baking powder
1 ½ cups almond flour

Directions

Combine the cream cheese, cinnamon, and swerve with a hand mixer until smooth. Cover and chill until ready to use.

To make the waffles, whisk the butter, milk, and eggs in a medium bowl. Add the stevia and baking powder and mix. Stir in the almond flour and combine until no lumps exist. Let the batter sit for 5 minutes to thicken. Spritz a waffle iron with a non-stick cooking spray.

Ladle a ¼ cup of the batter into the waffle iron and cook according to the manufacturer's instructions until golden, about 10 minutes in total. Repeat with the remaining batter.

Slice the waffles into quarters; apply the cinnamon spread in between each of two waffles and snap. Sprinkle with cinnamon powder and serve.

Smoked Salmon Rolls with Dill Cream Cheese

Ready in about: 10 minutes + time refrigeration | Serves: 3
Per serving: Kcal 250, Fat 16g, Net Carbs 7g, Protein 18g

Ingredients

3 tbsp cream cheese, softened
1 small lemon, zested and juiced
3 tsp chopped fresh dill
Salt and black pepper to taste
3 (7-inch) low carb tortillas
6 slices smoked salmon

Directions

In a bowl, mix the cream cheese, lemon juice, zest, dill, salt, and black pepper.

Lay each tortilla on a plastic wrap (just wide enough to cover the tortilla), spread with cream cheese mixture, and top each (one) with two salmon slices. Roll up the tortillas and secure both ends by twisting. Refrigerate for 2 hours, remove plastic, cut off both ends of each wrap, and cut wraps into wheels.

Egg Tofu Scramble with Kale & Mushrooms

Ready in about: 30 minutes | Serves: 4
Per serving: Kcal 469, Fat 39g, Net Carbs 5g, Protein 25g

Ingredients

2 tbsp ghee
1 cup sliced white mushrooms
2 cloves garlic, minced
16 oz firm tofu, pressed and crumbled
Salt and black pepper to taste
½ cup thinly sliced kale
6 fresh eggs

Directions

Melt the ghee in a non-stick skillet over medium heat, and sauté the mushrooms for 5 minutes until they lose their liquid. Add the garlic and cook for 1 minute. Crumble the tofu into the skillet, season with salt and black pepper. Cook with continuous stirring for 6 minutes. Introduce the kale in batches and cook to soften for about 7 minutes.

Crack the eggs into a bowl, whisk until well combined and creamy in color, and pour all over the kale. Use a spatula to immediately stir the eggs while cooking until scrambled and no more runny, about 5 minutes. Plate, and serve with low carb crusted bread.

Egg in a Cheesy Spinach Nests

Ready in about: 35 minutes | Serves: 4
Per serving: Kcal 230, Fat 17.5g, Net Carbs 4g, Protein 12g

Ingredients

2 tbsp olive oil
1 clove garlic, grated
½ lb spinach, chopped
Salt and black pepper to taste
2 tbsp shredded Parmesan cheese
2 tbsp shredded gouda cheese
4 eggs

Directions

Preheat oven to 350ºF. Warm the oil in a non-stick skillet over medium heat; add the garlic and sauté until softened for 2 minutes. Add the spinach to wilt for about 5 minutes, and season with salt and black pepper. Allow cooling.

Grease a baking sheet with cooking spray, mold 4 (firm and separate) spinach nests on the sheet, and crack an egg into each nest. Sprinkle with Parmesan and gouda cheese.

Bake for 15 minutes just until the egg whites have set and the yolks are still runny. Plate the nests and serve right away with low carb toasts and coffee.

Breakfast Almond Muffins

Ready in about: 30 minutes | Serves: 4
Per serving: Kcal 320, Fat 30.6g, Net Carbs 6g,
Protein 4g

Ingredients

2 drops liquid stevia
2 cups almond flour
2 tsp baking powder
½ tsp salt
8 oz cream cheese, softened
¼ cup melted butter
1 egg
1 cup unsweetened almond milk

Directions

Preheat oven to 400ºF and grease a 12-cup muffin tray with cooking spray. Mix the flour, baking powder, and salt in a large bowl.

In a separate bowl, beat the cream cheese, stevia, and butter using a hand mixer and whisk in the egg and milk. Fold in the flour, and spoon the batter into the muffin cups two-thirds way up.

Bake for 20 minutes until puffy at the top and golden brown, remove to a wire rack to cool slightly for 5 minutes before serving. Serve with tea.

Kale Frittata with Crispy Pancetta Salad

Ready in about: 22 minutes | Serves: 4
Per serving: Kcal 453, Fat 30.3g, Net Carbs 4.6g,
Protein 26.4g

Ingredients

6 slices pancetta
4 tomatoes, cut into 1-inch chunks
1 large cucumber, seeded and sliced
1 small red onion, sliced
¼ cup balsamic vinegar
Salt and black pepper to taste
8 eggs
1 bunch kale, chopped
Salt and black pepper to taste
6 tbsp grated Parmesan cheese
4 tbsp olive oil
1 large white onion, sliced
3 oz beef salami, thinly sliced
1 clove garlic, minced

Directions

Place the pancetta in a skillet and fry over medium heat until crispy, about 4 minutes. Remove to a cutting board and chop.

Then, in a small bowl, whisk the vinegar, 2 tbsp of olive oil, salt, and pepper to make the dressing.

Next, combine the tomatoes, red onion, and cucumber in a salad bowl, drizzle with the dressing and toss the veggies. Sprinkle with the pancetta and set aside.

Reheat the broiler to 400ºF.

Crack the eggs into a bowl and whisk together with half of the Parmesan, salt, and pepper. Set aside.

Next, heat the remaining olive oil in the cast iron pan over medium heat. Sauté the onion and garlic for 3 minutes. Add the kale to the skillet, season with salt and pepper, and cook for 2 minutes. Top with the salami, stir and cook further for 1 minute. Pour the egg mixture all over the kale, reduce the heat to medium-low, cover, and cook the ingredients for 4 minutes.

Sprinkle the remaining cheese on top and transfer the pan to the oven. Broil to brown on top for 1 minute. When ready, remove the pan and run a spatula around the edges of the frittata; slide it onto a warm platter. Cut the frittata into wedges and serve with the pancetta salad.

Giant Egg Quiche

Ready in about: 60 minutes | Serves: 6
Per serving: Kcal 485, Fat 39.7g, Net Carbs 6.3g,
Protein 24.5g

Ingredients

12 eggs
1 ½ cups shredded cheddar cheese
1 ½ cups almond milk
½ tsp dried thyme
Salt to taste
¼ cup sliced mushrooms
½ cup chopped broccoli
1 clove garlic, minced
For the Quiche Pastry
¾ cup almond flour
A pinch of salt
2 oz cold butter
½ tsp baking powder
1 tbsp cold water
2 eggs
Cooking spray

Directions

Preheat the oven to 370ºF.

In a large bowl, mix all the crust ingredients until dough is formed. Press it into a greased baking dish and bake for 20-25 minutes until lightly golden.

Spread the cheddar cheese in the pie crust. Beat the eggs with the almond milk, thyme, and salt, then, stir in the mushrooms, broccoli, and garlic.

Pour the ingredients into the pie crust and bake in the oven for 35 minutes until the quiche is set.

Remove and serve sliced with a tomato and avocado salad.

Zesty Ginger Pancakes with Lemon Sauce

Ready in about: 15 minutes | Serves: 4
Per serving: Kcal 324, Fat 24.2g, Net Carbs 5.8g, Protein 7.3g

2 cups almond flour
1 tsp baking powder
1 ½ tsp cinnamon powder
⅓ cup swerve brown sugar
¼ tsp baking soda
1 tsp ginger powder
⅓ tsp salt
2 eggs
1 ¼ cups almond milk
½ cup lemon juice
½ tsp lemon zest
3 ½ tbsp olive oil

Lemon Sauce:

½ cup swerve
1 tsp arrowroot starch
1 ¼ cup hot water
2 tbsp lemon juice
2 ½ tbsp butter
Lemon zest to taste

Directions

In a bowl, mix the almond flour, baking powder, cinnamon powder, swerve brown sugar, baking soda, ginger powder, salt, eggs, almond milk, lemon juice, lemon zest, and olive oil.

Heat oil in a skillet over medium heat and spoon 4 to 5 tablespoons of the mixture into the skillet. Cook the batter for 1 minute, flip it and cook the other side for another minute. Remove the pancake onto a plate after and repeat the cooking process until the batter is exhausted.

Mix the swerve and arrowroot starch in a medium saucepan. Set the pan over medium heat and gradually stir the water until it thickens, about 1 minute.

Turn the heat off and add the butter, lemon juice, and lemon zest. Stir the mixture until the butter melts. After, drizzle the sauce on the pancakes immediately and serve them warm.

Chocolate Crepes with Caramel Cream

Ready in about: 35 minutes | Serves: 4
Per serving: Kcal 330, Fat 21g, Net Carbs 5.1g, Protein 11g

Ingredients

4 tbsp coconut flour
4 tbsp unsweetened cocoa powder
½ tsp baking powder
4 egg whites
½ cup + 4 tbsp flax milk
2 tbsp erythritol
2 tbsp olive oil

Caramel Cream:

½ cup salted butter
4 tbsp swerve brown sugar
1 tsp vanilla extract
1 cup heavy cream

Directions

In a bowl, mix the coconut flour, cocoa powder, and baking powder together. Set aside.

Then, in another bowl, whisk the egg whites, ½ cup flax milk, erythritol, and the olive oil. Pour the wet ingredients into the dry ingredients, and whisk until smooth.

Set a skillet over medium heat, grease with cooking spray, and pour in a ladleful of the batter. Swirl the pan quickly to spread the dough all around the skillet and cook the crepe for 2-3 minutes.

When it is firm enough to touch and cooked through, slide the crepe into a flat plate. Wipe the pan with a napkin and continue cooking until the remaining batter has finished.

Put the butter and brown sugar in a pot and melt the butter over medium heat while stirring continually. Keep cooking for 4 minutes after the butter has melted; be careful not to burn.

Stir in the cream, reduce the heat to low, and let the sauce simmer for 10 minutes while stirring continually. Turn the heat off and stir in the vanilla extract. Once the crepes are ready, drizzle the caramel sauce over them, and serve with a cup of coffee.

Carrot Zucchini Bread

Ready in about: 70 minutes | Serves: 4
Per serving: Kcal 175, Fat 10.5g, Net Carbs 1.8g, Protein 11.6g

Ingredients

1 cup shredded carrots
1 cup shredded zucchini, squeezed
⅓ cup coconut flour
1 tsp vanilla extract
6 eggs
1 tbsp coconut oil
¾ tsp baking soda
1 tbsp cinnamon powder
½ tsp salt
½ cup Greek yogurt
1 tsp apple cider vinegar
½ tsp nutmeg powder

Directions

Preheat the oven to 350ºF and grease the loaf pan with cooking spray. Set aside.

Mix the carrots, zucchini, coconut flour, vanilla extract, eggs, coconut oil, baking soda, cinnamon powder, salt, Greek yogurt, vinegar, and nutmeg. Pour the batter into the loaf pan and bake for 55 minutes.

Remove the bread after and let cool for 5 minutes. Preserve the bread and use it for toasts, sandwiches, or served with soups and salads.

Smoked Ham and Egg Muffins

Ready in about: 40 minutes | Serves: 9
Per serving: Kcal 367, Fat: 28g, Net Carbs: 1g, Protein: 13.5g

Ingredients

2 cups chopped smoked ham
⅓ cup grated Parmesan cheese
¼ cup almond flour
9 eggs
⅓ cup mayonnaise, sugar-free
¼ tsp garlic powder
¼ cup chopped onion
Sea salt to taste

Directions

Preheat your oven to 370ºF.

Lightly grease nine muffin pans with cooking spray and set aside. Place the onion, ham, garlic powder, and salt, in a food processor, and pulse until ground. Stir in the mayonnaise, almond flour, and Parmesan cheese. Press this mixture into the muffin cups.

Make sure it goes all the way up the muffin sides so that there will be room for the egg. Bake for 5 minutes. Crack an egg into each muffin cup. Return to the oven and bake for 20 more minutes or until the tops are firm to the touch and eggs are cooked. Leave to cool slightly before serving.

Sausage & Squash Omelet with Swiss Chard

Ready in about: 10 minutes | Serves: 1
Per serving: Kcal 558, Fat 51.7g, Net Carbs 7.5g, Protein 32.3g

Ingredients

2 eggs
1 cup Swiss chard, chopped
4 oz sausage, chopped
2 tbsp ricotta cheese
4 ounces roasted squash
1 tbsp olive oil
Salt and black pepper, to taste
Fresh parsley to garnish

Directions

Beat the eggs in a bowl, season with salt and pepper; stir in the swiss chard and the ricotta cheese.

In another bowl, mash the squash and add to the egg mixture. Heat ¼ tbsp of olive oil in a pan over medium heat. Add sausage and cook until browned on all sides, turning occasionally.

Drizzle the remaining olive oil. Pour the egg mixture over. Cook for about 2 minutes per side until the eggs are thoroughly cooked and lightly browned. Remove the pan and run a spatula around the edges of the omelet; slide it onto a warm platter. Fold in half, and serve sprinkled with fresh parsley.

Coconut Flour Bagels

Ready in about: 25 minutes | Serves: 4
Per serving: Kcal 426, Fat 19.1g, Net Carbs 0.4g, Protein 33.1g

Ingredients

½ cup coconut flour
6 eggs, beaten in a bowl
½ cup vegetable broth
¼ cup flax seed meal
¼ cup chia seed meal
1 tsp onion powder
1 tsp garlic powder
1 tsp dried parsley
1 tsp chia seeds
1 tsp sesame seeds
1 chopped onion

Directions

Preheat the oven to 350ºF.

Mix the coconut flour, eggs, broth, flax seed meal, chia seed meal, onion powder, garlic powder, and parsley. Spoon the mixture into a donut tray.

In a small bowl, mix the chia seeds, sesame seeds, and onion, and sprinkle on the batter. Bake the bagels for 20 minutes. Serve the bagels with creamy pumpkin soup.

Bacon Tomato Cups

Ready in about: 33 minutes | Serves: 6
Per serving: Kcal 425, Fat 45.2g, Net Carbs 4.3g, Protein 16.2g

Ingredients

12 bacon slices
2 tomatoes, diced
1 onion, diced
1 cup shredded cheddar cheese
1 cup mayonnaise
12 low carb crepes/pancakes
1 tsp dried basil
Chopped chives to garnish

Directions

Fry the bacon in a skillet over medium heat for 5 minutes. Remove and chop with a knife. Transfer to a bowl. Add in cheddar cheese, tomatoes, onion, mayonnaise, and basil. Mix well set aside.

Place the crepes on a flat surface and use egg rings to cut a circle out of each crepe. Grease the muffin cups with cooking spray and fit the circled crepes into them to make a cup.

Now, fill the cups with 3 tbsp of bacon-tomato mixture. Place the muffin cups on a baking sheet, and bake for 18 minutes. Garnish with the chives, and serve with a tomato or cheese sauce.

Cheesy Sausage Quiche

Ready in about: 55 minutes | Serves: 6
Per serving: Kcal 340, Fat: 28g, Net Carbs: 3g, Protein: 17g

Ingredients

6 eggs
12 ounces raw sausage roll
10 cherry tomatoes, halved
2 tbsp heavy cream
2 tbsp Parmesan cheese
¼ tsp salt
A pinch of black pepper

2 tbsp chopped parsley
5 eggplant slices
Directions
Preheat your oven to 370ºF.
Grease a pie dish with cooking spray. Press the sausage roll at the bottom of a pie dish. Arrange the eggplant slices on top of the sausage. Top with cherry tomatoes.
Whisk the eggs along with the heavy cream, salt, Parmesan cheese, and black pepper. Spoon the mixture over the sausage. Bake for about 40 minutes until browned around the edges. Serve warm, sprinkled with parsley.

Ricotta Cloud Pancakes with Whipped Cream
Ready in about: 10 minutes | Serves: 4
Per serving: Kcal 407, Fat 30.6g, Net Carbs 6.6g, Protein 11.5g
Ingredients
1 cup almond flour
1 tsp baking powder
2 ½ tbsp swerve
⅓ tsp salt
1 ¼ cups ricotta cheese
⅓ cup coconut milk
2 large eggs
1 cup heavy whipping cream
Directions
In a medium bowl, whisk the almond flour, baking powder, swerve, and salt. Set aside.
Crack the eggs into the blender and process on medium speed for 30 seconds. Add the ricotta cheese, continue processing it, and gradually pour the coconut milk in while you keep on blending. In about 90 seconds, the mixture will be creamy and smooth. Pour it into the dry ingredients and whisk to combine.
Set a skillet over medium heat and let it heat for a minute. Then, fetch a soup spoonful of mixture into the skillet and cook it for 1 minute.
Flip the pancake and cook further for 1 minute. Remove onto a plate and repeat the cooking process until the batter is exhausted. Serve the pancakes with whipping cream.

Mushroom & Cheese Lettuce Wraps
Ready in about: 20 minutes | Serves: 4
Per serving: Kcal 472; Fat: 44g, Net Carbs: 5.4g, Protein: 19.5g
Ingredients
For the Wraps:
6 eggs
2 tbsp almond milk
1 tbsp olive oil
Sea salt, to taste
For the Filling:
1 tsp olive oil
1 cup mushrooms, chopped
Salt and black pepper, to taste
½ tsp cayenne pepper

8 fresh lettuce leaves
4 slices gruyere cheese
2 tomatoes, sliced
Directions
Mix all the ingredients for the wraps thoroughly.
Set a frying pan over medium heat. Add in ¼ of the mixture and cook for 4 minutes on both sides. Do the same thrice and set the wraps aside, they should be kept warm.
In a separate pan over medium heat, warm 1 teaspoon of olive oil. Cook the mushrooms for 5 minutes until soft; add cayenne pepper, black pepper, and salt. Set 1-2 lettuce leaves onto every wrap, split the mushrooms among the wraps and top with tomatoes and cheese.

Bacon & Cheese Pesto Mug Cakes
Ready in about: 8 minutes | Serves: 2
Per serving: Kcal 511, Fat: 38.2g, Net Carbs: 4.5g, Protein: 16.4g
Ingredients
¼ cup flax meal
1 egg
2 tbsp heavy cream
2 tbsp pesto
¼ cup almond flour
¼ tsp baking soda
Salt and black pepper, to taste
Filling:
2 tbsp cream cheese
4 slices bacon
½ medium avocado, sliced
Directions
Mix together the dry muffin ingredients in a bowl. Add egg, heavy cream, and pesto, and whisk well with a fork. Season with salt and pepper. Divide the mixture between two ramekins.
Place in the microwave and cook for 60-90 seconds. Leave to cool slightly before filling.
Meanwhile, in a skillet, over medium heat, cook the bacon slices until crispy. Transfer to paper towels to soak up excess fat; set aside. Invert the muffins onto a plate and cut in half, crosswise. To assemble the sandwiches: spread cream cheese and top with bacon and avocado slices.

Mascarpone & Vanilla Breakfast Cups
Ready in about: 20 minutes | Serves: 6
Per serving: Kcal 181; Fat: 13.5g, Net Carbs: 3.7g, Protein: 10.5g
Ingredients
¾ cup mascarpone cheese
¼ cup natural yogurt
3 eggs, beaten
1 tbsp walnuts, ground
4 tbsp erythritol
½ tsp vanilla essence
⅓ tsp ground cinnamon
Directions

Set oven to 360ºF and grease a muffin pan. Mix all ingredients in a bowl. Split the batter into the muffin cups. Bake for 12 to 15 minutes. Remove and set on a wire rack to cool slightly before serving.

Quickly Blue Cheese Omelet

Ready in about: 15 minutes | Serves: 2
Per serving: Kcal 307; Fat: 25g, Net Carbs: 2.5g, Protein: 18.5g

Ingredients

4 eggs
Salt, to taste
1 tbsp sesame oil
½ cup blue cheese, crumbled
1 tomato, thinly sliced

Directions

In a mixing bowl, beat the eggs and season with salt. Set a sauté pan over medium heat and warm the oil. Add in the eggs and cook as you swirl the eggs around the pan using a spatula. Cook eggs until partially set. Top with cheese; fold the omelet in half to enclose filling. Decorate with tomato and serve while warm.

Breakfast Buttered Eggs

Ready in about: 15 minutes | Serves: 2
Per serving: Kcal 321, Fat: 21.5g, Net Carbs: 2.5g, Protein: 12.8g

Ingredients

1 tbsp coconut oil
2 tbsp butter
1 tsp fresh thyme
4 eggs
2 garlic cloves, minced
½ cup chopped parsley
½ cup chopped cilantro
¼ tsp cumin
¼ tsp cayenne pepper
Salt and black pepper, to taste

Directions

Drizzle the coconut oil into a non-stick skillet over medium heat. Once the oil is warm, add the butter, and melt. Add garlic and thyme and cook for 30 seconds. Sprinkle with parsley and cilantro; and cook for another 2 minutes, until crisp.
Carefully crack the eggs into the skillet. Lower the heat and cook for 4-6 minutes. Season with salt, black pepper, cumin, and cayenne pepper. When the eggs are just set, turn the heat off and transfer to a serving plate.

Bacon & Cheese Zucchini Balls

Ready in about: 3 hours 20 minutes | Serves: 6
Per serving: Kcal 407; Fat: 26.8g, Net Carbs: 5.8g, Protein: 33.4g

Ingredients

4 cups zoodles
½ pound bacon, chopped
6 ounces cottage cheese, curds
6 ounces cream cheese
1 cup fontina cheese

½ cup dill pickles, chopped, squeezed
2 cloves garlic, crushed
1 cup grated Parmesan cheese
½ tsp caraway seeds
¼ tsp dried dill weed
½ tsp onion powder
Salt and black pepper, to taste
1 cup crushed pork rinds
Cooking oil

Directions

Thoroughly mix zoodles, cottage cheese, dill pickles, ½ cup of Parmesan cheese, garlic, cream cheese, bacon, and fontina cheese until well combined. Shape the mixture into balls. Refrigerate for 3 hours.
In a mixing bowl, mix the remaining ½ cup of Parmesan cheese, crushed pork rinds, dill, black pepper, onion powder, caraway seeds, and salt. Roll cheese ball in Parmesan mixture to coat.
Set a skillet over medium heat and warm 1-inch of oil. Fry cheeseballs until browned on all sides. Set on a paper towel to soak up any excess oil.

Chorizo and Mozzarella Omelet

Ready in about: 15 minutes | Serves: 1
Per serving: Kcal 451, Fat: 36.5g, Net Carbs: 3g, Protein: 30g

Ingredients

2 eggs
6 basil leaves
2 ounces mozzarella cheese
1 tbsp butter
1 tbsp water
4 thin slices chorizo
1 tomato, sliced
Salt and black pepper, to taste

Directions

Whisk the eggs along with the water and some salt and pepper. Melt the butter in a skillet and cook the eggs for 30 seconds. Spread the chorizo slices over. Arrange the tomato and mozzarella over the chorizo. Cook for about 3 minutes. Cover the skillet and cook for 3 minutes until omelet is set.
When ready, remove the pan from heat; run a spatula around the edges of the omelet and flip it onto a warm plate, folded side down. Serve garnished with basil leaves and green salad.

Hashed Zucchini & Bacon Breakfast

Ready in about: 25 minutes | Serves: 1
Per serving: Kcal 340, Fat: 26.8g, Net Carbs: 6.6g, Protein: 17.4g

Ingredients

1 medium zucchini, diced
2 bacon slices
1 egg
1 tbsp coconut oil
½ small onion, chopped
1 tbsp chopped parsley
¼ tsp salt

Directions

Place the bacon in a skillet and cook for a few minutes, until crispy. Remove and set aside.

Warm the coconut oil and cook the onion until soft, for about 3-4 minutes, occasionally stirring. Add the zucchini, and cook for 10 more minutes until zucchini is brown and tender, but not mushy. Transfer to a plate and season with salt.

Crack the egg into the same skillet and fry over medium heat. Top the zucchini mixture with the bacon slices and a fried egg. Serve hot, sprinkled with parsley.

Morning Almond Shake

Ready in about: 4 minutes | Serves: 1
Per serving: Kcal 326, Fat: 27g, Net Carbs: 6g, Protein: 19g

Ingredients

1 ½ cups almond milk
2 tbsp almond butter
½ tsp almond extract
½ tsp cinnamon
2 tbsp flax meal
1 tbsp collagen peptides
A pinch of salt
15 drops of stevia
A handful of ice cubes

Directions

Add almond milk, almond butter, flax meal, almond extract, collagen peptides, a pinch of salt, and stevia to the bowl of a blender. Blitz until uniform and smooth, for about 30 seconds. Add a bit more almond milk if it's very thick.

Then taste, and adjust flavor as needed, adding more stevia for sweetness or almond butter to the creaminess. Pour in a smoothie glass, add the ice cubes and sprinkle with cinnamon.

Egg Omelet Roll with Cream Cheese & Salmon

Ready in about: 15 minutes | Serves: 1
Per serving: Kcal 514, Fat: 47.9g, Net Carbs: 5.8g, Protein: 36.9g

Ingredients

½ avocado, sliced
2 tbsp chopped chives
½ package smoked salmon, cut into strips
1 spring onions, sliced
3 eggs
2 tbsp cream cheese
1 tbsp butter
Salt and black pepper, to taste

Directions

In a small bowl, combine the chives and cream cheese; set aside. Beat the eggs in a large bowl and season with salt and black pepper.

Melt the butter in a pan over medium heat. Add the eggs to the pan and cook for about 3 minutes. Flip the omelet over and continue cooking for another 2 minutes until golden.

Remove the omelet to a plate and spread the chive mixture over. Arrange the salmon, avocado, and onion slices. Wrap the omelet and serve immediately.

Traditional Spinach and Feta Frittata

Ready in about: 40 minutes | Serves: 4
Per serving: Kcal 461, Fat: 35g, Net Carbs: 6g, Protein: 26g

Ingredients

5 ounces spinach
8 ounces crumbled feta cheese
1 pint halved cherry tomatoes
10 eggs
3 tbsp olive oil
4 scallions, diced
Salt and black pepper, to taste

Directions

Preheat your oven to 350ºF.

Drizzle the oil in a casserole and place in the oven until heated. In a bowl, whisk the eggs along with the black pepper and salt, until thoroughly combined. Stir in the spinach, feta cheese, and scallions.

Pour the mixture into the casserole, top with the cherry tomatoes and place back in the oven. Bake for 25 minutes until your frittata is set in the middle.

When done, remove the casserole from the oven and run a spatula around the edges of the frittata; slide it onto a warm platter. Cut the frittata into wedges and serve with salad.

Chocolate Protein Coconut Shake

Ready in about: 4 minutes | Serves: 4
Per serving: Kcal 265, Fat: 15.5g, Net Carbs: 4g, Protein: 12g

Ingredients

3 cups flax milk, chilled
3 tsp unsweetened cocoa powder
1 medium avocado, pitted, peeled, sliced
1 cup coconut milk, chilled
3 mint leaves + extra to garnish
3 tbsp erythritol
1 tbsp low carb Protein powder
Whipping cream for topping

Directions

Combine the flax milk, cocoa powder, avocado, coconut milk, 3 mint leaves, erythritol, and protein powder into the smoothie maker, and blend for 1 minute to smooth.

Pour the drink into serving glasses, lightly add some whipping cream on top, and garnish with 1 or 2 mint leaves. Serve immediately.

Broccoli & Colby Cheese Frittata

Ready in about: 20 minutes | Serves: 4
Per serving: Kcal 248; Fat: 17.1g, Net Carbs: 6.2g, Protein: 17.6g
Ingredients
2 tbsp olive oil
½ cup onions, chopped
1 cup broccoli, chopped
8 eggs, beaten
½ tsp jalapeño pepper, minced
Salt and red pepper, to taste
¾ cup colby cheese, grated
¼ cup fresh cilantro, to serve
Directions
Set an ovenproof frying pan over medium heat and warm the oil. Add onions and sauté until caramelized. Place in the broccoli and cook until tender. Add in jalapeno pepper and eggs; season with red pepper and salt. Cook until the eggs are set.
Scatter colby cheese over the frittata. Set oven to 370ºF and cook for approximately 12 minutes, until frittata is set in the middle. Slice into wedges and decorate with fresh cilantro before serving.

Baked Eggs in Avocados

Ready in about: 13 minutes | Serves: 4
Per serving: Kcal 234, Fat 19.1g, Net Carbs 2.2g, Protein 8.2g
Ingredients
2 large avocados, halved and pitted
4 small eggs
Salt and black pepper to season
Chopped parsley to garnish
Directions
Preheat the oven to 400ºF.
Crack each egg into each avocado half and place them on a greased baking sheet. Bake the filled avocados in the oven for 8 or 10 minutes or until eggs are cooked. Season with salt and pepper, and garnish with parsley.

Ham and Vegetable Frittata

Ready in about: 25 minutes | Serves: 4
Per serving: Kcal 310; Fat: 26.2g, Net Carbs: 3.9g, Protein: 15.4g
Ingredients
2 tbsp butter, at room temperature
½ cup green onions, chopped
2 garlic cloves, minced
1 jalapeño pepper, chopped
1 carrot, chopped
8 ham slices
8 eggs, whisked
Salt and black pepper, to taste
½ tsp dried thyme
Directions
Set a pan over medium heat and warm the butter. Stir in green onions and sauté for 4 minutes.

Place in garlic and cook for 1 minute. Stir in carrot and jalapeño pepper, and cook for 4 more minutes. Remove the mixture to a lightly greased baking pan, with cooking spray, and top with ham slices.
Place in the eggs over vegetables and ham; add thyme, black pepper, and salt for seasoning. Bake in the oven for about 18 minutes at 360ºF. Serve warm alongside a dollop of full-fat natural yogurt.

Eggs & Crabmeat with Creme Fraiche Salsa

Ready in about: 15 minutes | Serves: 3
Per serving: Kcal 334; Fat: 26.2g, Net Carbs: 4.4g, Protein: 21.1g
Ingredients
1 tbsp olive oil
6 eggs, whisked
1 (6 oz) can crabmeat, flaked
Salt and black pepper to taste
For the Salsa:
¾ cup crème fraiche
½ cup scallions, chopped
½ tsp garlic powder
Salt and black pepper to taste
½ tsp fresh dill, chopped
Directions
Set a sauté pan over medium heat and warm olive oil. Crack in eggs and scramble them. Stir in crabmeat and season with salt and black pepper; cook until cooked thoroughly.
In a mixing dish, combine all salsa ingredients. Equally, split the egg/crabmeat mixture among serving plates; serve alongside the scallions and salsa to the side.

Fontina Cheese and Chorizo Waffles

Ready in about: 30 minutes | Serves: 6
Per serving: Kcal 316; Fat: 25g, Net Carbs: 1.5g, Protein: 20.2g
Ingredients
6 eggs
6 tbsp almond milk
1 tsp Spanish spice mix or allspice
Sea salt and black pepper, to taste
3 chorizo sausages, cooked, chopped
1 cup fontina cheese, shredded
Directions
Using a mixing bowl, beat the eggs, Spanish spice mix, black pepper, salt, and almond milk. Add in shredded cheese and chopped sausage. Use a nonstick cooking spray to spray a waffle iron.
Cook the egg mixture for 5 minutes. Serve alongside homemade sugar-free tomato ketchup.

Cheesy Turkey Sausage Egg Muffins

Ready in about: 15 minutes | Serves: 3
Per serving: Kcal 423; Fat: 34.1g, Net Carbs: 2.2g, Protein: 26.5g

Ingredients

1 tsp butter
6 eggs
Salt and black pepper, to taste
½ tsp dried rosemary
1 cup pecorino romano cheese, grated
3 turkey sausages, chopped

Directions

Preheat oven to 400ºF and grease muffin cups with cooking spray.
In a skillet over medium heat add the butter and cook the turkey sausages for 4-5 minutes.
Beat 3 eggs with a fork. Add in sausages, cheese, and seasonings. Divide between the muffin cups and bake for 4 minutes. Crack in an egg to each of the cups. Bake for an additional 4 minutes. Allow cooling before serving.

Cheese & Aioli Eggs

Ready in about: 20 minutes | Serves: 8
Per serving: Kcal: 355; Fat 22.5g, Net Carbs 1.8g, Protein 29.5g

Ingredients

8 eggs, hard-boiled, chopped
28 ounces tuna in brine, drained
½ cup lettuces, torn into pieces
½ cup green onions, finely chopped
½ cup feta cheese, crumbled
⅓ cup sour cream
½ tbsp mustard

For Aioli:

1 cup mayonnaise
2 cloves garlic, minced
1 tbsp lemon juice
Salt and black pepper, to taste

Directions

Set the eggs in a serving bowl. Place in tuna, onion, mustard, cheese, lettuce, and sour cream.
To prepare aioli, mix in a bowl mayonnaise, lemon juice, and garlic. Add in black pepper and salt. Stir in the prepared aioli to the bowl to incorporate everything. Serve with pickles.

Duo-Cheese Omelet with Pimenta and Basil

Ready in about: 15 minutes | Serves: 2
Per serving: Kcal: 490; Fat: 44.6g, Net Carbs: 4.5g, Protein: 22.7g

Ingredients

3 tbsp olive oil
4 eggs, beaten
Salt and black pepper, to taste
¼ tsp paprika
¼ tsp cayenne pepper
½ cup asiago cheese, shredded
½ cup cheddar cheese, shredded
2 tbsp fresh basil, roughly chopped

Directions

Set a pan over medium heat and warm the oil. Season eggs with cayenne pepper, salt, paprika, and black pepper. Transfer to the pan and ensure they are evenly spread. Top with the asiago and cheddar cheeses. Slice the omelet into two halves. Decorate with fresh basil, to serve.

Cheese Stuffed Avocados

Ready in about: 20 minutes | Serves: 4
Per serving: Kcal 342; Fat: 30.4g, Net Carbs: 7.5g, Protein: 11.1g

Ingredients

3 avocados, halved and pitted, skin on
½ cup feta cheese, crumbled
½ cup cheddar cheese, grated
2 eggs, beaten
Salt and black pepper, to taste
1 tbsp fresh basil, chopped

Directions

Set oven to 360ºF and lay the avocado halves in an ovenproof dish. In a mixing dish, mix both types of cheeses, black pepper, eggs, and salt. Split the mixture equally into the avocado halves. Bake thoroughly for 15 to 17 minutes. Decorate with fresh basil before serving.

Cauliflower & Cheese Burgers

Ready in about: 35 minutes | Serves: 6
Per serving: Kcal 416; Fat: 33.8g, Net Carbs: 7.8g, Protein: 13g

Ingredients

1 ½ tbsp olive oil
1 onion, chopped
1 garlic clove, minced
1 pound cauliflower, grated
6 tbsp coconut flour
½ cup gruyere cheese, shredded
1 cup Parmesan cheese
2 eggs, beaten
½ tsp dried rosemary
Sea salt and ground black pepper, to taste

Directions

Set a cast iron skillet over medium heat and warm oil. Add in garlic and onion and cook until soft, about 3 minutes. Stir in grated cauliflower and cook for a minute; allow cooling and set aside.
To the cooled cauliflower, add the rest of the ingredients; form balls from the mixture, then, press each ball to form burger patty.
Set oven to 400ºF and bake the burgers for 20 minutes. Flip and bake for another 10 minutes or until the top becomes golden brown.

Kielbasa and Roquefort Waffles

Ready in about: 20 minutes | Serves: 2
Per serving: Kcal 470; Fat: 40.3g, Net Carbs: 2.9g,
Protein: 24.4g

Ingredients

2 tbsp butter, melted
Salt and black pepper, to taste
½ tsp parsley flakes
½ tsp chili pepper flakes
4 eggs
½ cup Roquefort cheese, crumbled
4 slices kielbasa, chopped
2 tbsp fresh chives, chopped

Directions

In a mixing bowl, combine all ingredients except fresh chives. Preheat waffle iron and spray with a cooking spray. Pour in the batter and close the lid.
Cook for 5 minutes or until golden-brown, do the same with the rest of the batter. Decorate with fresh chives and serve while warm.

Coconut & Walnut Chia Pudding

Ready in about: 10 minutes | Serves: 1
Per serving: Kcal 334, Fat: 29g, Net Carbs: 1.5g
Protein: 15g

Ingredients

½ tsp vanilla extract
½ cup water
1 tbsp chia seeds
2 tbsp hemp seeds
1 tbsp flax seed meal
2 tbsp almond meal
2 tbsp shredded coconut
¼ tsp granulated stevia
1 tbsp walnuts, chopped

Directions

Put chia seeds, hemp seeds, flaxseed meal, almond meal, granulated stevia, and shredded coconut in a nonstick saucepan and pour over the water. Simmer over medium heat, occasionally stirring, until creamed and thickened, for about 3-4 minutes. Stir in vanilla.
When the pudding is ready, spoon into a serving bowl, sprinkle with walnuts and serve warm.

Cheese Ciabatta with Pepperoni

Ready in about: 30 minutes | Serves: 6
Per serving: Kcal 464, Fat: 33.6g, Net Carbs: 9.1g,
Protein: 31.1g

INGREDIENTS

10 ounces cream cheese, melted
2 ½ cups mozzarella cheese, shredded
4 large eggs, beaten
3 tbsp Romano cheese, grated
½ cup pork rinds, crushed
2 ½ tsp baking powder
½ cup tomato puree
12 large slices pepperoni

DIRECTIONS

Combine eggs, mozzarella cheese and cream cheese. Place in baking powder, pork rinds, and Romano cheese. Form into 6 chiabatta shapes. Set a nonstick pan over medium heat. Cook each ciabatta for 2 minutes per side. Sprinkle tomato puree over each one and top with pepperoni slices to serve.

POULTRY RECIPES

Bacon Wrapped Chicken with Grilled Asparagus

Ready in about: 48 minutes | Serves: 4
Per serving: Kcal 468, Fat 38g, Net Carbs 2g, Protein 26g

Ingredients

6 chicken breasts
Pink salt and black pepper to taste
8 bacon slices
3 tbsp olive oil
1 lb asparagus spears
3 tbsp olive oil
2 tbsp fresh lemon juice
Manchego cheese for topping

Directions

Preheat the oven to 400ºF.
Season chicken breasts with salt and black pepper, and wrap 2 bacon slices around each chicken breast. Arrange on a baking sheet that is lined with parchment paper, drizzle with oil and bake for 25-30 minutes until bacon is brown and crispy.
Preheat your grill to high heat.
Brush the asparagus spears with olive oil and season with salt. Grill for 8-10 minutes, frequently turning until slightly charred. Remove to a plate and drizzle with lemon juice. Grate over Manchego cheese so that it melts a little on contact with the hot asparagus and forms a cheesy dressing.

Spinach Chicken Cheesy Bake

Ready in about: 45 minutes | Serves: 6
Per serving: Kcal 340, Fat 30.2g, Net Carbs 3.1g, Protein 15g

Ingredients

6 chicken breasts, skinless and boneless
1 tsp mixed spice seasoning
Pink salt and black pepper to season
2 loose cups baby spinach
3 tsp olive oil
4 oz cream cheese, cubed
1 ¼ cups shredded mozzarella cheese
4 tbsp water

Directions

Preheat oven to 370ºF.
Season chicken with spice mix, salt, and black pepper. Pat with your hands to have the seasoning stick on the chicken. Put in the casserole dish and layer spinach over the chicken. Mix the oil with cream cheese, mozzarella, salt, and black pepper and stir in water a tablespoon at a time. Pour the mixture over the chicken and cover the pot with aluminium foil.
Bake for 20 minutes, remove foil and continue cooking for 15 minutes until a nice golden brown color is formed on top. Take out and allow sitting for 5 minutes. Serve warm with braised asparagus.

Cilantro Chicken Breasts with Mayo-Avocado Sauce

Ready in about: 22 minutes | Serves: 4
Per serving: Kcal 398, Fat 32g, Net Carbs 4g, Protein 24g

Ingredients

For the Sauce
1 avocado, pitted
½ cup mayonnaise
Salt to taste
For the Chicken
3 tbsp ghee
4 chicken breasts
Pink salt and black pepper to taste
1 cup chopped cilantro leaves
½ cup chicken broth

Directions

Spoon the avocado, mayonnaise, and salt into a small food processor and puree until a smooth sauce is derived. Pour sauce into a jar and refrigerate while you make the chicken.
Melt ghee in a large skillet, season chicken with salt and black pepper and fry for 4 minutes on each side to golden brown. Remove chicken to a plate.
Pour the broth in the same skillet and add the cilantro. Bring to simmer covered for 3 minutes and add the chicken. Cover and cook on low heat for 5 minutes until the liquid has reduced and chicken is fragrant. Dish chicken only into serving plates and spoon the mayo-avocado sauce over.

Parmesan Wings with Yogurt Sauce

Ready in about: 25 minutes | Serves: 6
Per serving: Kcal 452, Fat 36.4g, Net Carbs 4g, Protein 24g

Ingredients

For the Dipping Sauce
1 cup plain yogurt
1 tsp fresh lemon juice
Salt and black pepper to taste
For the Wings
2 lb chicken wings
Salt and black pepper to taste
Cooking spray
½ cup melted butter
½ cup Hot sauce
¼ cup grated Parmesan cheese

Directions

Mix the yogurt, lemon juice, salt, and black pepper in a bowl. Chill while making the chicken.
Preheat oven to 400ºF and season wings with salt and black pepper. Line them on a baking sheet and grease lightly with cooking spray. Bake for 20 minutes until golden brown. Mix butter, hot sauce, and Parmesan cheese in a bowl. Toss chicken in the sauce to evenly coat and plate. Serve with yogurt dipping sauce and celery strips.

Sweet Garlic Chicken Skewers

Ready in about: 17 minutes + time refrigeration | Serves: 4

Per serving: Kcal 225, Fat 17.4g, Net Carbs 2g, Protein 15g

Ingredients

For the Skewers

3 tbsp soy sauce
1 tbsp ginger-garlic paste
2 tbsp swerve brown sugar
Chili pepper to taste
2 tbsp olive oil
3 chicken breasts, cut into cubes

For the Dressing

½ cup tahini
½ tsp garlic powder
Pink salt to taste
¼ cup warm water

Directions

In a small bowl, whisk the soy sauce, ginger-garlic paste, brown sugar, chili pepper, and olive oil.

Put the chicken in a zipper bag, pour the marinade over, seal and shake for an even coat. Marinate in the fridge for 2 hours.

Preheat a grill to 400ºF and thread the chicken on skewers. Cook for 10 minutes in total with three to four turnings to be golden brown; remove to a plate.

Mix the tahini, garlic powder, salt, and warm water in a bowl. Pour into serving jars.

Serve the chicken skewers and tahini dressing with cauli fried rice.

Roasted Chicken Breasts with Capers

Ready in about: 65 minutes | Serves: 6

Per serving: Kcal 430, Fat 23g, Net Carbs 3g, Protein 33g

Ingredients

3 medium lemons, sliced
½ tsp salt
1 tsp olive oil
3 chicken breasts, halved
Salt and black pepper to season
¼ cup almond flour
2 tsp olive oil
2 tbsp capers, rinsed
1 ¼ cup chicken broth
2 tsp butter
1 ½ tbsp chopped fresh parsley
Parsley for garnish

Directions

Preheat the oven to 350ºF and lay a piece of parchment paper on a baking sheet.

Lay the lemon slices on the baking sheet, drizzle with olive oil and sprinkle with salt. Roast in the oven for 25 minutes to brown the lemon rinds.

Cover the chicken with plastic wrap, place them on a flat surface, and gently pound with the rolling pin to flatten to about ½ -inch thickness. Remove the plastic wraps and season with salt and pepper.

Next, dredge the chicken in the almond flour on each side, and shake off any excess flour. Set aside.

Heat the olive oil in a skillet over medium heat and fry the chicken on both sides to a golden brown, for about 8 minutes in total. Pour the chicken broth in, shake the skillet, and let the broth boil and reduce to a thick consistency, about 12 minutes.

Lightly stir in the capers, roasted lemon, pepper, butter, and parsley, and simmer on low heat for 10 minutes. Turn the heat off and serve the chicken with the sauce hot, an extra garnish of parsley with a creamy squash mash.

Eggplant & Tomato Braised Chicken Thighs

Ready in about: 45 minutes | Serves: 4

Per serving: Kcal 468, Fat 39.5g, Net Carbs 2g, Protein 26g

Ingredients

2 tbsp ghee
1 lb chicken thighs
Salt and black pepper to taste
2 cloves garlic, minced
1 (14 oz) can whole tomatoes
1 eggplant, diced
10 fresh basil leaves, chopped + extra to garnish

Directions

Melt ghee in a saucepan over medium heat, season the chicken with salt and black pepper and fry for 4 minutes on each side until golden brown. Remove to a plate.

Sauté the garlic in the ghee for 2 minutes, pour in the tomatoes, and cook covered for 8 minutes. Add in the eggplant and basil. Cook for 4 minutes. Season the sauce with salt and black pepper, stir and add the chicken. Coat with sauce and simmer for 3 minutes.

Serve chicken with sauce on a bed of squash pasta. Garnish with extra basil.

Poulet en Papillote

Ready in about: 48 minutes | Serves: 4

Per serving: Kcal 364, Fat 16.5g, Net Carbs 4.8g, Protein 25g

Ingredients

4 chicken breasts, skinless, scored
4 tbsp white wine
2 tbsp olive oil + extra for drizzling
4 tbsp butter
3 cups mixed mushrooms, teared up
1 medium celeriac, peeled, chopped
2 cups water
3 cloves garlic, minced
4 sprigs thyme, chopped
3 lemons, juiced
Salt and black pepper to taste
2 tbsp Dijon mustard

Directions

Preheat the oven to 450ºF.

Arrange the celeriac on a baking sheet, drizzle it with a little oil, and bake for 20 minutes; set aside.

In a bowl, evenly mix the chicken, roasted celeriac, mushrooms, garlic, thyme, lemon juice, salt, black pepper, and mustard. Make 4 large cuts of foil, fold them in half, and then fold them in half again. Tightly fold the two open edges together to create a bag.

Now, share the chicken mixture into each bag, top with the white wine, olive oil, and a tablespoon of butter. Seal the last open end securely making sure not to pierce the bag. Put the bag on a baking tray and bake the chicken in the middle of the oven for 25 minutes.

Chicken Paella with Chorizo

Ready in about: 63 minutes | Serves: 6
Per serving: Kcal 440, Fat 28g, Net Carbs 3g, Protein 22g
Ingredients
18 chicken drumsticks
12 oz chorizo, chopped
1 white onion, chopped
4 oz jarred piquillo peppers, finely diced
2 tbsp olive oil
½ cup chopped parsley
1 tsp smoked paprika
2 tbsp tomato puree
½ cup white wine
1 cup chicken broth
2 cups cauli rice
1 cup chopped green beans
1 lemon, cut in wedges
Salt and pepper, to taste
Directions
Preheat the oven to 350ºF.
Heat the olive oil in a cast iron pan over medium heat, meanwhile season the chicken with salt and black pepper, and fry in the hot oil on both sides for 10 minutes to lightly brown. After, remove onto a plate with a perforated spoon.
Then, add the chorizo and onion to the hot oil, and sauté for 4 minutes. Include the tomato puree, piquillo peppers, and paprika, and let simmer for 2 minutes. Add the broth, and bring the ingredients to boil for 6 minutes until slightly reduced.
Stir in the cauli rice, white wine, green beans, half of the parsley, and lay the chicken on top. Transfer the pan to the oven and continue cooking for 20-25 minutes. Let the paella sit to cool for 10 minutes before serving garnished with the remaining parsley and lemon wedges.

Lemon Threaded Chicken Skewers

Ready in about: 2 hours 17 minutes | Serves: 4
Per serving: Kcal 350, Fat 11g, Net Carbs 3.5g, Protein 34g
Ingredients
3 chicken breasts, cut into cubes
2 tbsp olive oil, divided
2/3 jar preserved lemon, flesh removed, drained
2 cloves garlic, minced
½ cup lemon juice

Salt and black pepper to taste
1 tsp rosemary leaves to garnish
2 to 4 lemon wedges to garnish
Directions
First, thread the chicken onto skewers and set aside.
In a wide bowl, mix half of the oil, garlic, salt, pepper, and lemon juice, and add the chicken skewers, and lemon rind. Cover the bowl and let the chicken marinate for at least 2 hours in the refrigerator.
When the marinating time is almost over, preheat a grill to 350ºF, and remove the chicken onto the grill. Cook for 6 minutes on each side.
Remove and serve warm garnished with rosemary leaves and lemons wedges.

Chicken Cauliflower Bake

Ready in about: 58 minutes | Serves: 6
Per serving: Kcal 390, Fat 27g, Net Carbs 3g, Protein 22g
Ingredients
3 cups cubed leftover chicken
3 cups spinach
2 cauliflower heads, cut into florets
3 cups water
3 eggs, lightly beaten
2 cups grated sharp cheddar cheese
1 cup pork rinds, crushed
½ cup unsweetened almond milk
3 tbsp olive oil
3 cloves garlic, minced
Salt and black pepper to taste
Cooking spray
Directions
Preheat the oven to 350ºF and grease a baking dish with cooking spray. Set aside.
Pour the cauli florets and water in a pot; bring to boil over medium heat. Cover and steam the cauli florets for 8 minutes. Drain them through a colander and set aside.
Also, combine the cheddar cheese and pork rinds in a large bowl and mix in the chicken. Set aside.
Heat the olive oil in a skillet and cook the garlic and spinach until the spinach has wilted, about 5 minutes. Season with salt and black pepper, and add the spinach mixture and cauli florets to the chicken bowl. Top with the eggs and almond milk, mix and transfer everything to the baking dish. Layer the top of the ingredients and place the dish in the oven to bake for 30 minutes.
By this time the edges and top must have browned nicely, then remove the chicken from the oven, let rest for 5 minutes, and serve. Garnish with steamed and seasoned green beans.

Creamy Stuffed Chicken with Parma Ham

Ready in about: 40 minutes | Serves: 4
Per serving: Kcal 485, Fat 35g, Net Carbs 2g, Protein 26g

Ingredients

4 chicken breasts
2 tbsp olive oil
3 cloves garlic, minced
3 shallots, finely chopped
4 tbsp dried mixed herbs
8 slices Parma ham
8 oz cream cheese
2 lemons, zested
Salt to taste

Directions

Preheat the oven to 350ºF.

Heat the oil in a small skillet and sauté the garlic and shallots with a pinch of salt and lemon zest for 3 minutes; let it cool. After, stir the cream cheese and mixed herbs into the shallot mixture.

Score a pocket in each chicken breast, fill the holes with the cream cheese mixture and cover with the cut-out chicken. Wrap each breast with two Parma ham and secure the ends with a toothpick. Lay the chicken parcels on a greased baking sheet and cook in the oven for 20 minutes. Remove to rest for 4 minutes before serving with green salad and roasted tomatoes.

Chicken Drumsticks in Tomato Sauce

Ready in about: 1 ½ hours | Serves: 4
Per serving: Kcal 515, Fat 34.2g, Net Carbs 7.3g, Protein 50.8g

Ingredients

8 chicken drumsticks
1 ½ tbsp olive oil
1 medium white onion, diced
3 medium turnips, peeled and diced
2 medium carrots, chopped in 1-inch pieces
2 green bell peppers, seeded, cut into chunks
2 cloves garlic, minced
¼ cup coconut flour
1 cup chicken broth
1 (28 oz) can sugar-free tomato sauce
2 tbsp dried Italian herbs
Salt and black pepper to taste

Directions

Preheat oven to 400ºF.

Heat the oil in a large skillet over medium heat, meanwhile season the drumsticks with salt and pepper, and fry in the oil to brown on both sides for 10 minutes. Remove to a baking dish. Sauté the onion, turnips, bell peppers, carrots, and garlic in the same oil and for 10 minutes with continuous stirring.

In a bowl, combine the broth, coconut flour, tomato paste, and Italian herbs together, and pour it over the vegetables in the pan. Stir and cook to thicken for 4

minutes. Pour the mixture on the chicken in the baking dish. Bake for around 1 hour. Remove from the oven and serve with steamed cauli rice.

Garlic & Ginger Chicken with Peanut Sauce

Ready in about: 1 hour and 50 minutes | Serves: 6
Per serving: Kcal 492, Fat: 36g, Net Carbs: 3g, Protein: 35g

Ingredients

1 tbsp wheat-free soy sauce
1 tbsp sugar-free fish sauce
1 tbsp lime juice
1 tsp cilantro
1 tsp minced garlic
1 tsp minced ginger
1 tbsp olive oil
1 tbsp rice wine vinegar
1 tsp cayenne pepper
1 tsp erythritol
6 chicken thighs

Peanut sauce:

½ cup peanut butter
1 tsp minced garlic
1 tbsp lime juice
2 tbsp water
1 tsp minced ginger
1 tbsp chopped jalapeño
2 tbsp rice wine vinegar
2 tbsp erythritol
1 tbsp fish sauce

Directions

Combine all chicken ingredients in a large Ziploc bag. Seal the bag and shake to combine. Refrigerate for 1 hour. Remove from fridge about 15 minutes before cooking.

Preheat the grill to medium heat and cook the chicken for 7 minutes per side. Whisk together all sauce ingredients in a mixing bowl. Serve the chicken drizzled with peanut sauce.

Chicken, Broccoli & Cashew Stir-Fry

Ready in about: 30 minutes | Serves: 4
Per serving: Kcal 286, Fat 10.1g, Net Carbs 3.4g, Protein 17.3g

Ingredients

2 chicken breasts, cut into strips
3 tbsp olive oil
2 tbsp soy sauce
2 tsp white wine vinegar
1 tsp erythritol
2 tsp xanthan gum
1 lemon, juiced
1 cup unsalted cashew nuts
2 cups broccoli florets
1 white onion, thinly sliced
Salt and black pepper to taste

Directions

In a bowl, mix the soy sauce, vinegar, lemon juice, erythritol, and xanthan gum. Set aside.

Heat the oil in a wok and fry the cashew for 4 minutes until golden-brown. Remove to a paper towel lined plate. Sauté the onion in the same oil for 4 minutes until soft and browned; add to the cashew nuts.

Add the chicken to the wok and cook for 4 minutes; include the broccoli, salt, and black pepper. Stir-fry and pour the soy sauce mixture in. Stir and cook the sauce for 4 minutes and pour in the cashews and onion. Stir once more, cook for 1 minute, and turn the heat off.

Serve the chicken stir-fry with some steamed cauli rice.

Cheese Stuffed Chicken Breasts with Spinach

Ready in about: 50 minutes | Serves: 4
Per serving: Kcal 491, Fat: 36g, Net Carbs: 3.5g, Protein: 38g

Ingredients
4 chicken breasts, boneless and skinless
½ cup mozzarella cheese
⅓ cup Parmesan cheese
6 ounces cream cheese
2 cups spinach, chopped
A pinch of nutmeg
½ tsp minced garlic
Breading:
2 eggs
⅓ cup almond flour
2 tbsp olive oil
½ tsp parsley
⅓ cup Parmesan cheese
A pinch of onion powder
Directions
Pound the chicken until it doubles in size. Mix the cream cheese, spinach, mozzarella, nutmeg, salt, black pepper, and Parmesan cheese in a bowl. Divide the mixture between the chicken breasts and spread it out evenly. Wrap the chicken in a plastic wrap. Refrigerate for 15 minutes.

Heat the oil in a pan and preheat the oven to 370ºF. Beat the eggs and combine all other breading ingredients in a bowl. Dip the chicken in egg first, then in the breading mixture. Cook in the pan until browned. Place on a lined baking sheet and bake for 20 minutes.

Chili Turkey Patties with Cucumber Salsa

Ready in about: 30 minutes | Serves: 4
Per serving: Kcal 475, Fat: 38g, Net Carbs: 5g, Protein: 26g

Ingredients
2 spring onions, thinly sliced
1 pound ground turkey
1 egg
2 garlic cloves, minced
1 tbsp chopped herbs
1 small chili pepper, deseeded and diced

2 tbsp ghee
Cucumber Salsa
1 tbsp apple cider vinegar
1 tbsp chopped dill
1 garlic clove, minced
2 cucumbers, grated
1 cup sour cream
1 jalapeño pepper, minced
2 tbsp olive oil
Directions
Place all turkey ingredients, except the ghee, in a bowl. Mix to combine. Make patties out of the mixture.

Melt the ghee in a skillet over medium heat. Cook the patties for 3 minutes per side. Place all salsa ingredients in a bowl and mix to combine. Serve the patties topped with salsa.

Lemon & Rosemary Chicken in a Skillet

Ready in about: 1 hour and 20 minutes | Serves: 4
Per serving: Kcal 477, Fat: 31g, Net Carbs: 2.5g, Protein: 31g

Ingredients
8 chicken thighs
1 tsp salt
2 tbsp lemon juice
1 tsp lemon zest
2 tbsp olive oil
1 tbsp chopped rosemary
¼ tsp black pepper
1 garlic clove, minced
Directions
Combine all ingredients in a bowl. Place in the fridge for one hour. Heat a skillet over medium heat. Add the chicken along with the juices and cook until crispy, about 7 minutes per side.

Chicken Wings with Thyme Chutney

Ready in about: 45 minutes | Serves: 4
Per serving: Kcal 243, Fat 15g, Net Carbs 3.5g, Protein 22g

Ingredients
12 chicken wings, cut in half
1 tbsp turmeric
1 tbsp cumin
3 tbsp fresh ginger, grated
1 tbsp cilantro, chopped
2 tbsp paprika
Salt and ground black pepper, to taste
3 tbsp olive oil
Juice of ½ lime
1 cup thyme leaves
¾ cup cilantro, chopped
1 tbsp water
1 jalapeño pepper
Directions
In a bowl, stir together 1 tbsp ginger, cumin, paprika, salt, 2 tbsp olive oil, black pepper, and turmeric. Place in the chicken wings pieces, toss to coat, and refrigerate for 20 minutes.

Heat the grill, place in the marinated wings, cook for 25 minutes, turning from time to time, remove and set to a serving plate.

Using a blender, combine thyme, remaining ginger, salt, jalapeno pepper, black pepper, lime juice, cilantro, remaining olive oil, and water, and blend well. Drizzle the chicken wings with the sauce to serve.

Oregano & Chili Flattened Chicken
Ready in about: 5 minutes | Serves: 6
Per serving: Kcal 265, Fat 9g, Net Carbs 3g, Protein 26g
Ingredients
6 chicken breasts
4 cloves garlic, minced
½ cup oregano leaves, chopped
½ cup lemon juice
2/3 cup olive oil
¼ cup erythritol
Salt and black pepper to taste
3 small chilies, minced
Directions
Preheat a grill to 350ºF.
In a bowl, mix the garlic, oregano, lemon juice, olive oil, chilies and erythritol. Set aside.
While the spices incorporate in flavor, cover the chicken with plastic wraps, and use the rolling pin to pound to ½ -inch thickness. Remove the wrap, and brush the mixture on the chicken on both sides.
Place on the grill, cover the lid and cook for 15 minutes. Baste the chicken with more of the spice mixture, and continue cooking for 15 more minutes.

Grilled Chicken Wings
Ready in about: 15 minutes + chilling time | Serves: 4
Per serving: Kcal 216, Fat 11.5g, Net Carbs 4.3g, Protein 18.5g
Ingredients
2 pounds chicken wings
Juice from 1 lemon
½ cup fresh parsley, chopped
2 garlic cloves, peeled and minced
1 serrano pepper, chopped
3 tbsp olive oil
Salt and black pepper, to taste
Lemon wedges, for serving
Ranch dip, for serving
½ tsp cilantro
Directions
In a bowl, stir together lemon juice, garlic, salt, serrano pepper, cilantro, olive oil, and black pepper. Place in the chicken wings and toss well to coat. Refrigerate for 2 hours.
Set a grill over high heat and add on the chicken wings; cook each side for 6 minutes. Remove to a plate and serve alongside lemon wedges and ranch dip.

Spicy Chicken Kabobs
Ready in about: 20 minutes + marinade time | Serves: 6
Per serving: Kcal 198, Fat: 13.5g, Net Carbs: 3.1g, Protein: 17.5g
Ingredients
2 pounds chicken breasts, cubed
1 tsp sesame oil
1 tbsp olive oil
1 cup red bell pepper pieces
2 tbsp five spice powder
2 tbsp granulated sweetener
1 tbsp fish sauce
Directions
Combine the sesame and olive oils, fish sauce, and seasonings in a bowl. Add the chicken, and let marinate for 1 hour in the fridge.
Preheat the grill. Take 12 skewers and thread the chicken and bell peppers. Grill for 3 minutes per side.

Roasted Stuffed Chicken with Tomato Basil Sauce
Ready in about: 35 minutes | Serves: 6
Per serving: Kcal 338, Fat: 28g, Net Carbs: 2.5g, Protein: 37g
Ingredients
4 ounces cream cheese
3 ounces mozzarella slices
10 ounces spinach
⅓ cup shredded mozzarella cheese
1 tbsp olive oil
1 cup tomato basil sauce
3 whole chicken breasts
Directions
Preheat your oven to 400ºF. Combine the cream cheese, shredded mozzarella cheese, and spinach in the microwave. Cut the chicken a couple of times horizontally and stuff with the spinach mixture. Brush with olive oil. place on a lined baking dish and bake in the oven for 25 minutes.
Pour the tomato basil sauce over and top with mozzarella slices. Return to the oven and cook for an additional 5 minutes.

Chicken in Creamy Spinach Sauce
Ready in about: 35 minutes | Serves: 4
Per serving: Kcal 446, Fat: 38g, Net Carbs: 2.6g, Protein: 18g
Ingredients
1 pound chicken thighs
2 tbsp coconut oil
2 tbsp coconut flour
2 cups spinach, chopped
1 tsp oregano
1 cup heavy cream
1 cup chicken broth
2 tbsp butter
Directions
Warm the coconut oil in a skillet and brown the chicken on all sides, about 6-8 minutes. Set aside.

Add and melt the butter and whisk in the flour over medium heat. Whisk in the heavy cream and chicken broth and bring to a boil. Stir in oregano. Add the spinach to the skillet and cook until wilted. Add the thighs in the skillet and cook for an additional 15 minutes.

Zucchini Spaghetti with Turkey Bolognese Sauce

Ready in about: 30 minutes | Serves: 6
Per serving: Kcal 273, Fat: 16g, Net Carbs: 3.8g, Protein: 19g

Ingredients
2 cups sliced mushrooms
2 tsp olive oil
1 pound ground turkey
3 tbsp pesto sauce
1 cup diced onion
2 cups broccoli florets
6 cups zucchini, spiralized

Directions
Heat the oil in a skillet. Add zucchini and cook for 2-3 minutes, stirring continuously; set aside.
Add turkey to the skillet and cook until browned, about 7-8 minutes. Transfer to a plate. Add onion and cook until translucent, about 3 minutes. Add broccoli and mushrooms, and cook for 7 more minutes. Return the turkey to the skillet. Stir in the pesto sauce. Cover the pan, lower the heat, and simmer for 15 minutes. Stir in zucchini pasta and serve immediately.

Roast Chicken with Herb Stuffing

Ready in about: 120 minutes | Serves: 8
Per serving: Kcal 432, Fat: 32g, Net Carbs: 5.1g, Protein: 30g

Ingredients
5-pound whole chicken
1 bunch oregano
1 bunch thyme
1 tbsp marjoram
1 tbsp parsley
1 tbsp olive oil
2 pounds Brussels sprouts
1 lemon
4 tbsp butter

Directions
Preheat your oven to 450ºF.
Stuff the chicken with oregano, thyme, and lemon. Roast for 15 minutes. Reduce the heat to 325ºF and cook for 40 minutes. Spread the butter over the chicken, and sprinkle parsley and marjoram. Add the brussels sprouts. Return to the oven and bake for 40 more minutes. Let sit for 10 minutes before carving.

Basil Turkey Meatballs

Ready in about: 15 minutes | Serves: 4
Per serving: Kcal 310, Fat: 26g, Net Carbs: 2g, Protein: 22g

Ingredients
1 pound ground turkey
2 tbsp chopped sun-dried tomatoes
2 tbsp chopped basil
½ tsp garlic powder
1 egg
½ tsp salt
¼ cup almond flour
2 tbsp olive oil
½ cup shredded mozzarella cheese
¼ tsp pepper

Directions
Place everything, except the oil in a bowl. Mix with your hands until combined. Form into 16 balls. Heat the olive oil in a skillet over medium heat. Cook the meatballs for 4-5 minutes per each side. Serve.

Lemon Chicken Wings

Ready in about: 30 minutes | Serves: 4
Per serving: Kcal 365, Fat: 25g, Net Carbs: 4g, Protein: 21g

Ingredients
1 cup omission ipa
A pinch of garlic powder
1 tsp lemon zest
3 tbsp lemon juice
½ tsp ground cilantro
1 tbsp fish sauce
2 tbsp butter
¼ tsp xanthan gum
3 tbsp swerve sweetener
20 chicken wings
Salt and black pepper, to taste

Directions
Combine lemon juice and zest, fish sauce, cilantro, omission ipa, sweetener, and garlic powder in a saucepan. Bring to a boil, cover, lower the heat, and let simmer for 10 minutes. Stir in the butter and xanthan gum. Set aside. Season the wings with some salt and pepper.
Preheat the grill and cook for 5 minutes per side. Serve topped with the sauce.

Chicken Garam Masala

Ready in about: 45 minutes | Serves: 4
Per serving: Kcal: 564, Fat: 50g, Net Carbs: 5g, Protein: 33g

Ingredients
1 lb chicken breasts, sliced lengthwise
2 tbsp butter
1 tbsp olive oil
1 yellow bell pepper, finely chopped
1 ¼ cups heavy whipping cream
1 tbsp fresh cilantro, finely chopped
Salt and pepper, to taste
For the garam masala
1 tsp ground cumin
2 tsp ground coriander
1 tsp ground cardamom
1 tsp turmeric
1 tsp ginger

1 tsp paprika
1 tsp cayenne, ground
1 pinch ground nutmeg

Set your oven to 400ºF. In a bowl, mix the garam masala spices. Coat the chicken with half of the masala mixture. Heat the olive oil and butter in a frying pan over medium-high heat, and brown the chicken for 3-5 minutes per side. Transfer to a baking dish.

To the remaining masala, add heavy cream and bell pepper. Season with salt and pepper and pour over chicken. Bake for 20 minutes until the mixture starts to bubble. Garnish with chopped cilantro to serve.

Easy Chicken Chili

Ready in about: 30 minutes | Serves: 4
Per serving: Kcal: 421, Fat: 21g, Net Carbs: 5.6g, Protein: 45g

Ingredients
4 chicken breasts, skinless, boneless, cubed
1 tbsp butter
½ onion, chopped
2 cups chicken broth
8 oz diced tomatoes
2 oz tomato puree
1 tbsp chili powder
1 tbsp cumin
½ tbsp garlic powder
1 serrano pepper, minced
½ cup shredded cheddar cheese
Salt and black pepper to taste

Directions
Set a large pan over medium-high heat and add the chicken. Cover with water and bring to a boil. Cook until no longer pink, for 10 minutes. Transfer the chicken to a flat surface to shred with forks.

In a large pot, pour in the butter and set over medium heat. Sauté onion until transparent for 5 minutes. Stir in the chicken, tomatoes, cumin, serrano pepper, garlic powder, tomato puree, broth, and chili powder. Adjust the seasoning and let the mixture boil. Reduce heat to simmer for about 10 minutes. Divide chili among bowls and top with shredded cheese to serve.

Thyme Chicken Thighs

Ready in about: 30 minutes | Serves: 4
Per serving: Kcal 528, Fat: 42g, Net Carbs: 4g, Protein: 33g

Ingredients
½ cup chicken stock
1 tbsp olive oil
½ cup chopped onion
4 chicken thighs
¼ cup heavy cream
2 tbsp Dijon mustard
1 tsp thyme
1 tsp garlic powder

Directions

Heat the olive oil in a pan. Cook the chicken for about 4 minutes per side. Set aside. Sauté the onion in the same pan for 3 minutes, add the stock, and simmer for 5 minutes. Stir in mustard and heavy cream, along with thyme and garlic powder. Pour the sauce over the chicken and serve.

Stuffed Chicken Breasts with Cucumber Noodle Salad

Ready in about: 60 minutes | Serves: 4
Per serving: Kcal: 453, Fat: 31g, Net Carbs: 6g, Protein: 43g

Ingredients
For the chicken
4 chicken breasts
1/3 cup baby spinach
1/4 cup goat cheese
1/4 cup shredded cheddar cheese
4 tbsp butter
Salt and black pepper, to taste
For the tomato sauce
1 tbsp butter
1 shallot, chopped
2 garlic cloves, chopped
½ tbsp red wine vinegar
2 tbsp tomato paste
14 oz canned crushed tomatoes
½ tsp salt
1 tsp dried basil
1 tsp dried oregano
Black pepper, to taste
For the salad
2 cucumbers, spiralized
2 tbsp olive oil
1 tbsp rice vinegar

Directions
Set oven to 400ºF and grease a baking dish. Set aside. Place a pan over medium heat. Melt 2 tbsp of butter and sauté spinach until it shrinks; season with salt and pepper. Transfer to a bowl containing goat cheese, stir and set aside. Cut the chicken breasts lengthwise and stuff with the cheese mixture and set into the baking dish. On top, spread the grated cheddar cheese, add 2 tbsp of butter then set into the oven. Bake until cooked through for 20-30 minutes.

Set a pan over medium-high heat and warm 1 tbsp of butter. Add in garlic and shallot and cook until soft. Place in herbs, tomato paste, vinegar, tomatoes, salt, and pepper. Bring the mixture to a boil. Set heat to low and simmer for 15 minutes. Arrange the cucumbers on a serving platter, season with salt, pepper, olive oil, and vinegar, Top with the chicken and pour over the sauce.

Chicken Goujons with Tomato Sauce

Ready in about: 50 minutes | Serves: 8
Per serving: Kcal 415, Fat 36g, Net Carbs 5g, Protein 28g

Ingredients

1½ pounds chicken breasts, skinless, boneless, cubed
Salt and ground black pepper, to taste
1 egg
1 cup almond flour
¼ cup Parmesan cheese, grated
½ tsp garlic powder
1½ tsp dried parsley
½ tsp dried basil
4 tbsp avocado oil
4 cups spaghetti squash, cooked
6 oz gruyere cheese, shredded
1½ cups tomato sauce
Fresh basil, chopped, for serving

Directions

In a bowl, combine the almond flour with 1 teaspoon parsley, Parmesan cheese, black pepper, garlic powder, and salt. In a separate bowl, combine the egg with black pepper and salt. Dip the chicken in the egg, and then in almond flour mixture.

Set a pan over medium heat and warm 3 tablespoons avocado oil, add in the chicken, cook until golden, and remove to paper towels. In a bowl, combine the spaghetti squash with salt, dried basil, rest of the parsley, 1 tablespoon avocado oil, and black pepper. Sprinkle this into a baking dish, top with the chicken pieces, followed by the tomato sauce. Scatter shredded gruyere cheese on top, and bake for 30 minutes at 360ºF. Remove, and sprinkle with fresh basil before serving.

Spanish Chicken

Ready in about: 60 minutes | Serves: 4
Per serving: Kcal 415, Fat 33g, Net Carbs 4g, Protein 25g

Ingredients

1/2 cup mushrooms, chopped
1 pound chorizo sausages, chopped
2 tbsp avocado oil
4 cherry peppers, chopped
1 red bell pepper, seeded, chopped
1 onion, peeled and sliced
2 tbsp garlic, minced
2 cups tomatoes, chopped
4 chicken thighs
Salt and black pepper, to taste
½ cup chicken stock
1 tsp turmeric
1 tbsp vinegar
2 tsp dried oregano
Fresh parsley, chopped, for serving

Directions

Set a pan over medium heat and warm half of the avocado oil, stir in the chorizo sausages, and cook for 5-6 minutes until browned; remove to a bowl. Heat the rest of the oil, place in the chicken thighs, and apply pepper and salt for seasoning. Cook each side for 3 minutes and set aside on a bowl.

In the same pan, add the onion, bell pepper, cherry peppers, and mushrooms, and cook for 4 minutes. Stir in the garlic and cook for 2 minutes. Pour in the stock, turmeric, salt, tomatoes, pepper, vinegar, and oregano. Stir in the chorizo sausages and chicken, place everything to the oven at 400ºF, and bake for 30 minutes. Ladle into serving bowls and garnish with chopped parsley to serve.

Cheesy Chicken Bake with Zucchini

Ready in about: 45 minutes | Serves: 6
Per serving: Kcal: 489, Fat: 37g, Net Carbs: 4.5g, Protein: 21g

Ingredients

2 lb chicken breasts, cubed
1 tbsp butter
1 cup green bell peppers, sliced
1 cup yellow onions, sliced
1 zucchini, cubed
2 garlic cloves, divided
2 tsp Italian seasoning
½ tsp salt
½ tsp black pepper
8 oz cream cheese, softened
½ cup mayonnaise
2 tbsp Worcestershire sauce (sugar-free)
2 cups cheddar cheese, shredded

Directions

Set oven to 370ºF and grease and line a baking dish.

Set a pan over medium heat. Place in the butter and let melt, then add in the chicken. Cook until lightly browned, about 5 minutes. Place in onions, zucchini, black pepper, garlic, bell peppers, salt, and 1 tsp of Italian seasoning. Cook until tender and set aside.

In a bowl, mix cream cheese, garlic, remaining seasoning, mayonnaise, and Worcestershire sauce. Stir in meat and sauteed vegetables. Place the mixture into the prepared baking dish, sprinkle with the shredded cheddar cheese and insert into the oven. Cook until browned for 30 minutes.

Chicken Skewers with Celery Fries

Ready in about: 60 minutes | Serves: 4
Per serving: Kcal: 579, Fat: 43g, Net Carbs: 6g, Protein: 39g

Ingredients

2 chicken breasts
½ tsp salt
¼ tsp ground black pepper
2 tbsp olive oil
1/4 cup chicken broth

For the fries

1 lb celery root
2 tbsp olive oil
½ tsp salt
¼ tsp ground black pepper

Set oven to 400ºF. Grease and line a baking sheet. In a bowl, mix oil, spices and the chicken; set in the fridge for 10 minutes while covered. Peel and chop celery root to form fry shapes and place into a separate bowl. Apply oil to coat and add pepper and salt for seasoning. Arrange to the baking tray in an even layer and bake for 10 minutes.

Take the chicken from the refrigerator and thread onto the skewers. Place over the celery, pour in the chicken broth, then set in the oven for 30 minutes. Serve with lemon wedges.

One Pot Chicken with Mushrooms

Ready in about: 35 minutes | Serves: 6
Per serving: Kcal 447, Fat: 37g, Net Carbs: 1g, Protein: 31g

Ingredients

2 cups sliced mushrooms
½ tsp onion powder
½ tsp garlic powder
¼ cup butter
1 tsp Dijon mustard
1 tbsp tarragon, chopped
2 pounds chicken thighs
Salt and black pepper, to taste

Directions

Season the thighs with salt, pepper, garlic, and onion powder. Melt the butter in a skillet, and cook the chicken until browned; set aside. Add mushrooms to the same fat and cook for about 5 minutes.

Stir in Dijon mustard and ½ cup of water. Return the chicken to the skillet. Season to taste with salt and pepper, reduce the heat and cover, and let simmer for 15 minutes. Stir in tarragon. Serve warm.

Chicken in Creamy Tomato Sauce

Ready in about: 20 minutes | Serves: 6
Per serving: Kcal 456, Fat 38.2g, Net Carbs 2g, Protein 24g

Ingredients

2 tbsp butter
6 chicken thighs
Pink salt and black pepper to taste
14 oz canned tomato sauce
2 tsp Italian seasoning
½ cup heavy cream
1 cup shredded Parmesan cheese
Parmesan cheese to garnish.

Directions

In a saucepan, melt the butter over medium heat, season the chicken with salt and black pepper, and cook for 5 minutes on each side to brown. Plate the chicken.

Pour the tomato sauce and Italian seasoning in the pan and cook covered for 8 minutes. Adjust the taste with salt and black pepper and stir in the heavy cream and Parmesan cheese.

Once the cheese has melted, return the chicken to the pot, and simmer for 4 minutes. Dish the chicken with sauce, garnish with more Parmesan cheese, and serve with zoodles.

Sticky Cranberry Chicken Wings

Ready in about: 50 minutes | Serves: 6
Per serving: Kcal 152, Fat 8.5g, Net Carbs 1.6g, Protein 17.6g

Ingredients

2 lb chicken wings
4 tbsp unsweetened cranberry puree
2 tbsp olive oil
Salt to taste
Sweet chili sauce to taste
Lemon juice from 1 lemon

Directions

Preheat oven to 400ºF. In a bowl, mix cranberry puree, olive oil, salt, sweet chili sauce, and lemon juice. Add in the wings and toss to coat. Place the chicken under the broiler, and cook for 45 minutes, turning once halfway. Remove the chicken after and serve warm with a cranberry and cheese dipping sauce.

Pacific Chicken

Ready in about: 50 minutes | Serves: 6
Per serving: Kcal: 465, Fat: 31g, Net Carbs: 2.6g, Protein: 33g

Ingredients

4 chicken breasts
Salt and black pepper, to taste
½ cup mayonnaise
3 tbsp Dijon mustard
1 tsp xylitol
¾ cup pork rinds
¾ cup grated Grana-Padano cheese
2 tsp garlic powder
1 tsp onion powder
¼ tsp salt
¼ tsp black pepper
8 pieces ham, sliced
4 slices gruyere cheese

Directions

Set oven to 350ºF and grease a baking dish. Using a small bowl, place in the pork rinds and crush. Add chicken to a plate and season well.

In a separate bowl, mix mustard, mayonnaise, and xylitol. Take about ¼ of this mixture and spread over the chicken. Take ½ pork rinds, seasonings, most of Grana-Padano cheese, and place to the bottom of the baking dish. Add the chicken to the top. Cover with the remaining Grana-Padano, pork rinds, and seasonings. Place in the oven for about 40 minutes until the chicken is cooked completely. Take out from the oven and top with gruyere cheese and ham. Place back in the oven and cook until golden brown.

Greek Chicken with Capers

Ready in about: 30 minutes | Serves: 4
Per serving: Kcal 387, Fat 21g, Net Carbs 2.2g,
Protein 25g

Ingredients

¼ cup olive oil
1 onion, chopped
4 chicken breasts, skinless and boneless
4 garlic cloves, minced
Salt and ground black pepper, to taste
½ cup kalamata olives, pitted and chopped
1 tbsp capers
1 pound tomatoes, chopped
½ tsp red chili flakes

Directions

Sprinkle black pepper and salt on the chicken, and rub with half of the oil. Add the chicken to a pan set over high heat, cook for 2 minutes, flip to the other side, and cook for 2 more minutes. Set the chicken breasts in the oven at 450ºF and bake for 8 minutes. Split the chicken into serving plates.

Set the same pan over medium heat and warm the remaining oil, place in the onion, olives, capers, garlic, and chili flakes, and cook for 1 minute. Stir in the tomatoes, black pepper, and salt, and cook for 2 minutes. Sprinkle over the chicken breasts and enjoy.

Grilled Paprika Chicken with Steamed Broccoli

Ready in about: 17 minutes | Serves: 6
Per serving: Kcal 422, Fat 35.3g, Net Carbs 2g,
Protein 26g

Ingredients

3 tbsp smoked paprika
Salt and black pepper to taste
2 tsp garlic powder
1 tbsp olive oil
6 chicken breasts
1 head broccoli, cut into florets

Directions

Place broccoli florets onto the steamer basket over the boiling water; steam approximately 8 minutes or until crisp-tender. Set aside. Grease grill grate with cooking spray and preheat to 400ºF.
Combine paprika, salt, black pepper, and garlic powder in a bowl. Brush chicken with olive oil and sprinkle spice mixture over and massage with hands. Grill chicken for 7 minutes per side until well-cooked, and plate. Serve warm with steamed broccoli.

Chicken with Anchovy Tapenade

Ready in about: 30 minutes | Serves: 2
Per serving: Kcal 155, Fat 13g, Net Carbs 3g, Protein 25g

Ingredients

1 chicken breast, cut into 4 pieces
2 tbsp coconut oil
3 garlic cloves, crushed

For the tapenade
1 cup black olives, pitted
1 oz anchovy fillets, rinsed
1 garlic clove, crushed
Salt and ground black pepper, to taste
2 tbsp olive oil
¼ cup fresh basil, chopped
1 tbsp lemon juice

Directions

Using a food processor, combine the olives, salt, olive oil, basil, lemon juice, anchovy, and black pepper, blend well. Set a pan over medium heat and warm coconut oil, stir in the garlic, and sauté for 2 minutes. Place in the chicken pieces and cook each side for 4 minutes. Split the chicken among plates and apply a topping of the anchovy tapenade.

Bacon & Cheese Chicken

Ready in about: 30 minutes | Serves: 4
Per serving: Kcal 423, Fat 21g, Net Carbs 3.3g,
Protein 34g

Ingredients

4 bacon strips
4 chicken breasts
3 green onions, chopped
4 ounces ranch dressing
1 ounce coconut aminos
2 tbsp coconut oil
4 oz Monterey Jack cheese, grated

Directions

Set a pan over high heat and warm the oil. Place in the chicken breasts, cook for 7 minutes, then flip to the other side; cook for an additional 7 minutes. Set another pan over medium heat, place in the bacon, cook until crispy, remove to paper towels, drain the grease, and crumble.
Add the chicken breast to a baking dish. Place the green onions, coconut aminos, cheese, and crumbled bacon on top, set in an oven, turn on the broiler, and cook for 5 minutes at high temperature. Split among serving plates and serve.

Chicken Stroganoff

Ready in about: 4 hours 15 minutes | Serves: 4
Per serving: Kcal 365, Fat 22g, Net Carbs 4g, Protein 26g

Ingredients

2 garlic cloves, minced
8 oz mushrooms, chopped
¼ tsp celery seeds, ground
1 cup chicken stock
1 cup sour cream
1 cup leeks, chopped
1 pound chicken breasts
1½ tsp dried thyme
2 tbsp fresh parsley, chopped
Salt and black pepper, to taste
4 zucchinis, spiralized

Directions

Place the chicken in a slow cooker. Place in the salt, leeks, sour cream, half of the parsley, celery seeds, garlic, black pepper, mushrooms, stock, and thyme. Cook on high for 4 hours while covered.

Uncover the pot and add the rest of the parsley. Heat a pan with water over medium heat, place in some salt, bring to a boil, stir in the zucchini pasta, cook for 1 minute, and drain. Place in serving bowls, top with the chicken mixture, and serve.

Chicken in Creamy Mushroom Sauce

Ready in about: 36 minutes | Serves: 4
Per serving: Kcal 448, Fat 38.2g, Net Carbs 2g, Protein 22g

Ingredients

1 tbsp ghee
4 chicken breasts, cut into chunks
Salt and black pepper to taste
1 packet white onion soup mix
2 cups chicken broth
15 baby bella mushrooms, sliced
1 cup heavy cream
1 small bunch parsley, chopped

Directions

Melt ghee in a saucepan over medium heat, season the chicken with salt and black pepper, and brown on all sides for 6 minutes in total. Put in a plate.

In a bowl, stir the onion soup mix with chicken broth and add to the saucepan. Simmer for 3 minutes and add the mushrooms and chicken. Cover and simmer for another 20 minutes. Stir in heavy cream and parsley, cook on low heat for 3 minutes, and season with salt and pepper. Ladle the chicken with creamy sauce and mushrooms over beds of cauli mash. Garnish with parsley to serve.

Yummy Chicken Nuggets

Ready in about: 25 minutes | Serves: 2
Per serving: Kcal 417, Fat 37g, Net Carbs 4.3g, Protein 35g

Ingredients

½ cup almond flour
1 egg
2 tbsp garlic powder
2 chicken breasts, cubed
Salt and black pepper, to taste
½ cup butter

Directions

In a bowl, combine salt, garlic powder, flour, and pepper, and stir. In a separate bowl, beat the egg. Add the chicken breast cubes in egg mixture, then in the flour mixture. Set a pan over medium-high heat and warm butter, add in the chicken nuggets, and cook for 6 minutes on each side. Remove to paper towels, drain the excess grease and serve.

Herby Chicken Meatballs

Ready in about: 25 minutes | Serves: 3
Per serving: Kcal 456, Fat 31g, Net Carbs 2.1g, Protein 32g

Ingredients

1 pound ground chicken
Salt and black pepper, to taste
2 tbsp ranch dressing
½ cup almond flour
¼ cup mozzarella cheese, grated
1 tbsp dry Italian seasoning
¼ cup hot sauce + more for serving
1 egg

Directions

In a bowl, combine chicken meat, pepper, ranch dressing, Italian seasoning, flour, hot sauce, mozzarella cheese, salt, and the egg. Form 9 meatballs, arrange them on a lined baking tray and cook for 16 minutes at 480ºF. Place the chicken meatballs in a bowl and serve with the hot sauce.

Chicken & Squash Traybake

Ready in about: 60 minutes | Serves: 4
Per serving: Kcal: 411, Fat: 15g, Net Carbs: 5.5g, Protein: 31g

Ingredients

2 lb chicken thighs
1 pound butternut squash, cubed
½ cup black olives, pitted
¼ cup olive oil
5 garlic cloves, sliced
1 tbsp dried oregano
Salt and black pepper, to taste

Directions

Set oven to 400ºF and grease a baking dish. Place in the chicken with the skin down. Set the garlic, olives and butternut squash around the chicken then drizzle with oil.

Spread black pepper, salt, and oregano over the mixture then add into the oven. Cook for 45 minutes.

One-Pot Chicken with Mushrooms and Spinach

Ready in about: 40 minutes | Serves: 4
Per serving: Kcal 453, Fat 23g, Net Carbs 1g, Protein 32g

Ingredients

4 chicken thighs
2 cups mushrooms, sliced
1 cup spinach, chopped
¼ cup butter
Salt and black pepper, to taste
½ tsp onion powder
½ tsp garlic powder
½ cup water
1 tsp Dijon mustard
1 tbsp fresh tarragon, chopped

Directions

Set a pan over medium heat and warm half of the butter, place in the thighs, and sprinkle with onion powder, pepper, garlic powder, and salt. Cook each side for 3 minutes and set on a plate.

Place the remaining butter to the same pan and warm. Stir in mushrooms and cook for 5 minutes. Place in water and mustard, take the chicken pieces back to the pan, and cook for 15 minutes while covered. Stir in the tarragon and spinach, and cook for 5 minutes.

Cheddar Chicken Tenders

Ready in about: 40 minutes | Serves: 4
Per serving: Kcal 507, Fat 54g, Net Carbs 1.3g, Protein 42g

Ingredients
2 eggs
3 tbsp butter, melted
3 cups coarsely crushed cheddar cheese
½ cup pork rinds, crushed
1 lb chicken tenders
Pink salt to taste

Directions
Preheat oven to 350ºF and line a baking sheet with parchment paper. Whisk the eggs with the butter in one bowl and mix the cheese and pork rinds in another bowl.

Season chicken with salt, dip in egg mixture, and coat generously in cheddar mixture. Place on the baking sheet, cover with aluminium foil and bake for 25 minutes. Remove foil and bake further for 12 minutes to golden brown. Serve chicken with mustard dip.

Fried Chicken with Coconut Sauce

Ready in about: 30 minutes | Serves: 6
Per serving: Kcal 491, Fat 35g, Net Carbs 3.2g, Protein 58g

Ingredients
1 tbsp coconut oil
3 ½ pounds chicken breasts
1 cup chicken stock
1¼ cups leeks, chopped
1 tbsp lime juice
¼ cup coconut cream
2 tsp paprika
1 tsp red pepper flakes
2 tbsp green onions, chopped for garnishing
Salt and ground black pepper, to taste

Directions
Set a pan over medium heat and warm oil, place in the chicken, cook each side for 2 minutes, set to a plate, and set aside. Set heat to medium, place the leeks to the pan and cook for 4 minutes.

Stir in the black pepper, stock, pepper flakes, salt, paprika, coconut cream, and lime juice. Take the chicken back to the pan, season with some more pepper and salt, and cook covered for 15 minutes.

Lemon Chicken Bake

Ready in about: 55 minutes | Serves: 6
Per serving: Kcal 274, Fat 9g, Net Carbs 4.5g, Protein 25g

Ingredients
6 skinless chicken breasts
1 parsnip, cut into wedges
Salt and ground black pepper, to taste
Juice from 2 lemons
Zest from 2 lemons
Lemon rinds from 2 lemons

Directions
In a baking dish, add the chicken alongside pepper and salt. Sprinkle with lemon juice. Toss well to coat, place in parsnip, lemon rinds and lemon zest, set in an oven at 370ºF, and bake for 45 minutes.

Get rid of the lemon rinds, split the chicken onto plates, sprinkle sauce from the baking dish over.

Bacon and Chicken Cottage Pie

Ready in about: 55 minutes | Serves: 4
Per serving: Kcal 571, Fat 45g, Net Carbs 8.2g, Protein 41g

Ingredients
½ cup onion, chopped
4 bacon slices
3 tbsp butter
1 carrot, chopped
3 garlic cloves, minced
Salt and ground black pepper, to taste
¾ cup crème fraîche
½ cup chicken stock
12 ounces chicken breasts, cubed
2 tbsp Dijon mustard
¾ cup cheddar cheese, shredded
For the dough
¾ cup almond flour
3 tbsp cream cheese
1½ cup mozzarella cheese, shredded
1 egg
1 tsp onion powder
1 tsp garlic powder
1 tsp Italian seasoning
Salt and ground black pepper, to taste

Directions
Set a pan over medium heat and warm butter and sauté the onion, garlic, black pepper, bacon, and carrot, for 5 minutes. Add in the chicken, and cook for 3 minutes. Stir in the crème fraîche, salt, mustard, black pepper, and stock, cook for 7 minutes. Add in the cheddar and set aside.

In a bowl, combine the mozzarella cheese with the cream cheese, and heat in a microwave for 1 minute. Stir in the garlic powder, salt, flour, black pepper, Italian seasoning, onion powder, and egg. Knead the dough well, split into 4 pieces, and flatten each into a circle. Set the chicken mixture into 4 ramekins, top each with a dough circle, place in an oven at 370º F for 25 minutes.

Quattro Formaggi Chicken

Ready in about: 40 minutes | Serves: 8
Per serving: Kcal 565, Fat 37g, Net Carbs 2g, Protein 51g

Ingredients

3 pounds chicken breasts
2 ounces mozzarella cheese, cubed
2 ounces mascarpone cheese
4 ounces cheddar cheese, cubed
2 ounces provolone cheese, cubed
1 zucchini, shredded
Salt and ground black pepper, to taste
1 tsp garlic, minced
½ cup pancetta, cooked and crumbled

Directions

Sprinkle black pepper and salt to the zucchini, squeeze well, and place to a bowl. Stir in the pancetta, mascarpone, cheddar cheese, provolone cheese, mozzarella, black pepper, and garlic.
Cut slits into chicken breasts, apply black pepper and salt, and stuff with the zucchini and cheese mixture. Set on a lined baking sheet, place in the oven at 400ºF, and bake for 45 minutes.

Pancetta & Chicken Casserole

Ready in about: 40 minutes | Serves: 3
Per serving: Kcal 313, Fat 18g, Net Carbs 3g, Protein 26g

Ingredients

8 pancetta strips, chopped
⅓ cup Dijon mustard
Salt and black pepper, to taste
1 onion, chopped
1 tbsp olive oil
1½ cups chicken stock
3 chicken breasts, skinless and boneless
¼ tsp sweet paprika

Directions

In a bowl, combine paprika, black pepper, salt, and mustard. Sprinkle this on chicken breasts and massage. Set a pan over medium heat, stir in the pancetta, cook until it browns, and remove to a plate. Place oil in the same pan and heat over medium heat, add in the chicken breasts, cook for each side for 2 minutes and set aside. Put in the stock, and bring to a simmer. Stir in black pepper, pancetta, salt, and onion. Return the chicken to the pan as well, stir gently, and simmer for 20 minutes over medium heat, turning the meat halfway through. Split the chicken on serving plates, sprinkle the sauce over it to serve.

Chicken in White Wine Sauce

Ready in about: 50 minutes | Serves: 4
Per serving: Kcal 345, Fat 12g, Net Carbs 4g, Protein 24g

Ingredients

8 chicken thighs
Salt and black pepper, to taste
1 onion, peeled and chopped
1 tbsp coconut oil
4 pancetta strips, chopped
4 garlic cloves, minced
10 oz white mushrooms, halved
2 cups white wine
1 cup whipping cream
½ cup fresh parsley, chopped

Directions

Set a pan over medium heat and warm oil, cook the pancetta until crispy, about 4-5 minutes and remove to paper towels. To the pancetta fat, add the chicken, sprinkle with black pepper and salt, cook until brown, and remove to paper towels too.
In the same pan, sauté the onion and garlic for 4 minutes. Then, mix in the mushrooms and cook for another 5 minutes. Return the pancetta and browned chicken to the pan.
Stir in the wine and bring to a boil, reduce the heat, and simmer for 20 minutes. Pour in the whipping cream and warm without boiling. Split among serving bowls and enjoy. Scatter over the parsley and serve with steamed green beans.

Chicken and Zucchini Bake

Ready in about: 45 minutes | Serves: 4
Per serving: Kcal 235, Fat 11g, Net Carbs 2g, Protein 35g

Ingredients

1 zucchini, chopped
Salt and black pepper, to taste
1 tsp garlic powder
1 tbsp avocado oil
2 chicken breasts, skinless, boneless, sliced
1 tomato, cored and chopped
½ tsp dried oregano
½ tsp dried basil
½ cup mozzarella cheese, shredded

Directions

Apply pepper, garlic powder and salt to the chicken. Set a pan over medium heat and warm avocado oil, add in the chicken slices, cook until golden; remove to a baking dish. To the same pan add the zucchini, tomato, pepper, basil, oregano, and salt, cook for 2 minutes, and spread over chicken.
Bake in the oven at 330ºF for 20 minutes. Sprinkle the mozzarella over the chicken, return to the oven, and bake for 5 minutes until the cheese is melted and bubbling. Serve with green salad.

Almond-Crusted Chicken Breasts

Ready in about: 60 minutes | Serves: 4
Per serving: Kcal 485, Fat 32g, Net Carbs 1g, Protein 41g

Ingredients

4 bacon slices, cooked and crumbled
4 chicken breasts
1 tbsp water
½ cup olive oil
1 egg, whisked
Salt and black pepper, to taste
1 cup asiago cheese, shredded
¼ tsp garlic powder
1 cup ground almonds

Directions

In a bowl, combine almonds with pepper, salt, and garlic. Place egg in a separate bowl and combine with water. Season with pepper and salt and dip each piece into the egg, and then into the almond mixture. Set a pan over medium heat and warm oil, add in the chicken breasts, cook until are golden-brown, and remove to a baking pan. Bake in the oven at 360ºF for 20 minutes. Scatter with Asiago cheese and bacon and return to the oven. Roast for a few minutes until the cheese melts.

Chicken with Asparagus & Root Vegetables

Ready in about: 35 minutes | Serves: 4
Per serving: Kcal 497, Fat 31g, Net Carbs 7.4g, Protein 37g

Ingredients

2 cups whipping cream
3 chicken breasts, boneless, skinless, chopped
3 tbsp butter
½ cup onion, chopped
¾ cup carrot, chopped
5 cups chicken stock
Salt and black pepper, to taste
1 bay leaf
1 turnip, chopped
1 parsnip, chopped
17 ounces asparagus, trimmed
3 tsp fresh thyme, chopped

Directions

Set a pan over medium heat and add whipping cream, allow simmering, and cook until it's reduced by half, about 7 minutes.
Set another pan over medium heat and warm butter, sauté the onion for 3 minutes. Pour in the chicken stock, carrots, turnip, and parsnip, chicken, and bay leaf, bring to a boil, and simmer for 20 minutes.
Add in the asparagus and cook for 7 minutes. Discard the bay leaf, stir in the reduced whipping cream, adjust the seasoning and ladle the stew into serving bowls. Scatter with fresh thyme.

Stuffed Mushrooms with Chicken

Ready in about: 40 minutes | Serves: 5
Per serving: Kcal 261, Fat 16g, Net Carbs 6g, Protein 14g

Ingredients

3 cups cauliflower florets
Salt and black pepper, to taste
1 onion, chopped
1½ pounds ground chicken
3 tsp fajita seasoning
2 tbsp butter
10 portobello mushrooms, stems removed
½ cup vegetable broth

Directions

In a food processor, add the cauliflower florets, pepper and salt, blend for a few times, and transfer to a plate. Set a pan over medium heat and warm butter, stir in onion and cook for 3 minutes. Add in the cauliflower rice, and cook for 3 minutes.
Stir in the seasoning, pepper, chicken, broth, and salt and cook for a further 2 minutes. Arrange the mushrooms on a lined baking sheet, stuff each one with chicken mixture, put in the oven at 350ºF, and bake for 30 minutes. Serve in serving plates and enjoy.

Chicken with Monterey Jack Cheese

Ready in about: 30 minutes | Serves: 3
Per serving: Kcal 445, Fat 34g, Net Carbs 4g, Protein 39g

Ingredients

2 tbsp butter
1 tsp garlic, minced
1 pound chicken breasts
1 tsp creole seasoning
¼ cup scallions, chopped
½ cup tomatoes, chopped
½ cup chicken stock
¼ cup whipping cream
½ cup Monterey Jack cheese, grated
¼ cup fresh cilantro, chopped
Salt and black pepper, to taste
4 ounces cream cheese
8 eggs
A pinch of garlic powder

Directions

Set a pan over medium heat and warm 1 tbsp butter. Add chicken, season with creole seasoning and cook each side for 2 minutes; remove to a plate. Melt the rest of the butter and stir in garlic and tomatoes; cook for 4 minutes. Return the chicken to the pan and pour in stock; cook for 15 minutes. Place in whipping cream, scallions, salt, Monterey Jack cheese, and pepper; cook for 2 minutes.
In a blender, combine the cream cheese with garlic powder, salt, eggs, and pepper, and pulse well. Place the mixture into a lined baking sheet, and then bake for 10 minutes in the oven at 325ºF. Allow the cheese sheet to cool down, place on a cutting board, roll, and slice into medium slices. Split the slices among bowls

and top with chicken mixture. Sprinkle with chopped cilantro to serve.

Chicken Gumbo
Ready in about: 40 minutes | Serves: 5
Per serving: Kcal 361, Fat 22g, Net Carbs 6g, Protein 26g
Ingredients
2 sausages, sliced
3 chicken breasts, cubed
1 cup celery, chopped
2 tbsp dried oregano
2 bell peppers, seeded and chopped
1 onion, peeled and chopped
2 cups tomatoes, chopped
4 cups chicken broth
3 tbsp dried thyme
2 tbsp garlic powder
2 tbsp dry mustard
1 tsp cayenne powder
1 tbsp chili powder
Salt and black pepper, to taste
6 tbsp cajun seasoning
3 tbsp olive oil
Directions
In a pot over medium heat warm olive oil. Add the sausages, chicken, pepper, onion, dry mustard, chili, tomatoes, thyme, bell peppers, salt, oregano, garlic powder, cayenne, and cajun seasoning.
Cook for 10 minutes. Add the remaining ingredients and bring to a boil. Reduce the heat and simmer for 20 minutes covered. Serve hot divided between bowls.

Baked Chicken with Acorn Squash and Goat's Cheese
Ready in about: 60 minutes | Serves: 6
Per serving: Kcal 235, Fat 16g, Net Carbs 5g, Protein 12g
Ingredients
6 chicken breasts, butterflied
1 lb acorn squash, cubed
Salt and black pepper, to taste
1 cup goat's cheese, shredded
1 tbsp dried parsley
3 tbsp olive oil
Directions
Arrange the chicken breasts and squash in a baking dish. Season with salt, black pepper, and parsley. Drizzle with olive oil and pour a cup of water. Cover with aluminium foil and bake in the oven for 30 minutes at 420ºF. Discard the foil, scatter goat's cheese, and bake for 15-20 minutes. Remove to a serving plate and enjoy.

Baked Pecorino Toscano Chicken
Ready in about: 50 minutes | Serves: 4
Per serving: Kcal 346, Fat 24g, Net Carbs 6g, Protein 20g
Ingredients
4 chicken breasts, halved
½ cup mayonnaise
½ cup buttermilk
Salt and black pepper, to taste
¾ cup Pecorino Toscano cheese, grated
8 mozzarella cheese slices
1 tsp garlic powder
1 tbsp parsley, chopped
Directions
Spray a baking dish with cooking spray and add in the chicken breasts.
In a bowl, combine mayonnaise, buttermilk, Pecorino Toscano cheese, garlic powder, salt, and black pepper. Spread half of the mixture over the chicken, arrange the mozzarella over, and finish with a layer of the remaining mixture. Bake in the oven for 35-40 minutes at 370ºF. Sprinkle with parsley to serve.

Habanero Chicken Wings
Ready in about: 40 minutes | Serves: 4
Per serving: Kcal 416, Fat 25g, Net Carbs 2g, Protein 26g
Ingredients
2 pounds chicken wings
Salt and black pepper, to taste
3 tbsp coconut aminos
3 tbsp rice vinegar
3 tbsp stevia
¼ cup chives, chopped
½ tsp xanthan gum
5 dried habanero peppers, chopped
Directions
Spread the chicken wings on a lined baking sheet and sprinkle with 2 tbsp of water, black pepper and salt. Bake in the oven at 370ºF for 35 minutes. Put a small pan over medium heat and add in the remaining ingredients. Bring the mixture to a boil and cook for 2 minutes.
Pour the sauce over the chicken and bake for 10 more minutes. Serve warm.

Chicken with Green Sauce
Ready in about: 35 minutes | Serves: 4
Per serving: Kcal 236, Fat 9g, Net Carbs 2.3g, Protein 18g
Ingredients
2 tbsp butter
4 scallions, chopped
4 chicken breasts, skinless and boneless
Salt and black pepper, to taste
6 ounces sour cream
2 tbsp fresh dill, chopped
Directions
Heat a pan with the butter over medium heat, add in the chicken, season with pepper and salt, and fry for 2-3 per side until golden. Transfer to a baking dish and cook in the oven for 15 minutes at 390ºF, until no longer pink.
To the pan add scallions, and cook for 2 minutes. Pour in the sour cream, warm through without boil.

Slice the chicken and serve on a platter with green sauce spooned over and fresh dill.

Chicken and Green Cabbage Casserole
Ready in about: 55 minutes | Serves: 4
Per serving: Kcal 231, Fat 15g, Net Carbs 6g, Protein 25g
Ingredients
3 cups cheddar cheese, grated
10 ounces green cabbage, shredded
3 chicken breasts, skinless, boneless, cooked, cubed
1 cup mayonnaise
1 tbsp coconut oil, melted
⅓ cup chicken stock
Salt and ground black pepper, to taste
Juice of 1 lemon
Directions
Apply oil to a baking dish, and set chicken pieces to the bottom. Spread green cabbage, followed by half of the cheese. In a bowl, combine the mayonnaise with pepper, stock, lemon juice, and salt.
Pour this mixture over the chicken, spread the rest of the cheese, cover with aluminum foil, and bake for 30 minutes in the oven at 350ºF. Open the aluminum foil, and cook for 20 more minutes.

Homemade Chicken Pizza Calzone
Ready in about: 60 minutes | Serves: 4
Per serving: Kcal 425, Fat 15g, Net Carbs 4.6g, Protein 28g
Ingredients
2 eggs
1 low carb pizza crust
½ cup Pecorino cheese, grated
1 lb chicken breasts, skinless, boneless, halved
½ cup sugar-free marinara sauce
1 tsp Italian seasoning
1 tsp onion powder
1 tsp garlic powder
Salt and black pepper, to taste
¼ cup flax seed, ground
6 ounces provolone cheese
Directions
In a bowl, combine the Italian seasoning with onion powder, salt, Pecorino cheese, pepper, garlic powder, and flax seed. In a separate bowl, combine the eggs with pepper and salt.
Dip the chicken pieces in eggs, and then in seasoning mixture, lay all parts on a lined baking sheet, and bake for 25 minutes in the oven at 390º F.
Place the pizza crust dough on a lined baking sheet and spread half of the provolone cheese on half. Remove chicken from oven, chop it, and scatter it over the provolone cheese. Spread over the marinara sauce and top with the remaining cheese.
Cover with the other half of the dough and shape the pizza in a calzone. Seal the edges, set in the oven and bake for 20 minutes. Allow the calzone to cool down before slicing and enjoy.

Easy Chicken Meatloaf
Ready in about: 50 minutes | Serves: 8
Per serving: Kcal 273, Fat 14g, Net Carbs 4g, Protein 28
Ingredients
1 cup sugar-free marinara sauce
2 lb ground chicken
2 tbsp fresh parsley, chopped
3 garlic cloves, minced
2 tsp onion powder
2 tsp Italian seasoning
Salt and ground black pepper, to taste
For the filling
½ cup ricotta cheese
1 cup Grana Padano cheese, grated
1 cup Colby cheese, shredded
2 tsp fresh chives, chopped
2 tbsp fresh parsley, chopped
1 garlic clove, minced
Directions
In a bowl, combine the chicken with half of the marinara sauce, pepper, onion powder, Italian seasoning, salt, and 2 garlic cloves. In a separate bowl, combine the ricotta cheese with half of the Grana Padano cheese, chives, pepper, 1 garlic clove, half of the Colby cheese, salt, and 2 tablespoons parsley.
Place half of the chicken mixture into a loaf pan, and spread evenly. Top with cheese filling. Cover with the rest of the meat mixture and spread again. Set the meatloaf in the oven at 380ºF and bake for 25 minutes.
Remove meatloaf from the oven, spread the rest of the marinara sauce, Grana Padano cheese and Colby cheese, and bake for 18 minutes. Allow meatloaf cooling and serve in slices sprinkled with 2 tbsp of chopped parsley.

Chicken, Eggplant and Gruyere Gratin
Ready in about: 55 minutes | Serves: 4
Per serving: Kcal 412, Fat 37g, Net Carbs 5g, Protein 34g
Ingredients
3 tbsp butter
1 eggplant, chopped
2 tbsp gruyere cheese, grated
Salt and black pepper, to taste
2 garlic cloves, minced
6 chicken thighs
Directions
Set a pan over medium heat and warm 1 tablespoon butter, place in the chicken thighs, season with pepper and salt, cook each side for 3 minutes and lay them in a baking dish. In the same pan melt the rest of the butter and cook the garlic for 1 minute.
Stir in the eggplant, pepper, and salt, and cook for 10 minutes. Ladle this mixture over the chicken, spread with the cheese, set in the oven at 350ºF, and bake for 30 minutes. Turn on the oven's broiler, and broil everything for 2 minutes. Split among serving plates and enjoy.

Coconut Chicken Soup

Ready in about: 30 minutes | Serves: 4 Per serving:
Kcal 387, Fat 23g, Net Carbs 5g, Protein 31g

Ingredients

3 tbsp butter
4 ounces cream cheese
2 chicken breasts, diced
4 cups chicken stock
Salt and black pepper, to taste
½ cup coconut cream
¼ cup celery, chopped

Directions

In the blender, mix stock, butter, coconut cream, salt, cream cheese, and pepper. Remove to a pot, heat over medium heat, and stir in the chicken and celery. Simmer for 15 minutes, share into bowls to serve.

Chicken Breasts with Cheddar & Pepperoni

Ready in about: 40 minutes | Serves: 4
Per serving: Kcal 387, Fat 21g, Net Carbs 4.5g, Protein 32g

Ingredients

12 oz canned tomato sauce
1 tbsp olive oil
4 chicken breast halves, skinless and boneless
Salt and ground black pepper, to taste
1 tsp dried oregano
4 oz cheddar cheese, sliced
1 tsp garlic powder
2 oz pepperoni, sliced

Directions

Preheat your oven to 390ºF. In a bowl, combine chicken with oregano, salt, garlic, and pepper.

Heat a pan with the olive oil over medium heat, add in the chicken, cook each side for 2 minutes, and remove to a baking dish. Top with the cheddar cheese slices spread the sauce, then cover with pepperoni slices. Bake for 30 minutes. Serve warm garnished with fresh oregano if desired

Red Wine Chicken

Ready in about: 30 minutes | Serves: 4
Per serving: Kcal 314, Fat 12g, Net Carbs 4g, Protein 27g

Ingredients

3 tbsp coconut oil
2 lb chicken breast halves, skinless and boneless
3 garlic cloves, minced
Salt and black pepper, to taste
1 cup chicken stock
3 tbsp stevia
½ cup red wine
2 tomatoes, sliced
6 mozzarella slices
Fresh basil, chopped, for serving

Directions

Set a pan over medium heat and warm oil, add the chicken, season with pepper and salt, cook until brown. Stir in the stevia, garlic, stock, and red wine, and cook for 10 minutes.

Remove to a lined baking sheet and arrange mozzarella cheese slices on top. Broil in the oven over medium heat until cheese melts and lay tomato slices over chicken pieces.

Sprinkle with chopped basil to serve.

Spinach & Ricotta Stuffed Chicken Breasts

Ready in about: 25 minutes | Serves: 3
Per serving: Kcal 305, Fat 12g, Net Carbs 4g, Protein 23g

Ingredients

1 cup spinach, cooked and chopped
3 chicken breasts
Salt and ground black pepper, to taste
4 ounces cream cheese, softened
1/2 cup ricotta cheese, crumbled
1 garlic clove, peeled and minced
1 tbsp coconut oil
½ cup white wine

Directions

In a bowl, combine the ricotta cheese with cream cheese, salt, garlic, pepper, and spinach. Add the chicken breasts on a working surface, cut a pocket in each, stuff them with the spinach mixture, and add more pepper and salt.

Set a pan over medium heat and warm oil, add the stuffed chicken, cook each side for 5 minutes. Put in a baking tray, drizzle with white wine and 2 tablespoons of water and then place in the oven at 420ºF. Bake for 10 minutes, arrange on a serving plate and serve.

Slow-Cooked Mexican Turkey Soup

Ready in about: 4 hours 15 minutes | Serves: 4
Per serving: Kcal 387, Fat 24g, Net Carbs 6g, Protein 38g

Ingredients

1 ½ lb turkey breasts, skinless, boneless, cubed
4 cups chicken stock
1 chopped onion
1 cup canned chunky salsa
8 ounces cheddar cheese, into chunks
¼ tsp cayenne red pepper
4 oz canned diced green chilies
1 tsp fresh cilantro, chopped

Directions

In a slow cooker, combine the turkey with salsa, onion, green chilies, cayenne pepper, chicken stock, and cheese, and cook for 4 hours on High while covered. Open the slow cooker, sprinkle with fresh cilantro and ladle in bowls to serve.

Chicken Thighs with Broccoli & Green Onions

Ready in about: 25 minutes | Serves: 2
Per serving: Kcal 387, Fat 23g, Net Carbs 5g, Protein 27g

Ingredients

2 chicken thighs, skinless, boneless, cut into strips
1 tbsp olive oil
1 tsp red pepper flakes
1 tsp onion powder
1 tbsp fresh ginger, grated
¼ cup tamari sauce
½ tsp garlic powder
½ cup water
½ cup erythritol
½ tsp xanthan gum
½ cup green onions, chopped
1 small head broccoli, cut into florets

Directions

Set a pan over medium heat and warm oil, cook in the chicken and ginger for 4 minutes. Stir in the water, onion powder, pepper flakes, garlic powder, tamari sauce, xanthan gum, and erythritol, and cook for 15 minutes. Add in the green onions and broccoli, cook for 6 minutes. Serve hot.

Chicken with Parmesan Topping

Ready in about: 45 minutes | Serves: 4
Per serving: Kcal 361, Fat 15g, Net Carbs 5g, Protein 25g

Ingredients

4 chicken breast halves, skinless and boneless
Salt and black pepper, to taste
¼ cup green chilies, chopped
5 bacon slices, chopped
6 ounces cream cheese
¼ cup onion, chopped
½ cup mayonnaise
½ cup Grana Padano cheese, grated
1 cup cheddar cheese, grated
2 ounces pork rinds, crushed
2 tbsp olive oil
½ cup Parmesan cheese, shredded

Directions

Season the chicken with salt and pepper. Heat the olive oil in a pan over medium heat and fry the chicken for approximately 4-6 minutes until cooked through with no pink showing. Remove to a baking dish.

In the same pan, fry bacon until crispy and remove to a plate. Sauté the onion for 3 minutes, until soft. Remove from heat, add in the fried bacon, cream cheese, 1 cup of water, Grana Padano cheese, mayonnaise, chilies, and cheddar cheese, and spread over the chicken.

Bake in the oven for 10-15 minutes at 370ºF. Remove and sprinkle with mixed Parmesan cheese and pork rinds and return to the oven. Bake for another 10-15 minutes until the cheese melts. Serve immediately.

Zesty Grilled Chicken

Ready in about: 35 minutes | Serves: 8
Per serving: Kcal 375, Fat 12g, Net Carbs 3g, Protein 42g

Ingredients

2½ pounds chicken thighs and drumsticks
1 tbsp coconut aminos
1 tbsp apple cider vinegar
A pinch of red pepper flakes
Salt and black pepper, to taste
½ tsp ground ginger
⅓ cup butter
1 garlic clove, minced
1 tsp lime zest
½ cup warm water

Directions

In a blender, combine the butter with water, salt, ginger, vinegar, garlic, pepper, lime zest, aminos, and pepper flakes. Pat the chicken dry, lay on a pan, and top with zesty marinade. Refrigerate for 1 hour.

Set the chicken pieces skin side down on a preheated grill over medium heat, cook for 10 minutes, turn, brush with some marinade, and cook for 10 minutes. Split among serving plates and enjoy.

Chicken Stew with Sun-Dried Tomatoes

Ready in about: 60 minutes | Serves: 4
Per serving: Kcal 224, Fat 11g, Net Carbs 6g, Protein 23g

Ingredients

2 carrots, chopped
2 tbsp olive oil
2 celery stalks, chopped
2 cups chicken stock
1 shallot, chopped
28 oz chicken thighs, skinless, boneless
3 garlic cloves, peeled and minced
½ tsp dried rosemary
2 oz sun-dried tomatoes, chopped
1 cup spinach
¼ tsp dried thyme
½ cup heavy cream
Salt and ground black pepper, to taste
A pinch of xanthan gum

Directions

In a pot, heat the olive oil over medium heat and add garlic, carrots, celery, and shallot; season with salt and pepper and sauté for 5-6 minutes until tender. Stir in the chicken and cook for 5 minutes.

Pour in the stock, tomatoes, rosemary, and thyme, and cook for 30 minutes covered. Stir in xanthan gum, cream, and spinach; cook for 5 minutes. Adjust the seasonings and separate into bowls.

Roasted Chicken with Herbs

Ready in about: 50 minutes | Serves: 12
Per serving: Kcal 367, Fat 15g, Net Carbs 1.1g, Protein 33g

Ingredients

1 (4-5 lb) whole chicken
½ tsp onion powder
Salt and black pepper, to taste
2 tbsp olive oil
1 tsp dry thyme
1 tsp dry rosemary
1 ½ cups chicken broth
2 tsp guar gum

Directions

Rub chicken with half of the oil, salt, rosemary, thyme, pepper, and onion powder. Place the rest of the oil into a baking dish, and add chicken. Place in the stock, and bake for 40 minutes at 380ºF. Remove the chicken to a platter, and set aside. Stir in the guar gum in a pan over medium heat, and cook until thickening. Place sauce over chicken to serve.

Stuffed Avocados with Chicken

Ready in about: 10 minutes | Serves: 2
Per serving: Kcal 511, Fat 40, Net Carbs 5g, Protein 24g

Ingredients

2 avocados, cut in half and pitted
¼ cup pesto
2 tbsp cream cheese
1½ cups chicken, cooked and shredded
¼ tsp cayenne pepper
½ tsp onion powder
½ tsp garlic powder
1 tsp paprika
Salt and black pepper, to taste
2 tbsp lemon juice

Directions

Scoop the insides of the avocado halves, and place the flesh in a bowl. Add in the chicken and stir in the remaining ingredients. Stuff the avocado cups with chicken mixture and enjoy.

Chicken Breasts with Walnut Crust

Ready in about: 30 minutes | Serves: 4
Per serving: Kcal 322, Fat 18g, Net Carbs 1.5g, Protein 35g

Ingredients

1 egg, whisked
Salt and black pepper, to taste
3 tbsp coconut oil
1½ cups walnuts, ground
4 chicken breast halves, boneless and skinless

Directions

In a bowl, add in walnuts and the whisked egg in another. Season the chicken, dip in the egg and then in pecans. Warm oil in a pan over medium heat and brown the chicken. Remove the chicken pieces to a baking sheet, set in the oven, and bake for 10 minutes at 350º F. Serve topped with lemon slices.

Fried Chicken Breasts

Ready in about: 20 minutes | Serves: 4
Per serving: Kcal 387, Fat 16g, Net Carbs 2.5g, Protein 23g

Ingredients

2 chicken breasts, cut into strips
4 ounces pork rinds, crushed
4 tbsp coconut oil
16 ounces jarred pickle juice
2 eggs, whisked

Directions

In a bowl, combine chicken and pickle juice; refrigerate for 12 hours. Set the eggs in one bowl, and pork rinds in a separate one. Dip the chicken in the eggs, and then in pork rinds. Put a pan over medium heat and warm oil. Fry the chicken for 3 minutes per side, and remove to a plate. Serve.

Chicken and Bacon Rolls

Ready in about: 45 minutes | Serves: 4
Per serving: Kcal 623, Fat 48g, Net Carbs 5g, Protein 38g

Ingredients

1 tbsp fresh chives, chopped
8 ounces blue cheese
2 pounds chicken breasts, skinless, boneless, halved
12 bacon slices
2 tomatoes, chopped
Salt and ground black pepper, to taste

Directions

Set a pan over medium heat, place in the bacon, cook until halfway done, remove to a plate. In a bowl, stir together blue cheese, chives, tomatoes, pepper and salt. Use a meat tenderizer to flatten the chicken breasts, season and lay blue cheese mixture on top. Roll them up, and wrap each in a bacon slice. Place the wrapped chicken breasts in a greased baking dish, and roast in the oven at 370ºF for 30 minutes. Serve on top of wilted kale.

Chicken Breasts with Spinach & Artichoke

Ready in about: 60 minutes | Serves: 4
Per serving: Kcal 431, Fat 21g, Net Carbs 3.5g, Protein 36g

Ingredients

4 ounces cream cheese
4 chicken breasts
8 oz canned artichoke hearts, chopped
1 cup spinach
½ cup Pecorino cheese, grated
1 tbsp onion powder
1 tbsp garlic powder
Salt and ground black pepper, to taste
4 ounces Monterrey Jack cheese, shredded

Directions

Lay the chicken breasts on a lined baking sheet, season with pepper and salt, set in the oven at 350ºF, and bake for 35 minutes. In a bowl, combine the artichokes with onion powder, Pecorino cheese, salt, spinach, cream cheese, garlic powder, and pepper. Remove the chicken from the oven, cut each piece in half, divide artichokes mixture on top, spread with Monterrey cheese, set in the oven at 350ºF, and bake for 20 minutes.

Paprika Chicken with Cream Sauce

Ready in about: 50 minutes | Serves: 4
Per serving: Kcal 381, Fat 33g, Net Carbs 2.6g, Protein 31.3g

Ingredients

1 pound chicken thighs
Salt and black pepper, to taste
1 tsp onion powder
¼ cup heavy cream
2 tbsp butter
2 tbsp sweet paprika

Directions

In a bowl, combine paprika with onion powder, pepper, and salt. Season chicken with this mixture and lay on a lined baking sheet; bake for 40 minutes in the oven at 400ºF. Set aside.

Add the cooking juices to a skillet over medium heat, and mix with the heavy cream and butter. Cook for 5-6 minutes until the sauce is thickened. Sprinkle the sauce over the chicken and serve.

Roasted Chicken with Tarragon

Ready in about: 50 minutes | Serves: 4
Per serving: Kcal: 415, Fat: 23g, Net Carbs: 5.5g, Protein: 42g

Ingredients

2 lb chicken thighs
2 lb radishes, sliced
4 ¼ oz butter
1 tbsp tarragon
Salt and black pepper, to taste
1 cup mayonnaise

Directions

Set oven to 400ºF and grease a baking dish. Add in the chicken, radishes, tarragon, pepper, and salt. Place in butter then set into the oven and cook for 40 minutes at 360ºF. Remove to a serving plate and serve with mayonnaise.

Turkey Enchilada Bowl

Ready in about: 30 minutes | Serves: 4
Per serving: Kcal: 568, Fat: 40.2g, Net Carbs: 5.9g, Protein: 38g

Ingredients

2 tbsp coconut oil
1 lb boneless, skinless turkey thighs, cut into pieces
¾ cup red enchilada sauce (sugar-free)
¼ cup water
¼ cup chopped onion
3 oz canned diced green chilis
1 avocado, diced
1 cup shredded mozzarella cheese
¼ cup chopped pickled jalapeños
½ cup sour cream
1 tomato, diced

Directions

Set a large pan over medium heat. Add coconut oil and warm. Place in the turkey and cook until browned on the outside. Stir in onion, chillis, water, and enchilada sauce, then close with a lid.

Allow simmering for 20 minutes until the turkey is cooked through. Spoon the turkey on a serving bowl and top with the sauce, cheese, sour cream, tomato, and avocado.

Cheesy Turkey and Broccoli Traybake

Ready in about: 30 minutes | Serves: 4
Per serving: Kcal: 365, Fat: 28g, Net Carbs: 2.6g, Protein: 29g

Ingredients

1 lb turkey breasts, cooked
2 tbsp olive oil
1 head broccoli, cut into florets
½ cup sour cream
½ cup heavy cream
1 cup Monterrey Jack cheese, grated
4 tbsp pork rinds, crushed
Salt and black pepper, to taste
½ tsp paprika
1 tsp oregano

Directions

Set oven to 450ºF and grease and line a baking tray. Boil water in a pan. Add in broccoli and cook for 8 minutes. Use two forks to shred the turkey.

Place turkey into a large bowl with sour cream, olive oil, and broccoli and stir. Transfer the mixture to the baking tray. Sprinkle heavy cream over the dish, top with seasonings; coat with grated cheese. Cover with pork rinds. Place in the oven and cook for 20-25 minutes. Ladle to a serving plate and serve.

Turkey & Cheese Stuffed Mushrooms

Ready in about: 20 minutes | Serves: 5
Per serving: Kcal 486, Fat 17g, Net Carbs 8.6g, Protein 51g

Ingredients

12 ounces button mushroom caps
3 ounces cream cheese
¼ cup carrot, chopped
1 tsp ranch seasoning mix
4 tbsp hot sauce
¾ cup blue cheese, crumbled
¼ cup onion, chopped
½ cup turkey breasts, cooked, chopped
Salt and black pepper, to taste
Cooking spray

Directions

In a bowl, combine cream cheese, blue cheese, ranch seasoning, turkey, onion, carrot, salt, hot sauce, and pepper. Stuff each mushroom cap with this mixture, set on a lined baking sheet, spray with cooking spray, place in the oven at 425ºF, and bake for 10 minutes.

Broccoli and Turkey Bacon Crepes

Ready in about: 40 minutes | Serves: 8
Per serving: Kcal 371, Fat 32g, Net Carbs 7g, Protein 25g

Ingredients

6 eggs
1 cup cream cheese
1 tsp erythritol
1½ tbsp coconut flour
⅓ cup Parmesan cheese, grated
A pinch of xanthan gum
Cooking spray
1 cup broccoli florets
1 cup mushrooms, sliced
8 ounces turkey bacon, cubed
8 ounces cheese blend
1 garlic clove, minced
1 onion, chopped
2 tbsp red wine vinegar
2 tbsp butter
½ cup heavy cream
1 tsp Worcestershire sauce
¼ cup chicken stock
A pinch of nutmeg
Fresh parsley, chopped
Salt and black pepper, to taste

Directions

In a bowl, combine 3/4 cup of cream cheese, eggs, erythritol, coconut flour, xanthan, Parmesan cheese to obtain a crepe batter. Set a pan sprayed with cooking spray over medium heat, pour some of the batter, spread well into the pan, cook for 2 minutes, flip to the other side, and cook for 40 seconds more or until golden. Do the same with the rest of the batter, greasing the pan with cooking spray between each one. Stack all the crepes on a serving plate.

In the same pan, melt the butter and stir in the onion and garlic; sauté for 3 minutes, until tender. Stir in the mushrooms and cook for 5 minutes. Add in the turkey bacon, salt, vinegar, heavy cream, 6 ounces of the cheese blend, remaining cream cheese, nutmeg, black pepper, broccoli, stock, and Worcestershire sauce, and cook for 7 minutes. Fill each crepe with this mixture, roll up each one, and arrange on a baking dish. Scatter over the remaining cheese blend, set under a preheated broiler for 5 minutes. Set the crepes on serving plates, garnish with chopped parsley, and enjoy.

Rosemary Turkey Pie

Ready in about: 40 minutes | Serves: 4
Per serving: Kcal 325, Fat 23g, Net Carbs 5.6g, Protein 21g

Ingredients

2 cups chicken stock
1 cup turkey meat, cooked and chopped
Salt and ground black pepper, to taste

1 tsp fresh rosemary, chopped
½ cup kale, chopped
½ cup butternut squash, chopped
½ cup Monterey jack cheese, shredded
¼ tsp smoked paprika
¼ tsp garlic powder
¼ tsp xanthan gum
Cooking spray

For the crust:

¼ cup butter
¼ tsp xanthan gum
2 cups almond flour
A pinch of salt
1 egg
¼ cup cheddar cheese

Directions

Set a greased pot over medium heat. Place in turkey and squash, and cook for 10 minutes. Stir in stock, Monterey Jack cheese, garlic powder, rosemary, black pepper, smoked paprika, kale, and salt.

In a bowl, combine ½ cup stock from the pot with ¼ teaspoon xanthan gum, and transfer everything to the pot; set aside. In a separate bowl, stir together salt, ¼ teaspoon xanthan gum, and flour.

Stir in the butter, cheddar cheese, egg, until a pie crust dough forms. Form into a ball and refrigerate. Spray a baking dish with cooking spray and sprinkle pie filling on the bottom. Set the dough on a working surface, roll into a circle, and top filling with this. Ensure well pressed and seal edges, set in an oven at 350ºF, and bake for 35 minutes. Allow the pie to cool, and enjoy.

Turkey Burgers with Fried Brussels Sprouts

Ready in about: 30 minutes | Serves: 4
Per serving: Kcal: 443, Fat: 25g, Net Carbs: 5.8g, Protein: 31g

Ingredients

For the burgers

1 pound ground turkey
1 free-range egg
½ onion, chopped
1 tsp salt
½ tsp ground black pepper
1 tsp dried thyme
2 oz butter

For the fried Brussels sprouts

1 ½ lb Brussels sprouts, halved
3 oz butter
1 tsp salt
½ tsp ground black pepper

Directions

Combine the burger ingredients in a mixing bowl. Create patties from the mixture. Set a large pan over medium heat, warm butter, and fry the patties until cooked completely.

Place on a plate and cover with aluminium foil to keep warm. Fry brussels sprouts in butter, season to your preference, then set to a bowl. Plate the burgers and brussels sprouts and serve.

Turkey Breast Salad

Ready in about: 25 minutes | Serves: 4
Per serving: Kcal 451, Fat 33g, Net Carbs 6g, Protein 28g

Ingredients

1 tbsp swerve
1 red onion, chopped
¼ cup vinegar
¼ cup olive oil
¼ cup water
1¾ cups raspberries
1 tbsp Dijon mustard
Salt and ground black pepper, to taste
10 ounces baby spinach
2 medium turkey breasts, boneless
4 ounces goat cheese, crumbled
½ cup pecans halves

Directions

In a blender, combine swerve, vinegar, 1 cup raspberries, black pepper, mustard, water, onion, oil, and salt, and ensure well blended. Strain this into a bowl, and set aside. Cut the turkey breast in half, add black pepper and salt, and place skin side down into a pan.

Cook for 8 minutes flipping to the other side and cooking for 5 minutes. Split the spinach among plates, spread with the remaining raspberries, pecan halves, and goat cheese. Slice the turkey breasts, put over the salad and top with raspberries vinaigrette and enjoy.

Turkey Stew with Salsa Verde

Ready in about: 30 minutes | Serves: 6
Per serving: Kcal 193, Fat 11g, Net Carbs 2g, Protein 27g

Ingredients

4 cups leftover turkey meat, chopped
2 cups green beans
6 cups chicken stock
Salt and ground black pepper, to taste
1 fresh chipotle pepper, chopped
½ cup salsa verde
1 tsp ground coriander
2 tsp cumin
¼ cup sour cream
1 tbsp fresh cilantro, chopped

Directions

Set a pan over medium heat. Add in the stock and heat. Stir in green beans, and cook for 10 minutes. Place in the turkey, ground coriander, salt, salsa verde, chipotle pepper, cumin, and black pepper, and cook for 10 minutes. Stir in the sour cream, kill the heat, and separate into bowls. Top with chopped cilantro to serve.

Turkey & Leek Soup

Ready in about: 45 minutes | Serves: 4
Per serving: Kcal 305, Fat 11g, Net Carbs 3g, Protein 15g

Ingredients

3 celery stalks, chopped
2 leeks, chopped
1 tbsp butter
6 cups chicken stock
Salt and ground black pepper, to taste
¼ cup fresh parsley, chopped
3 cups zoodles
3 cups turkey meat, cooked and chopped

Directions

Set a pot over medium heat, stir in leeks and celery and cook for 5 minutes. Place in the parsley, turkey meat, black pepper, salt, and stock, and cook for 20 minutes. Stir in the zoodles, and cook turkey soup for 5 minutes. Serve in bowls and enjoy.

Turkey Fajitas

Ready in about: 25 minutes | Serves: 4
Per serving: Kcal 448, Fat 32g, Net Carbs 5g, Protein 45g

Ingredients

2 lb turkey breasts, skinless, boneless, sliced
1 tsp garlic powder
1 tsp chili powder
2 tsp cumin
2 tbsp lime juice
Salt and black pepper, to taste
1 tsp sweet paprika
2 tbsp coconut oil
1 tsp ground coriander
1 green bell pepper, seeded, sliced
1 red bell pepper, seeded, sliced
1 onion, sliced
1 tbsp fresh cilantro, chopped
1 avocado, sliced
2 limes, cut into wedges

Directions

In a bowl, combine lime juice, cumin, garlic powder, coriander, paprika, salt, chili powder, and black pepper. Toss in the turkey pieces to coat well. Set a pan over medium heat and warm oil, place in the turkey, cook each side for 3 minutes and set to a plate.

Add the remaining oil to the pan and stir in the bell peppers and onion, and cook for 6 minutes. Take the turkey back to the pan. Add a topping of fresh cilantro, lime wedges, and avocado and serve.

Turkey & Mushroom Bake

Ready in about: 55 minutes | Serves: 8
Per serving: Kcal 245, Fat 15g, Net Carbs 3g, Protein 25g

Ingredients

4 cups mushrooms, sliced
1 egg, whisked
3 cups green cabbage, shredded
3 cups turkey meat, cooked and chopped
½ cup chicken stock
½ cup cream cheese
1 tsp poultry seasoning
2 cups cheddar cheese, grated
½ cup Parmesan cheese, grated
Salt and ground black pepper, to taste
¼ tsp garlic powder

Directions

Set a pan over medium-low heat. Stir in chicken broth, egg, Parmesan cheese, black pepper, garlic powder, poultry seasoning, cheddar cheese, cream cheese, and salt, and simmer. Place in the cabbage and turkey meat, and set away from the heat.

Add the mushrooms, pepper, turkey mixture and salt in a baking dish and spread. Place aluminum foil to cover, set in an oven at 390ºF, and bake for 35 minutes. Allow cooling and enjoy.

Turkey, Coconut and Kale Chili

Ready in about: 30 minutes | Serves: 5
Per serving: Kcal 295, Fat 15.2g, Net Carbs 4.2g, Protein 25g

Ingredients

18 ounces turkey breasts, cubed
1 cup kale, chopped
20 ounces canned diced tomatoes
2 tbsp coconut oil
2 tbsp coconut cream
2 garlic cloves, minced
2 onions, sliced
1 tbsp ground coriander
2 tbsp fresh ginger, grated
1 tbsp turmeric
1 tbsp cumin
Salt and ground black pepper, to taste
2 tbsp chili powder

Directions

Set a pan over medium heat and warm the coconut oil, stir in the turkey and onion, and cook for 5 minutes. Place in garlic and ginger, and cook for 1 minute. Stir in the tomatoes, pepper, turmeric, coriander, salt, cumin, and chili powder. Place in the coconut cream, and cook for 10 minutes.

Transfer to an immersion blender alongside kale; blend well. Allow simmering, cook for 15 minutes.

Buttered Duck Breast

Ready in about: 30 minutes | Serves: 1
Per serving: Kcal 547, Fat 46g, Net Carbs 2g, Protein 35g

Ingredients

1 medium duck breast, skin scored
1 tbsp heavy cream
2 tbsp butter
Salt and black pepper, to taste
1 cup kale
¼ tsp fresh sage

Directions

Set the pan over medium heat and warm half of the butter. Place in sage and heavy cream, and cook for 2 minutes. Set another pan over medium heat. Place in the remaining butter and duck breast as the skin side faces down, cook for 4 minutes, flip, and cook for 3 more minutes.

Place the kale to the pan containing the sauce, cook for 1 minute. Set the duck breast on a flat surface and slice. Arrange the duck slices on a platter and drizzle over the sauce.

Duck & Vegetable Casserole

Ready in about: 20 minutes | Serves: 2
Per serving: Kcal 433, Fat 21g, Net Carbs 8g, Protein 53g

Ingredients

2 duck breasts, skin on and sliced
2 zucchinis, sliced
1 tbsp coconut oil
1 green onion bunch, chopped
1 carrot, chopped
2 green bell peppers, seeded and chopped
Salt and ground black pepper, to taste

Directions

Set a pan over medium heat and warm oil, stir in the green onions, and cook for 2 minutes. Place in the zucchini, bell peppers, black pepper, salt, and carrot, and cook for 10 minutes.

Set another pan over medium heat, add in duck slices and cook each side for 3 minutes. Pour the mixture into the vegetable pan. Cook for 3 minutes. Set in bowls and enjoy.

PORK, BEEF & LAMB RECIPES

Baked Pork Meatballs in Pasta Sauce

Ready in about: 45 minutes | Serves: 6
Per serving: Kcal 590, Fat 46.8g, Net Carbs 4.1g,
Protein 46.2g

Ingredients

2 lb ground pork
1 tbsp olive oil
1 cup pork rinds, crushed
3 cloves garlic, minced
½ cup coconut milk
2 eggs, beaten
½ cup grated Parmesan cheese
½ cup grated asiago cheese
Salt and black pepper to taste
¼ cup chopped parsley
2 jars sugar-free marinara sauce
½ tsp Italian seasoning
1 cup Italian blend kinds of cheeses
Chopped basil to garnish

Directions

Preheat the oven to 400ºF, line a cast iron pan with foil and oil it with cooking spray. Set aside.
Combine the coconut milk and pork rinds in a bowl. Mix in the ground pork, garlic, Asiago cheese, Parmesan cheese, eggs, salt, and pepper, just until combined. Form balls of the mixture and place them in the prepared pan. Bake in the oven for 20 minutes at a reduced temperature of 370ºF.
Transfer the meatballs to a plate. Pour half of the marinara sauce in the baking pan. Place the meatballs back in the pan and pour the remaining marinara sauce all over them. Sprinkle with the Italian blend cheeses, drizzle with the olive oil, and then sprinkle with Italian seasoning.
Cover the pan with foil and put it back in the oven to bake for 10 minutes. After, remove the foil, and cook for 5 minutes. Once ready, take out the pan and garnish with basil. Serve on a bed of squash spaghetti.

Grilled Pork Loin Chops with Barbecue Sauce

Ready in about: 2 hours 15 minutes | Serves: 4
Per serving: Kcal 363, Fat 26.6g, Net Carbs 0g,
Protein 34.1g

Ingredients

4 (6 oz) thick-cut pork loin chops, boneless
½ cup sugar-free BBQ sauce
1 tsp black pepper
1 tbsp erythritol
½ tsp ginger powder
2 tsp sweet paprika

Directions

In a bowl, mix pepper, erythritol, ginger powder, and sweet paprika, and rub the pork on all sides with the mixture. Cover the pork chops with plastic wraps and place it in the fridge to marinate for 2 hours.
Preheat the grill to 450ºF. Unwrap the meat, place on the grill grate, and cook for 2 minutes per side.

Reduce the heat and brush the BBQ sauce on the meat, cover and grill them for 5 minutes.
Open the lid, turn the meat and brush again with barbecue sauce. Continue cooking covered for 5 minutes. Remove the meat to a serving platter and serve with mixed steamed vegetables.

Pork Sausage Bake

Ready in about: 50 minutes | Serves: 4
Per serving: Kcal 465, Fat 41.6g, Net Carbs 4.4g,
Protein 15.1g

Ingredients

12 pork sausages
5 large tomatoes, cut in rings
1 red bell pepper, seeded and sliced
1 yellow bell pepper, seeded and sliced
1 green bell pepper, seeded and sliced
1 sprig thyme, chopped
1 sprig rosemary, chopped
4 cloves garlic, minced
2 bay leaves
1 tbsp olive oil
2 tbsp balsamic vinegar

Directions

Preheat the oven to 350ºF.
In the cast iron pan, add the tomatoes, bell peppers, thyme, rosemary, garlic, bay leaves, olive oil, and balsamic vinegar. Toss everything and arrange the sausages on top of the veggies.
Put the pan in the oven and bake for 20 minutes. After, remove the pan shake it a bit and turn the sausages over with a spoon. Continue cooking for 25 minutes or until the sausages have browned to your desired color. Serve with the veggie and cooking sauce with cauli rice.

Pork Pie with Cauliflower

Ready in about: 1 hour and 30 minutes | Serves: 8
Per serving: Kcal 485, Fat: 41g, Net Carbs: 4g, Protein: 29g

Ingredients

Crust:

1 egg
¼ cup butter
2 cups almond flour
¼ tsp xanthan gum
¼ cup shredded mozzarella
A pinch of salt

Filling:

2 pounds ground pork
½ cup water
⅓ cup pureed onion
¾ tsp allspice
1 cup cooked and mashed cauliflower
1 tbsp ground sage
2 tbsp butter

Directions

Preheat your oven to 350ºF.
Whisk together all crust ingredients in a bowl. Make two balls out of the mixture and refrigerate for 10

minutes. Combine the water, meat, and salt, in a pot over medium heat. Cook for about 15 minutes, place the meat along with the other ingredients in a bowl. Mix with your hands to combine.

Roll out the pie crusts and place one at the bottom of a greased pie pan. Spread the filling over the crust. Top with the other coat. Bake in the oven for 50 minutes then serve.

Pork Osso Bucco

Ready in about: 1 hour 55 minutes | Serves: 6
Per serving: Kcal 590, Fat 40g, Net Carbs 6.1g, Protein 34g

Ingredients

4 tbsp butter, softened
6 (16 oz) pork shanks
2 tbsp olive oil
3 cloves garlic, minced
1 cup diced tomatoes
Salt and black pepper to taste
½ cup chopped onions
½ cup chopped celery
½ cup chopped carrots
2 cups Cabernet Sauvignon
5 cups vegetable broth
½ cup chopped parsley + extra to garnish
2 tsp lemon zest

Directions

Melt the butter in a large saucepan over medium heat. Season the pork with salt and black pepper and brown it for 12 minutes; remove to a plate.

In the same pan, sauté 2 cloves of garlic and onions in the oil, for 3 minutes; return the pork shanks. Stir in the Cabernet, carrots, celery, tomatoes, and vegetable broth; season with salt and pepper. Cover the pan and let simmer on low heat for 1 ½ hours basting the pork every 15 minutes with the sauce.

In a bowl, mix the remaining garlic, parsley, and lemon zest to make a gremolata, and stir the mixture into the sauce when it is ready. Turn the heat off and dish the Osso Bucco. Garnish with parsley and serve with creamy turnip mash.

Charred Tenderloin with Lemon Chimichurri

Ready in about: 64 minutes | Serves: 4
Per serving: Kcal 388, Fat 18g, Net Carbs 2.1g, Protein 28g

Ingredients

Lemon Chimichurri

1 lemon, juiced
¼ cup chopped mint leaves
¼ cup chopped oregano leaves
2 cloves garlic, minced
¼ cup olive oil
Salt to taste

Pork

1 (4 lb) pork tenderloin
Salt and black pepper to season
Olive oil for rubbing

Directions

Make the lemon chimichurri to have the flavors incorporate while the pork cooks.

In a bowl, mix the mint, oregano, and garlic. Then, add the lemon juice, olive oil, and salt, and combine well. Set the sauce aside at room temperature.

Preheat the charcoal grill to 450ºF in medium heat creating a direct heat area and indirect heat area. Rub the pork with olive oil, season with salt and pepper. Place the meat over direct heat and sear for 3 minutes on each side, after which, move to the indirect heat area.

Close the lid and cook for 25 minutes on one side, then open, turn the meat, and grill for 20 minutes on the other side. Remove the pork from the grill and let it sit for 5 minutes before slicing. Spoon lemon chimichurri over the pork and serve with fresh salad.

Pork Nachos

Ready in about: 15 minutes | Serves: 4
Per serving: Kcal 452, Fat 25g, Net Carbs 9.3g, Protein 22g

Ingredients

1 bag low carb tortilla chips
2 cups leftover pulled pork
1 red bell pepper, seeded and chopped
1 red onion, diced
2 cups shredded Monterey Jack cheese

Directions

Preheat oven to 350ºF. Arrange the chips in a medium cast iron pan, scatter pork over, followed by red bell pepper, and onion, and sprinkle with cheese. Place the pan in the oven and cook for 10 minutes until the cheese has melted. Allow cooling for 3 minutes and serve.

Herb Pork Chops with Raspberry Sauce

Ready in about: 17 minutes | Serves: 4
Per serving: Kcal 413, Fat 32.5g, Net Carbs 1.1g, Protein 26.3g

Ingredients

1 tbsp olive oil + extra for brushing
2 lb pork chops
Pink salt and black pepper to taste
2 cups raspberries
¼ cup water
1 ½ tbsp Italian Herb mix
3 tbsp balsamic vinegar
2 tsp sugar-free Worcestershire sauce

Directions

Heat oil in a skillet over medium heat, season the pork with salt and black pepper and cook for 5 minutes on each side. Put on serving plates and reserve the pork drippings.

Mash the raspberries with a fork in a bowl until jam-like. Pour into a saucepan, add the water, and herb mix. Bring to boil on low heat for 4 minutes. Stir in pork drippings, vinegar, and Worcestershire sauce. Simmer for 1 minute. Spoon sauce over the pork chops and serve with braised rapini.

Garlicky Pork with Bell Peppers

Ready in about: 40 minutes | Serves: 4
Per serving: Kcal 456, Fat 25g, Net Carbs 6g, Protein 40g

Ingredients

3 tbsp butter
4 pork steaks, bone-in
1 cup chicken stock
Salt and black pepper, to taste
A pinch of lemon pepper
3 tbsp olive oil
6 garlic cloves, minced
2 tbsp fresh parsley, chopped
4 bell peppers, sliced
1 lemon, sliced

Directions

Heat a pan with 2 tablespoons oil and 2 tablespoons butter over medium heat. Add in the pork steaks, season with black pepper and salt, and cook until browned; remove to a plate. In the same pan, warm the rest of the oil and butter, add garlic and bell peppers and cook for 4 minutes.

Pour the chicken stock, lemon slices, salt, lemon pepper, and black pepper, and cook everything for 5 minutes. Return the pork steaks to the pan and cook for 10 minutes. Split the sauce and steaks among plates and sprinkle with parsley to serve.

Pork Burgers with Caramelized Onion Rings

Ready in about: 20 minutes | Serves: 6
Per serving: Kcal 445, Fat 32g, Net Carbs 7.6g, Protein 26g

Ingredients

2 lb ground pork
Pink salt and chili pepper to taste
3 tbsp olive oil
1 tbsp butter
1 white onion, sliced into rings
1 tbsp balsamic vinegar
3 drops liquid stevia
6 low carb burger buns, halved
2 firm tomatoes, sliced into rings

Directions

Combine the pork, salt and chili pepper in a bowl and mold out 6 patties.

Heat the olive oil in a skillet over medium heat and fry the patties for 4 to 5 minutes on each side until golden brown on the outside. Remove onto a plate and sit for 3 minutes.

Melt butter in a skillet over medium heat, sauté onions for 2 minutes, and stir in the balsamic vinegar and liquid stevia. Cook for 30 seconds stirring once or twice until caramelized. In each bun, place a patty, top with some onion rings and 2 tomato rings. Serve the burgers with cheddar cheese dip.

Lemon Pork Chops with Buttered Brussels Sprouts

Ready in about: 27 minutes | Serves: 6

Per serving: Kcal 549, Fat 48g, Net Carbs 2g, Protein 26g

Ingredients

3 tbsp lemon juice
3 cloves garlic, pureed
1 tbsp olive oil
6 pork loin chops
1 tbsp butter
1 lb brussels sprouts, trimmed and halved
2 tbsp white wine
Salt and black pepper to taste

Directions

Preheat broiler to 400ºF and mix the lemon juice, garlic, salt, black pepper, and oil in a bowl.

Brush the pork with the mixture, place in a baking sheet, and cook for 6 minutes on each side until browned. Share into 6 plates and make the side dish.

Melt butter in a small wok or pan and cook in brussels sprouts for 5 minutes until tender. Drizzle with white wine, sprinkle with salt and black pepper and cook for another 5 minutes. Ladle brussels sprouts to the side of the chops and serve with a hot sauce.

Pork Chops with Cranberry Sauce

Ready in about: 2 hours 40 minutes | Serves: 4
Per serving: Kcal 450, Fat 34g, Net Carbs 6g, Protein 26g

Ingredients

4 pork chops
1 tsp garlic powder
Salt and black pepper, to taste
3 tsp fresh basil, chopped
A drizzle of olive oil
1 shallot, chopped
1 cup white wine
1 bay leaf
2 cups vegetable stock
Fresh parsley, chopped, for serving
2 cups cranberries
½ tsp fresh rosemary, chopped
½ cup swerve
Juice of 1 lemon
1 cup water
1 tsp harissa paste

Directions

In a bowl, combine the pork chops with 2 tsp of basil, salt, garlic powder and black pepper. Heat a pan with a drizzle of oil over medium heat, place in the pork and cook until browned; set aside.

Stir in the shallot, and cook for 2 minutes. Place in the bay leaf and wine, and cook for 4 minutes. Pour in juice from ½ lemon, and vegetable stock, and simmer for 5 minutes. Return the pork, and cook for 10 minutes. Cover the pan, and place in the oven to bake at 350ºF for 2 hours.

Set a pan over medium heat, add cranberries, rosemary, harissa paste, water, 1 tsp basil, swerve, and juice from ½ lemon, simmer for 15 minutes. Remove the pork chops from the oven, remove and discard the bay leaf. Split among plates, spread over with the cranberry sauce, sprinkle with parsley to serve.

Balsamic Grilled Pork Chops

Ready in about: 2 hours 20 minutes | Serves: 6
Per serving: Kcal 418, Fat 26.8g, Net Carbs 1.5g, Protein 38.1g

Ingredients

6 pork loin chops, boneless
2 tbsp erythritol
¼ cup balsamic vinegar
3 cloves garlic, minced
¼ cup olive oil
⅓ tsp salt
Black pepper to taste

Directions

Put the pork in a plastic bag. In a bowl, mix the erythritol, balsamic vinegar, garlic, olive oil, salt, pepper, and pour the sauce over the pork. Seal the bag, shake it, and place in the refrigerator.
Marinate the pork for 2 hours. Preheat the grill to medium heat, remove the pork when ready, and grill covered for 10 minutes on each side. Remove and let sit for 4 minutes, and serve with parsnip sauté.

Pork in White Wine

Ready in about: 1 hour 25 minutes | Serves: 6
Per serving: Kcal 514, Fat 32.5g, Net Carbs 6g, Protein 43g

Ingredients

2 tbsp olive oil
2 pounds pork stew meat, cubed
Salt and black pepper, to taste
2 tbsp butter
4 garlic cloves, minced
¾ cup vegetable stock
½ cup white wine
3 carrots, chopped
1 cabbage head, shredded
½ cup scallions, chopped
1 cup heavy cream

Directions

Set a pan over medium heat and warm butter and oil. Sear the pork until brown. Add garlic, scallions and carrots; sauté for 5 minutes. Pour in the cabbage, stock and wine, and bring to a boil. Reduce the heat and cook for 1 hour covered. Add in heavy cream as you stir for 1 minute, adjust seasonings and serve.

Stuffed Pork with Red Cabbage Salad

Ready in about: 40 minutes | Serves: 4
Per serving: Kcal 413, Fat 37g, Net Carbs 3g, Protein 26g

Ingredients

Zest and juice from 2 limes
2 garlic cloves, minced
¾ cup olive oil
1 cup fresh cilantro, chopped
1 cup fresh mint, chopped
1 tsp dried oregano

Salt and black pepper, to taste
2 tsp cumin
4 pork loin steaks
2 pickles, chopped
4 ham slices
6 Swiss cheese slices
2 tbsp mustard

For the Salad

1 head red cabbage, shredded
2 tbsp vinegar
3 tbsp olive oil
Salt to taste

Directions

In a food processor, blitz the lime zest, oil, oregano, black pepper, cumin, cilantro, lime juice, garlic, mint, and salt. Rub the steaks with the mixture and toss well to coat; set aside for some hours in the fridge.
Arrange the steaks on a working surface, split the pickles, mustard, cheese, and ham on them, roll, and secure with toothpicks. Heat a pan over medium heat, add in the pork rolls, cook each side for 2 minutes and remove to a baking sheet. Bake in the oven at 350ºF for 25 minutes. Prepare the red cabbage salad by mixing all salad ingredients and serve with the meat.

Spicy Mesquite Pork Ribs

Ready in about: 8 hours 45 minutes | Serves: 6
Per serving: Kcal 580, Fat 36.6g, Net Carbs 0g, Protein 44.5g

Ingredients

3 racks pork ribs, silver lining removed
2 cups sugar-free BBQ sauce
2 tbsp erythritol
2 tsp chili powder
2 tsp cumin powder
2 tsp onion powder
2 tsp smoked paprika
2 tsp garlic powder
Salt and black pepper to taste
1 tsp mustard powder

Directions

Preheat a smoker to 400ºF using mesquite wood to create flavor in the smoker.
In a bowl, mix the erythritol, chili powder, cumin powder, black pepper, onion powder, smoked paprika, garlic powder, salt, and mustard powder. Rub the ribs and let marinate for 30 minutes.
Place on the grill grate, and cook at reduced heat of 225ºF for 4 hours. Flip the ribs after and continue cooking for 4 hours. Brush the ribs with bbq sauce on both sides and sear them in increased heat for 3 minutes per side. Remove and let sit for 4 minutes before slicing. Serve with red cabbage coleslaw.

Paprika Pork Chops

Ready in about: 25 minutes | Serves: 4
Per serving: Kcal 349, Fat 18.5g, Net Carbs 4g,
Protein 41.8g

Ingredients

4 pork chops
Salt and black pepper, to taste
3 tbsp paprika
¾ cup cumin powder
1 tsp chili powder

Directions

In a bowl, combine the paprika with black pepper, cumin, salt, and chili. Place in the pork chops and rub them well. Heat a grill over medium temperature, add in the pork chops, cook for 5 minutes, flip, and cook for 5 minutes. Serve with steamed veggies.

Pork Casserole

Ready in about: 35 minutes | Serves: 4
Per serving: Kcal 495, Fat 29g, Net Carbs 2.7g,
Protein 36.5g

Ingredients

1 lb ground pork
1 large yellow squash, thinly sliced
Salt and black pepper to taste
1 clove garlic, minced
4 green onions, chopped
1 cup chopped cremini mushrooms
1 (15 oz) can diced tomatoes
½ cup pork rinds, crushed
¼ cup chopped parsley
1 cup cottage cheese
1 cup Mexican cheese blend
3 tbsp olive oil
⅓ cup water

Directions

Preheat the oven to 370ºF.
Heat the olive oil in a skillet over medium heat, add the pork, season it with salt and black pepper, and cook for 3 minutes or until no longer pink. Stir occasionally while breaking any lumps apart.
Add the garlic, half of the green onions, mushrooms, and 2 tablespoons of pork rinds. Cook for 3 minutes. Stir in the tomatoes, half of the parsley, and water. Cook further for 3 minutes, and then turn the heat off. Mix the remaining parsley, cottage cheese, and Mexican cheese blend. Set aside. Sprinkle the bottom of a baking dish with 3 tbsp of pork rinds; top with half of the squash and a season of salt, 2/3 of the pork mixture, and the cheese mixture. Repeat the layering process a second time to exhaust the ingredients.
Cover the baking dish with foil and bake for 20 minutes. After, remove the foil and brown the top of the casserole with the broiler side of the oven for 2 minutes. Remove the dish when ready and serve warm.

Spiced Pork Roast with Collard Greens

Ready in about: 60 minutes | Serves: 4
Per serving: Kcal 430, Fat 23g, Net Carbs 3g, Protein 45g

Ingredients

2 tbsp olive oil
Salt and black pepper, to taste
1 ½ pounds pork loin
A pinch of dry mustard
1 tsp hot red pepper flakes
½ tsp ginger, minced
1 cup collard greens, chopped
2 garlic cloves, minced
½ lemon sliced
¼ cup water

Directions

In a bowl, combine the ginger with salt, mustard, and black pepper. Add in the meat, toss to coat. Heat the oil in a saucepan over medium heat, brown the pork on all sides, for 10 minutes.
Transfer to the oven and roast for 40 minutes at 390ºF. To the saucepan, add collard greens, lemon slices, garlic, and water; cook for 10 minutes. Serve on a platter and sprinkle pan juices on top.

BBQ Pork Pizza with Goat Cheese

Ready in about: 30 minutes | Serves: 4
Per serving: Kcal 344, Fat 24g, Net Carbs 6,5g,
Protein 18g

Ingredients

1 low carb pizza bread
Olive oil for brushing
1 cup grated Manchego cheese
2 cups leftover pulled pork
½ cup sugar-free BBQ sauce
1 cup crumbled goat cheese

Directions

Preheat oven to 400ºF and put pizza bread on a pizza pan. Brush with olive oil and sprinkle the Manchego cheese all over. Mix the pork with BBQ sauce and spread over the cheese. Drop goat cheese on top and bake for 25 minutes until the cheese has melted. Slice the pizza with a cutter and serve.

Pork Wraps

Ready in about: 40 minutes | Serves: 6
Per serving: Kcal 435, Fat 37g, Net Carbs 2g, Protein 34g

Ingredients

6 bacon slices
2 tbsp fresh parsley, chopped
1 pound pork cutlets, sliced
⅓ cup ricotta cheese
1 tbsp coconut oil
¼ cup onions, chopped
3 garlic cloves, peeled and minced
2 tbsp Parmesan cheese, grated
15 ounces canned diced tomatoes
⅓ cup vegetable stock
Salt and black pepper, to taste

½ tsp Italian seasoning

Directions

Use a meat pounder to flatten the pork pieces. Set the bacon slices on top of each piece, then divide the parsley, ricotta cheese, and Parmesan cheese. Roll each pork piece and secure with a toothpick. Set a pan over medium heat and warm oil, cook the pork rolls until browned, and remove to a plate.

Add in onions and garlic, and cook for 5 minutes. Place in the stock and cook for 3 minutes. Get rid of the toothpicks from the rolls and return to the pan. Stir in the pepper, salt, tomatoes, and Italian seasoning, bring to a boil, set heat to medium-low, and cook for 20 minutes covered. Split among bowls to serve.

Oregano Pork Chops with Spicy Tomato Sauce

Ready in about: 50 minutes | Serves: 4
Per serving: Kcal 410, Fat 21g, Net Carbs 3.6g, Protein 39g

Ingredients

4 pork chops
1 tbsp fresh oregano, chopped
2 garlic cloves, minced
1 tbsp canola oil
15 ounces canned diced tomatoes
1 tbsp tomato paste
Salt and black pepper, to taste
¼ cup tomato juice
1 red chili, finely chopped

Directions

Set a pan over medium heat and warm oil, place in the pork, season with pepper and salt, cook for 6 minutes on both sides; remove to a bowl. Add in the garlic, and cook for 30 seconds. Stir in the tomato paste, tomatoes, tomato juice, and chili; bring to a boil, and reduce heat to medium-low.

Place in the pork chops, cover the pan and simmer everything for 30 minutes. Remove the pork to plates and sprinkle with fresh oregano to serve.

Zoodle, Bacon, Spinach, and Halloumi Gratin

Ready in about: 35 minutes | Serves: 4
Per serving: Kcal 350, Fat 27g, Net Carbs 5.3g, Protein 16g

Ingredients

2 large zucchinis, spiralized
4 slices bacon, chopped
2 cups baby spinach
4 oz halloumi cheese, cut into cubes
2 cloves garlic, minced
1 cup heavy cream
½ cup sugar-free tomato sauce
1 cup grated mozzarella cheese
½ tsp dried Italian mixed herbs
Salt and black pepper to taste

Directions

Preheat the oven to 350ºF. Place the cast iron pan over medium heat and fry the bacon for 4 minutes, then add garlic and cook for 1 minute.

In a bowl, mix the heavy cream, tomato sauce, and 1/6 cup water and add it to the pan. Stir in the zucchini, spinach, halloumi, Italian herbs, salt, and pepper. Sprinkle the mozzarella cheese on top, and transfer the pan to the oven. Bake for 20 minutes or until the cheese is golden. Serve the gratin warm.

Peanut Butter Pork Stir-Fry

Ready in about: 23 minutes | Serves: 4
Per serving: Kcal 571, Fat 49g, Net Carbs 1g, Protein 22.5g

Ingredients

1 ½ tbsp ghee
2 lb pork loin, cut into strips
Pink salt and chili pepper to taste
2 tsp ginger-garlic paste
¼ cup chicken broth
5 tbsp peanut butter
2 cups mixed stir-fry vegetables

Directions

Melt the ghee in a wok and mix the pork with salt, chili pepper, and ginger-garlic paste. Pour the pork into the wok and cook for 6 minutes until no longer pink.

Mix the peanut butter with some broth until smooth, add to the pork and stir; cook for 2 minutes. Pour in the remaining broth, cook for 4 minutes, and add the mixed veggies. Simmer for 5 minutes. Adjust the taste with salt and black pepper, and spoon the stir-fry to a side of cilantro cauli rice.

Pork Lettuce Cups

Ready in about: 20 minutes | Serves: 6
Per serving: Kcal 311, Fat 24.3g, Net Carbs 1g, Protein 19g

Ingredients

2 lb ground pork
1 tbsp ginger- garlic paste
Pink salt and chili pepper to taste
1 tsp ghee
1 head Iceberg lettuce
2 sprigs green onion, chopped
1 red bell pepper, seeded and chopped
½ cucumber, finely chopped

Directions

Put the pork with ginger-garlic paste, salt, and chili pepper seasoning in a saucepan. Cook for 10 minutes over medium heat while breaking any lumps until the pork is no longer pink. Drain liquid and add the ghee, melt and brown the meat for 4 minutes, continuously stirring. Turn the heat off.

Pat the lettuce dry with a paper towel and in each leaf, spoon two to three tablespoons of pork, top with green onions, bell pepper, and cucumber. Serve with soy drizzling sauce.

Pork and Mushroom Bake

Ready in about: 1 hour and 15 minutes | Serves: 6
Per serving: Kcal 403, Fat: 32.6g, Net Carbs: 8g,
Protein: 19.4g

Ingredients

1 onion, chopped
2 (10.5-oz) cans mushroom soup
6 pork chops
½ cup sliced mushrooms
Salt and ground pepper, to taste

Directions

Preheat the oven to 370ºF.
Season the pork chops with salt and black pepper,
and place in a baking dish. Combine the mushroom
soup, mushrooms, and onion, in a bowl. Pour this
mixture over the pork chops. Bake for 45 minutes.

Mustardy Pork Chops

Ready in about: 15 minutes | Serves: 4
Per serving: Kcal 382, Fat 21.5g, Net Carbs 1.2g,
Protein 38g

Ingredients

4 pork loin chops
1 tsp Dijon mustard
1 tbsp soy sauce
1 tsp lemon juice
1 tbsp water
Salt and black pepper, to taste
1 tbsp butter
A bunch of scallions, chopped

Directions

In a bowl, combine the water with lemon juice,
mustard and soy sauce. Set aside.
Set a pan over medium heat and melt butter, add in
the pork chops, season with salt, and black pepper.
Cook for 4 minutes, turn, and cook for an additional 4
minutes. Remove to a plate and keep warm.
In the same pan, pour mustard sauce, and simmer for
5 minutes. Drizzle the sauce over the pork, top with
scallions, and serve.

Greek Pork with Olives

Ready in about: 45 minutes | Serves: 4
Per serving: Kcal 415, Fat 25.2g, Net Carbs 2.2g,
Protein 36g

Ingredients

4 pork chops, bone-in
Salt and ground black pepper, to taste
1 tsp dried rosemary
3 garlic cloves, peeled and minced
½ cup kalamata olives, pitted and sliced
2 tbsp olive oil
¼ cup vegetable broth

Directions

Season pork chops with black pepper and salt, and
add in a roasting pan. Stir in the garlic, olives, olive
oil, broth, and rosemary, set in the oven at 425ºF, and
bake for 10 minutes. Reduce heat to 350ºF and roast

for 25 minutes. Slice the pork and sprinkle with pan
juices all over to serve.

Pork Goulash with Cauliflower

Ready in about: 15 minutes | Serves: 4
Per serving: Kcal 475, Fat 37g, Net Carbs 4.5g,
Protein 44g

Ingredients

1 red bell pepper, seeded and chopped
2 tbsp olive oil
1½ pounds ground pork
Salt and black pepper, to taste
2 cups cauliflower florets
1 onion, chopped
14 ounces canned diced tomatoes
¼ tsp garlic powder
1 tbsp tomato puree
1 ½ cups water

Directions

Heat olive oil in a pan over medium heat, stir in the
pork, and brown for 5 minutes. Place in the bell
pepper and onion, and cook for 4 minutes. Stir in the
water, tomatoes, and cauliflower, bring to a simmer
and cook for 5 minutes while covered. Place in the
black pepper, tomato paste, salt, and garlic powder.
Stir well, remove from the heat, split into bowls, and
enjoy.

Creamy Pork Chops

Ready in about: 50 minutes | Serves: 3
Per serving: Kcal 612, Fat 40g, Net Carbs 6.8g,
Protein 42g

Ingredients

8 ounces mushrooms, sliced
1 tsp garlic powder
1 onion, peeled and chopped
1 cup heavy cream
3 pork chops, boneless
1 tsp ground nutmeg
¼ cup coconut oil

Directions

Set a pan over medium heat and warm the oil, add in
the onion and mushrooms, and cook for 4 minutes.
Stir in the pork chops, season with garlic powder,
and nutmeg, and sear until browned.
Put the pan in the oven at 350ºF, and bake for 30
minutes. Remove pork chops to plates and maintain
warm. Place the pan over medium heat, pour in the
heavy cream over the mushroom mixture, and cook
for 5 minutes; remove from heat. Sprinkle sauce over
pork chops and enjoy.

Juicy Pork Medallions

Ready in about: 55 minutes | Serves: 4
Per serving: Kcal 325, Fat 18g, Net Carbs 6g, Protein 36g

Ingredients

2 onions, chopped
6 bacon slices, chopped
½ cup vegetable stock
Salt and black pepper, to taste
1 pound pork tenderloin, cut into medallions

Directions

Set a pan over medium heat, stir in the bacon, cook until crispy, and remove to a plate. Add onions, black pepper, and salt, and cook for 5 minutes; set to the same plate with bacon.

Add the pork medallions to the pan, season with black pepper and salt, brown for 3 minutes on each side, turn, reduce heat to medium, and cook for 7 minutes. Stir in the stock, and cook for 2 minutes. Return the bacon and onions to the pan and cook for 1 minute.

Pulled Pork with Avocado

Ready in about: 2 hours 55 minutes | Serves: 12
Per serving: Kcal 567, Fat 42.6g, Net Carbs 4.1g, Protein 42g

Ingredients

4 pounds pork shoulder
1 tbsp avocado oil
½ cup vegetable stock
¼ cup jerk seasoning
6 avocado, sliced

Directions

Rub the pork shoulder with jerk seasoning, and set in a greased baking dish. Pour in the stock, and cook for 1 hour 45 minutes in your oven at 350ºF covered with aluminium foil.

Discard the foil and cook for another 20 minutes. Leave to rest for 30 minutes, and shred it with 2 forks. Serve topped with avocado slices.

Garlic Pork Chops with Mint Pesto

Ready in about: 3 hours 10 minutes | Serves: 4
Per serving: Kcal 567, Fat 40g, Net Carbs 5.5g, Protein 37g

Ingredients

1 cup parsley
1 cup mint
1½ onions, chopped
⅓ cup pistachios
1 tsp lemon zest
5 tbsp avocado oil
Salt, to taste
4 pork chops
5 garlic cloves, minced
Juice from 1 lemon

Directions

In a food processor, combine the parsley with avocado oil, mint, pistachios, salt, lemon zest, and 1 onion. Rub the pork with this mixture, place in a bowl, and refrigerate for 1 hour while covered.

Remove the chops and set to a baking dish, place in ½ onion, and garlic; sprinkle with lemon juice, and bake for 2 hours in the oven at 250ºF. Split amongst plates and enjoy.

Jamaican Pork Oven Roast

Ready in about: 4 hours and 20 minutes | Serves: 12
Per serving: Kcal 282, Fat: 24g, Net Carbs: 0g, Protein: 23g

Ingredients

4 pounds pork roast
1 tbsp olive oil
¼ cup jerk spice blend
½ cup vegetable stock
Salt and black pepper, to taste

Directions

Rub the pork with olive oil and the spice blend. Heat a dutch oven over medium heat and sear the meat well on all sides; add in the stock. Cover the pot, reduce the heat, and let cook for 4 hours.

Hot Pork with Dill Pickles

Ready in about: 20 minutes | Serves: 4
Per serving: Kcal 315, Fat 18g, Net Carbs 2.3g, Protein 36g

Ingredients

¼ cup lime juice
4 pork chops
1 tbsp coconut oil, melted
2 garlic cloves, minced
1 tbsp chili powder
1 tsp ground cinnamon
2 tsp cumin
Salt and black pepper, to taste
½ tsp hot pepper sauce
4 dill pickles, cut into spears and squeezed

Directions

In a bowl, combine the lime juice with oil, cumin, salt, hot pepper sauce, black pepper, cinnamon, garlic, and chili powder. Place in the pork chops, toss to coat, and refrigerate for 4 hours.

Arrange the pork on a preheated grill over medium heat, cook for 7 minutes, turn, add in the dill pickles, and cook for another 7 minutes. Split among serving plates and enjoy.

Swiss-Style Italian Sausage

Ready in about: 25 minutes | Serves: 6
Per serving: Kcal 567, Fat 45g, Net Carbs 7.6g, Protein 34g

Ingredients

¼ cup olive oil
2 pounds Italian pork sausage, chopped
1 onion, sliced
4 sun-dried tomatoes, sliced thin
Salt and black pepper, to taste
½ pound Gruyere cheese, grated
3 yellow bell peppers, seeded and chopped
3 orange bell peppers, seeded and chopped

A pinch of red pepper flakes
½ cup fresh parsley, chopped
Directions
Set a pan over medium heat and warm oil, place in the sausage slices, cook each side for 3 minutes, remove to a bowl, and set aside. Stir in tomatoes, bell peppers, and onion, and cook for 5 minutes. Season with black pepper, pepper flakes, and salt and mix well. Cook for 1 minute, and remove from heat.
Lay sausage slices onto a baking dish, place the bell pepper mixture on top, scatter with the Gruyere cheese, set in the oven at 340º F. Bake for 10 minutes, until the cheese melts. Serve topped with parsley.

Bacon Smothered Pork Chops
Ready in about: 25 minutes | Serves: 6
Per serving: Kcal 435, Fat 37g, Net Carbs 3g, Protein 22g
Ingredients
7 strips bacon, chopped
6 pork chops
Pink salt and black pepper to taste
5 sprigs fresh thyme + extra to garnish
¼ cup chicken broth
½ cup heavy cream
Directions
Cook bacon in a large skillet on medium heat for 5 minutes. Remove with a slotted spoon onto a paper towel-lined plate to soak up excess fat.
Season pork chops with salt and black pepper, and brown in the bacon fat for 4 minutes on each side. Remove to the bacon plate. Stir in the thyme, chicken broth, and heavy cream and simmer for 5 minutes.
Return the chops and bacon, and cook further for another 2 minutes. Serve chops and a generous ladle of sauce with cauli mash. Garnish with thyme leaves.

Smoked Pork Sausages with Mushrooms
Ready in about: 1 hour 10 minutes | Serves: 6
Per serving: Kcal 525, Fat 32g, Net Carbs 7.3g, Protein 29g
Ingredients
3 yellow bell peppers, seeded and chopped
2 pounds smoked sausage, sliced
Salt and black pepper, to taste
2 pounds portobello mushrooms, sliced
2 sweet onions, chopped
1 tbsp swerve
2 tbsp olive oil
Arugula to garnish
Directions
In a baking dish, combine the sausages with swerve, oil, black pepper, onion, bell peppers, salt, and mushrooms. Pour in 1 cup of water and toss well to ensure everything is coated, set in the oven at 320ºF to bake for 1 hour. To serve, divide the sausages between plates and scatter over the arugula.

Pork Sausage with Spinach
Ready in about: 35 minutes | Serves: 6
Per serving: Kcal 352, Fat 28g, Net Carbs 6.2g, Protein 29g
Ingredients
1 onion, chopped
2 tbsp olive oil
2 pounds Italian pork sausage, sliced
1 red bell pepper, seeded and chopped
Salt and black pepper, to taste
4 pounds spinach, chopped
1 garlic, minced
¼ cup green chili peppers, chopped
1 cup water
Directions
Set pan over medium heat, warm oil and cook sausage for 10 minutes. Stir in onion, garlic and bell pepper and fry for 4 minutes. Place in spinach, salt, water, pepper, chili pepper, and cook for 10 minutes.

Sausage Links with Tomatoes & Pesto
Ready in about: 15 minutes | Serves: 8
Per serving: Kcal 365, Fat 26g, Net Carbs 6.8g, Protein 18g
Ingredients
8 pork sausage links, sliced
1 lb mixed cherry tomatoes, cut in half
4 cups baby spinach
1 tbsp olive oil
1 pound Monterrey Jack cheese, cubed
2 tbsp lemon juice
1 cup basil pesto
Salt and black pepper, to taste
Directions
Warm oil in a pan and cook sausage links for 4 minutes per side. In a salad bowl, combine spinach, cheese, salt, pesto, pepper, cherry tomatoes, and lemon juice, and toss to coat. Mix in the sausage.

Bacon Stew with Cauliflower
Ready in about: 40 minutes | Serves: 6
Per serving: Kcal 380, Fat 25g, Net Carbs 6g, Protein 33g
Ingredients
8 ounces mozzarella cheese, grated
2 cups chicken broth
½ tsp garlic powder
½ tsp onion powder
Salt and black pepper, to taste
4 garlic cloves, minced
¼ cup heavy cream
3 cups bacon, chopped
1 head cauliflower, cut into florets
Directions
In a pot, combine the bacon with broth, cauliflower, salt, heavy cream, black pepper, garlic powder, cheese, onion powder, and garlic, and cook for 35 minutes. Share into serving plates, and enjoy.

Pancetta Sausage with Kale

Ready in about: 30 minutes | Serves: 8
Per serving: Kcal 386, Fat 29g, Net Carbs 5.4g, Protein2 1g

Ingredients

2 cups kale
8 cups chicken broth
A drizzle of olive oil
1 cup heavy cream
6 pancetta slices, chopped
1 pound radishes, chopped
2 garlic cloves, minced
Salt and black pepper, to taste
A pinch of red pepper flakes
1 onion, chopped
1 ½ pounds hot pork sausage, chopped

Directions

Set a pot over medium heat. Add in a drizzle of olive oil and warm. Stir in garlic, onion, pancetta, and sausage; cook for 5 minutes. Pour in broth, radishes, and kale, and simmer for 10 minutes.
Stir in salt, red pepper flakes, black pepper, and heavy cream, and cook for about 5 minutes. Serve.

Sweet Chipotle Grilled Ribs

Ready in about: 32 minutes | Serves: 4
Per serving: Kcal 395, Fat 33g, Net Carbs 3g, Protein 21g

Ingredients

2 tbsp erythritol
Pink salt and black pepper to taste
1 tbsp olive oil
3 tsp chipotle powder
1 tsp garlic powder
1 lb beef spare ribs
4 tbsp sugar-free BBQ sauce + extra for serving

Directions

Mix the erythritol, salt, pepper, oil, chipotle, and garlic powder. Brush on the meaty sides of the ribs and wrap in foil. Sit for 30 minutes to marinate.
Preheat oven to 400ºF, place wrapped ribs on a baking sheet, and cook for 40 minutes to be cooked through. Remove ribs and aluminium foil, brush with BBQ sauce, and brown under the broiler for 10 minutes on both sides. Slice and serve with extra BBQ sauce and lettuce tomato salad.

Beef Mushroom Meatloaf

Ready in about: 1 hour and 15 minutes | Serves: 12
Per serving: Kcal 294, Fat: 19g, Net Carbs: 6g, Protein: 23g

Ingredients

3 pounds ground beef
½ cup chopped onions
½ cup almond flour
2 garlic cloves, minced
1 cup sliced mushrooms
3 eggs
¼ tsp pepper
2 tbsp chopped parsley
¼ cup chopped bell peppers
⅓ cup grated Parmesan cheese
1 tsp balsamic vinegar
1 tsp salt
Glaze:
2 cups balsamic vinegar
1 tbsp sweetener
2 tbsp sugar-free ketchup

Directions

Combine all meatloaf ingredients in a large bowl. Press this mixture into 2 greased loaf pans. Bake at 370ºF for about 30 minutes.
Meanwhile, make the glaze by combining all ingredients in a saucepan over medium heat. Simmer for 20 minutes, until the glaze is thickened. Pour ¼ cup of the glaze over the meatloaf. Save the extra for future use.
Put the meatloaf back in the oven and cook for 20 more minutes.

Zucchini Boats with Beef and Pimiento Rojo

Ready in about: 30 minutes | Serves: 4
Per serving: Kcal 335, Fat 24g, Net Carbs 7g, Protein 18g

Ingredients

4 zucchinis
2 tbsp olive oil
1 ½ lb ground beef
1 medium red onion, chopped
2 tbsp chopped pimiento
Pink salt and black pepper to taste
1 cup grated yellow cheddar cheese

Directions

Preheat oven to 350ºF.
Lay the zucchinis on a flat surface, trim off the ends and cut in half lengthwise. Scoop out the pulp from each half with a spoon to make shells. Chop the pulp.
Heat oil in a skillet; add the ground beef, red onion, pimiento, and zucchini pulp, and season with salt and black pepper. Cook for 6 minutes while stirring to break up lumps until beef is no longer pink. Turn the heat off. Spoon the beef into the boats and sprinkle with cheddar cheese.
Place on a greased baking sheet and cook to melt the cheese for 15 minutes until zucchini boats are tender. Take out, cool for 2 minutes, and serve warm with a mixed green salad.

Spicy Spinach Pinwheel Steaks

Ready in about: 40 minutes | Serves: 6
Per serving: Kcal 490, Fat 41g, Net Carbs 2g, Protein 28g

Ingredients

1 ½ lb beef flank steak
Salt and black pepper to taste
1 cup crumbled feta cheese
½ loose cup baby spinach
1 jalapeño pepper, chopped
¼ cup chopped basil leaves

Preheat oven to 400ºF and grease a baking sheet with cooking spray.

Wrap the steak in plastic wrap, place on a flat surface, and gently run a rolling pin over to flatten. Take off the wraps. Sprinkle with half of the feta cheese, top with spinach, jalapeno, basil leaves, and the remaining cheese. Roll the steak over on the stuffing and secure with toothpicks.

Place in the baking sheet and cook for 30 minutes, flipping once until nicely browned on the outside and the cheese melted within. Cool for 3 minutes, slice into pinwheels and serve with sautéed veggies.

Rib Roast with Roasted Red Shallots and Garlic

Ready in about: 55 minutes | Serves: 6
Per serving: Kcal 556, Fat 38.6g, Net Carbs 2.5g, Protein 58.4g

Ingredients

5 lb beef rib roast, on the bone
3 heads garlic, cut in half
3 tbsp olive oil
6 shallots, peeled and halved
2 lemons, zested and juiced
3 tbsp mustard seeds
3 tbsp swerve
Salt and black pepper to taste
3 tbsp thyme leaves

Directions

Preheat oven to 450ºF. Place garlic heads and shallots in a roasting dish, toss with olive oil, and bake for 15 minutes. Pour lemon juice on them. Score shallow crisscrosses patterns on the meat and set aside.

Mix swerve, mustard seeds, thyme, salt, pepper, and lemon zest to make a rub; and apply it all over the beef. Place the beef on the shallots and garlic; cook in the oven for 15 minutes. Reduce the heat to 400ºF, cover the dish with foil, and continue cooking for 5 minutes. Once ready, remove the dish, and let sit covered for 15 minutes before slicing.

Beef Tripe in Vegetable Sauté

Ready in about: 27 minutes + cooling time | Serves: 6
Per serving: Kcal 342, Fat 27g, Net Carbs 1g, Protein 22g

Ingredients

1 ½ lb beef tripe
4 cups buttermilk
Salt to taste
2 tsp creole seasoning
3 tbsp olive oil
2 large onions, sliced
3 tomatoes, diced

Directions

Put the tripe in a bowl and cover with buttermilk. Refrigerate for 3 hours to extract bitterness and gamey taste. Remove from buttermilk, pat dry with a paper towel, and season with salt and creole seasoning.

Heat 2 tbsp of oil in a skillet over medium heat and brown the tripe on both sides for 6 minutes in total. Set aside. Add the remaining oil and sauté the onions for 3 minutes until soft. Include the tomatoes and cook for 10 minutes. Pour in a few tablespoons of water if necessary. Put the tripe in the sauce and cook for 3 minutes. Adjust taste with salt and serve with low carb rice.

Beef Cauliflower Curry

Ready in about: 26 minutes | Serves: 6
Per serving: Kcal 374, Fat 33g, Net Carbs 2g, Protein 22g

Ingredients

1 tbsp olive oil
1 ½ lb ground beef
1 tbsp ginger-garlic paste
1 tsp garam masala
1 (7 oz) can whole tomatoes
1 head cauliflower, cut into florets
Pink salt and chili pepper to taste
¼ cup water

Directions

Heat oil in a saucepan over medium heat, add the beef, ginger-garlic paste and season with garam masala. Cook for 5 minutes while breaking any lumps. Stir in the tomatoes and cauliflower, season with salt and chili pepper, and cook covered for 6 minutes. Add the water and bring to a boil over medium heat for 10 minutes or until the water has reduced by half. Adjust taste with salt. Spoon the curry into serving bowls and serve with shirataki rice.

Easy Zucchini Beef Lasagna

Ready in about: 1 hour | Serves: 4
Per serving: Kcal 344, Fat 17.8g, Net Carbs 2.9g, Protein 40.4g

Ingredients

1 lb ground beef
2 large zucchinis, sliced lengthwise
3 cloves garlic
1 medium white onion, finely chopped
3 tomatoes, chopped
Salt and black pepper to taste
2 tsp sweet paprika
1 tsp dried thyme
1 tsp dried basil
1 cup shredded mozzarella cheese
1 tbsp olive oil
Cooking spray

Directions

Preheat the oven to 370ºF and lightly grease a baking dish with cooking spray.

Heat the olive oil in a skillet and cook the beef for 4 minutes while breaking any lumps as you stir. Top with onion, garlic, tomatoes, salt, paprika, and pepper. Stir and continue cooking for 5 minutes.

Then, lay ⅓ of the zucchini slices in the baking dish. Top with ⅓ of the beef mixture and repeat the layering process two more times with the same quantities. Season with basil and thyme.

Finally, sprinkle the mozzarella cheese on top and tuck the baking dish in the oven. Bake for 35 minutes. Remove the lasagna and let it rest for 10 minutes before serving.

Grilled Sirloin Steak with Sauce Diane

Ready in about: 25 minutes | Serves: 6
Per serving: Kcal 434, Fat 17g, Net Carbs 2.9g, Protein 36g

Ingredients
Sirloin Steak

1 ½ lb sirloin steak
Salt and black pepper to taste
1 tsp olive oil
Sauce Diane
1 tbsp olive oil
1 clove garlic, minced
1 cup sliced porcini mushrooms
1 small onion, finely diced
2 tbsp butter
1 tbsp Dijon mustard
2 tbsp Worcestershire sauce
¼ cup whiskey
2 cups double cream
Salt and black pepper to taste

Directions

Put a grill pan over high heat and as it heats, brush the steak with oil, sprinkle with salt and pepper, and rub the seasoning into the meat with your hands. Cook the steak in the pan for 4 minutes on each side for medium rare and transfer to a chopping board to rest for 4 minutes before slicing. Reserve the juice.

Heat the oil in a frying pan over medium heat and sauté the onion for 3 minutes. Add the butter, garlic, and mushrooms, and cook for 2 minutes.

Add the Worcestershire sauce, the reserved juice, and mustard. Stir and cook for 1 minute. Pour in the whiskey and cook further 1 minute until the sauce reduces by half. Swirl the pan and add the cream. Let it simmer to thicken for about 3 minutes. Adjust the taste with salt and pepper. Spoon the sauce over the steaks slices and serve with celeriac mash.

Italian Beef Ragout

Ready in about: 1 hour 52 minutes | Serves: 4
Per serving: Kcal 328, Fat 21.6g, Net Carbs 4.2g, Protein 36.6g

Ingredients

1 lb chuck steak, trimmed and cubed
2 tbsp olive oil
Salt and black pepper to taste
2 tbsp almond flour
1 medium onion, diced
½ cup dry white wine
1 red bell pepper, seeded and diced
2 tsp Worcestershire sauce
4 oz tomato puree
3 tsp smoked paprika
1 cup beef broth
Thyme leaves to garnish

Directions

First, lightly dredge the meat in the almond flour and set aside. Place a large skillet over medium heat, add 1 tablespoon of oil to heat and then sauté the onion, and bell pepper for 3 minutes. Stir in the paprika, and add the remaining olive oil.

Add the beef and cook for 10 minutes in total while turning them halfway. Stir in white wine, let it reduce by half, about 3 minutes, and add Worcestershire sauce, tomato puree, and beef broth.

Let the mixture boil for 2 minutes, then reduce the heat to lowest and let simmer for 1 ½ hours; stirring now and then. Adjust the taste and dish the ragout. Serve garnished with thyme leaves.

Beef Cotija Cheeseburger

Ready in about: 15 minutes | Serves: 4
Per serving: Kcal 386, Fat 32g, Net Carbs 2g, Protein 21g

Ingredients

1 lb ground beef
1 tsp dried parsley
½ tsp Worcestershire sauce
Salt and black pepper to taste
1 cup cotija cheese, shredded
4 low carb buns, halved

Directions

Preheat a grill to 400ºF and grease the grate with cooking spray.

Mix the beef, parsley, Worcestershire sauce, salt, and black pepper with your hands until evenly combined. Make medium sized patties out of the mixture, about 4 patties. Cook on the grill for 7 minutes one side to be cooked through and no longer pink.

Flip the patties and top with cheese. Cook for 7 minutes, until the cheese melts. Remove the patties and sandwich into two halves of a bun each. Serve with a tomato dipping sauce and zucchini fries.

Warm Rump Steak Salad

Ready in about: 40 minutes | Serves: 4
Per serving: Kcal 325, Fat 19g, Net Carbs 4g, Protein 28g

Ingredients

½ lb rump steak, excess fat trimmed
3 green onions, sliced
3 tomatoes, sliced
1 cup green beans, steamed and sliced
2 kohlrabi, peeled and chopped
½ cup water
2 cups mixed salad greens
Salt and black pepper to season
Salad Dressing
2 tsp Dijon mustard
1 tsp erythritol
Salt and black pepper to taste

3 tbsp olive oil + extra for drizzling
1 tbsp red wine vinegar

Directions

Preheat the oven to 400ºF. Place the kohlrabi on a baking sheet, drizzle with olive oil and bake in the oven for 25 minutes. After cooking, remove, and set aside to cool.

In a bowl, mix the Dijon mustard, erythritol, salt, black pepper, vinegar, and olive oil. Set aside.

Then, preheat a grill pan over high heat while you season the meat with salt and black pepper. Place the steak in the pan and brown on both sides for 4 minutes each. Remove to rest on a chopping board for 4 more minutes before slicing thinly.

In a salad bowl, add green onions, tomatoes, green beans, kohlrabi, salad greens, and steak slices. Drizzle the dressing over and toss with two spoons. Serve the steak salad warm with chunks of low carb bread.

Beef with Dilled Yogurt

Ready in about: 25 minutes | Serves: 6
Per serving: Kcal 408, Fat 22.4g, Net Carbs 8.3g, Protein 27g

Ingredients

¼ cup almond milk
2 pounds ground beef
1 onion, grated
5 zero carb bread slices, torn
1 egg, whisked
¼ cup fresh parsley, chopped
Salt and black pepper, to taste
2 garlic cloves, minced
¼ cup fresh mint, chopped
2 ½ tsp dried oregano
¼ cup olive oil
1 cup cherry tomatoes, halved
1 cucumber, sliced
1 cup baby spinach
1½ tbsp lemon juice
1 cup dilled Greek yogurt

Directions

Place the torn bread in a bowl, add in the milk, and set aside for 3 minutes. Squeeze the bread, chop, and place into a bowl. Stir in the beef, salt, mint, onion, parsley, pepper, egg, oregano, and garlic.

Form balls out of this mixture and place on a working surface. Set a pan over medium heat and warm half of the oil; fry the meatballs for 8 minutes. Flip occasionally, and set aside in a tray.

In a salad plate, combine the spinach with the cherry tomatoes and cucumber. Mix in the remaining oil, lemon juice, black pepper, and salt. Spread dilled yogurt over, and top with meatballs to serve.

Beef Stovies

Ready in about: 60 minutes | Serves: 4
Per serving: Kcal 316, Fat 18g, Net Carbs 3g, Protein 14g

Ingredients

1 lb ground beef

1 large onion, chopped
6 parsnips, peeled and chopped
1 large carrot, chopped
1 tbsp olive oil
1 clove garlic, minced
Salt and black pepper to taste
1 cup chicken broth
¼ tsp allspice
2 tsp rosemary leaves
1 tbsp sugar-free Worcestershire sauce
½ small cabbage, shredded

Directions

Heat the oil in a skillet over medium heat and cook the beef for 4 minutes. Season with salt and black pepper, and occasionally stir while breaking the lumps in it. Add in the onion, garlic, carrot, rosemary, and parsnips. Stir and cook for a minute, and pour the chicken broth, allspice, and Worcestershire sauce in it. Stir the mixture and cook the ingredients on low heat for 40 minutes.

Stir in the cabbage, season with salt and black pepper, and cook further for 2 minutes. After, turn the heat off, plate the stovies, and serve with wilted spinach and collards.

Beef with Grilled Vegetables

Ready in about: 30 minutes | Serves: 4
Per serving: Kcal 515, Fat 32.1g, Net Carbs 5.6g, Protein 66g

Ingredients

4 sirloin steaks
Salt and black pepper to taste
4 tbsp olive oil
3 tbsp balsamic vinegar

Vegetables

½ lb asparagus, trimmed
1 cup green beans
1 cup snow peas
1 red bell peppers, seeded, cut into strips
1 orange bell peppers, seeded, cut into strips
1 medium red onion, quartered

Directions

Set the grill pan over high heat.

Grab 2 separate bowls; put the beef in one and the vegetables in another. Mix salt, pepper, olive oil, and balsamic vinegar in a small bowl, and pour half of the mixture over the beef and the other half over the vegetables. Coat the ingredients in both bowls with the sauce and cook the beef first.

Place the steaks in the grill pan and sear both sides for 2 minutes each, then continue cooking for 6 minutes on each side. When done, remove the beef onto a plate; set aside.

Pour the vegetables and marinade in the pan; and cook for 5 minutes, turning once. Share the vegetables into plates. Top with each piece of beef, the sauce from the pan, and serve with a rutabaga mash.

Ribeye Steak with Shitake Mushrooms

Ready in about: 25 minutes | Serves: 1
Per serving: Kcal 478, Fat: 31g, Net Carbs: 3g, Protein: 33g

Ingredients

6 ounces ribeye steak
2 tbsp butter
1 tsp olive oil
½ cup shitake mushrooms, sliced
Salt and black pepper, to taste

Directions

Heat the olive oil in a pan over medium heat. Rub the steak with salt and black pepper and cook about 4 minutes per side; set aside. Melt the butter in the pan and cook the shitakes for 4 minutes. Pour the butter and mushrooms over the steak to serve.

Beef and Ale Pot Roast

Ready in about: 2 hours 20 minutes | Serves: 6
Per serving: Kcal 513, Fat 34g, Net Carbs 6g, Protein 26g

Ingredients

1 ½ lb brisket
1 tbsp olive oil
8 baby carrots, peeled
2 medium red onions, quartered
4 stalks celery, cut into chunks
Salt and black pepper to taste
2 bay leaves
1 ½ cups low carb beer (ale)

Directions

Preheat the oven to 370ºF. Heat the olive oil in a large skillet, while heating, season the brisket with salt and pepper. Brown the meat on both sides for 8 minutes. After, transfer to a deep casserole dish.
In the dish, arrange the carrots, onions, celery, and bay leaves around the brisket and pour the beer all over it. Cover the pot and cook the ingredients in the oven for 2 hours.
When ready, remove the casserole. Transfer the beef to a chopping board and cut it into thick slices. Serve the beef and vegetables with a drizzle of the sauce, and with steamed turnips.

Habanero and Beef Balls

Ready in about: 45 minutes | Serves: 6
Per serving: Kcal 455, Fat 31g, Net Carbs 8.3g, Protein 27g

Ingredients

3 garlic cloves, minced
1 pound ground beef
1 small onion, chopped
2 habanero peppers, chopped
1 tsp dried thyme
2 tsp cilantro
½ tsp allspice
2 tsp cumin
A pinch of ground cloves
Salt and black pepper, to taste
2 tbsp butter

3 tbsp butter, melted
6 ounces cream cheese
1 tsp turmeric
¼ tsp stevia
½ tsp baking powder
1½ cups flax meal
½ cup coconut flour

Directions

In a blender, mix onion with garlic, habaneros, and ½ cup water. Set a pan over medium heat, add in 2 tbsp butter and cook the beef for 3 minutes. Stir in the onion mixture, and cook for 2 minutes.
Stir in cilantro, cloves, salt, cumin, ½ teaspoon turmeric, thyme, allspice, and black pepper, and cook for 3 minutes. In a bowl, combine the remaining turmeric, with coconut flour, stevia, flax meal, and baking powder. In a separate bowl, combine the melted butter with the cream cheese.
Combine the 2 mixtures to obtain a dough. Form 12 balls from this mixture, set them on a parchment paper, and roll each into a circle. Split the beef mix on one-half of the dough circles, cover with the other half, seal edges, and lay on a lined sheet. Bake for 25 minutes in the oven at 350ºF.

Classic Italian Bolognese Sauce

Ready in about: 35 minutes | Serves: 5
Per serving: Kcal 318, Fat: 20g, Net Carbs: 5.9g, Protein: 26g

Ingredients

1 pound ground beef
2 garlic cloves
1 onion, chopped
1 tsp oregano
1 tsp sage
1 tsp rosemary
7 oz canned chopped tomatoes
1 tbsp olive oil

Directions

Heat olive oil in a saucepan. Add onion and garlic and cook for 3 minutes. Add beef and cook until browned, about 4-5 minutes. Stir in the herbs and tomatoes. Cook for 15 minutes. Serve with zoodles.

Beef Skewers with Ranch Dressing

Ready in about: 25 minutes | Serves: 4
Per serving: Kcal 230, Fat 14g, Net Carbs 3g, Protein 21g

Ingredients

1 lb sirloin steak, boneless, cubed
¼ cup ranch dressing, divided
Chopped scallions to garnish

Directions

Preheat the grill on medium heat to 400ºF and thread the beef cubes on the skewers, about 4 to 5 cubes per skewer. Brush half of the ranch dressing on the skewers (all around) and place them on the grill grate to cook for 6 minutes. Turn the skewers once and cook further for 6 minutes.

Brush the remaining ranch dressing on the meat and cook them for 1 more minute on each side. Plate, garnish with the scallions, and serve with a mixed veggie salad, and extra ranch dressing.

Adobo Beef Fajitas
Ready in about: 35 minutes + marinade time | Serves: 4
Per serving: Kcal 348, Fat 25g, Net Carbs 5g, Protein 18g

Ingredients
2 lb skirt steak
2 tbsp adobo seasoning
Salt to taste
2 tbsp olive oil
2 large white onion, chopped
1 cup mixed bell peppers, chopped
12 low carb tortillas

Directions
Season the steak with adobo seasoning and marinate in the fridge for one hour.
Preheat grill to 425ºF and cook steak for 6 minutes on each side, flipping once until lightly browned. Remove from heat and wrap in foil and let sit for 10 minutes. This allows the meat to cook in its heat for a few more minutes before slicing.
Heat olive oil in a skillet over medium heat and sauté onion and bell peppers for 5 minutes, until soft. Cut steak against the grain into strips and share on the tortillas. Top with the veggies and serve.

Mustard-Lemon Beef
Ready in about: 25 minutes | Serves: 4
Per serving: Kcal 435, Fat 30g, Net Carbs 5g, Protein 32g

Ingredients
2 tbsp olive oil
1 tbsp fresh rosemary, chopped
2 garlic cloves, minced
1 ½ pounds beef rump steak, thinly sliced
Salt and black pepper, to taste
1 shallot, chopped
½ cup heavy cream
½ cup beef stock
1 tbsp mustard
2 tsp Worcestershire sauce
2 tsp lemon juice
1 tsp erythritol
2 tbsp butter
A sprig of rosemary
A sprig of thyme

Directions
In a bowl, combine 1 tbsp of oil with black pepper, garlic, rosemary, and salt. Toss in the beef to coat, and set aside for some minutes. Heat a pan with the rest of the oil over medium heat, place in the beef steak, cook for 6 minutes, flipping halfway through; set aside and keep warm.
Set the pan to medium heat, stir in the shallot, and cook for 3 minutes; stir in the stock, Worcestershire

sauce, erythritol, thyme, cream, mustard, and rosemary, and cook for 8 minutes.
Stir in the butter, lemon juice, black pepper, and salt. Get rid of the rosemary and thyme, and remove from heat. Arrange the beef slices on serving plates, sprinkle over the sauce, and enjoy.

Beef and Egg Rice Bowls
Ready in about: 22 minutes | Serves: 4
Per serving: Kcal 320, Fat 26g, Net Carbs 4g, Protein 15g

Ingredients
2 cups cauli rice
3 cups frozen mixed vegetables
3 tbsp ghee
1 lb skirt steak
Salt and black pepper to taste
4 eggs
Hot sauce for topping

Directions
Mix the cauli rice and mixed vegetables in a bowl, sprinkle with a little water, and steam in the microwave for 1 minute until tender. Share into 4 serving bowls.
Melt the ghee in a skillet, season the beef with salt and black pepper, and brown for 5 minutes on each side. Use a perforated spoon to ladle the meat onto the vegetables.
Wipe out the skillet and return to medium heat, crack in an egg, season with salt and pepper and cook until the egg white has set, but the yolk is still runny 3 minutes. Remove egg onto the vegetable bowl and fry the remaining 3 eggs. Add to the other bowls. Drizzle the beef bowls with hot sauce and serve.

Soy-Glazed Meatloaf
Ready in about: 60 minutes | Serves: 6
Per serving: Kcal 474, Fat 21.4g, Net Carbs 7.5g, Protein 46g

Ingredients
1 cup white mushrooms, chopped
2 pounds ground beef
2 tbsp fresh parsley, chopped
2 garlic cloves, minced
1 onion, chopped
1 red bell pepper, seeded and chopped
½ cup almond flour
⅓ cup Parmesan cheese, grated
2 eggs
Salt and black pepper, to taste
1 tsp balsamic vinegar
1 tbsp swerve
1 tbsp soy sauce
2 tbsp sugar-free ketchup
2 cups balsamic vinegar

Directions
In a bowl, combine the beef with salt, mushrooms, bell pepper, Parmesan cheese, 1 teaspoon vinegar, parsley, garlic, black pepper, onion, almond flour, salt,

and eggs. Set this into a loaf pan, and bake for 30 minutes in the oven at 370ºF.

Meanwhile, heat a small pan over medium heat, add in the 2 cups vinegar, swerve, soy sauce, and ketchup, and cook for 20 minutes. Remove the meatloaf from the oven, spread the glaze over the meatloaf, and bake in the oven for 20 more minutes. Allow the meatloaf to cool, slice, and enjoy.

Homemade Classic Beef Burgers

Ready in about: 15 minutes | Serves: 4
Per serving: Kcal 664, Fat: 55g, Net Carbs: 7.9g, Protein: 39g

Ingredients

1 pound ground beef
½ tsp onion powder
½ tsp garlic powder
2 tbsp ghee
1 tsp Dijon mustard
4 low carb buns, halved
¼ cup mayonnaise
1 tsp sriracha sauce
4 tbsp cabbage slaw
Salt and black pepper to taste

Directions

Mix together the beef, onion powder, garlic powder, mustard, salt, and black pepper; create 4 burgers. Melt the ghee in a skillet and cook the burgers for about 3 minutes per side. Serve in buns topped with mayo, sriracha, and cabbage slaw.

Beef Zucchini Boats

Ready in about: 45 minutes | Serves: 4
Per serving: Kcal 422, Fat 33g, Net Carbs 7.8g, Protein 39g

Ingredients

2 garlic cloves, minced
1 tsp cumin
1 tbsp olive oil
1 pound ground beef
½ cup onions, chopped
1 tsp smoked paprika
Salt and black pepper, to taste
4 zucchinis
¼ cup fresh cilantro, chopped
½ cup Monterey Jack cheese, shredded
1 ½ cups enchilada sauce
1 avocado, chopped, for serving
Green onions, chopped, for serving
Tomatoes, chopped, for serving

Directions

Set a pan over high heat and warm the oil. Add the onions, and cook for 2 minutes. Stir in the beef, and brown for 4-5 minutes. Stir in the paprika, pepper, garlic, cumin, and salt; cook for 2 minutes.

Slice the zucchini in half lengthwise and scoop out the seeds. Set the zucchini in a greased baking pan, stuff each with the beef, scatter enchilada sauce on top, and spread with the Monterey cheese.

Bake in the oven at 350ºF for 20 minutes while covered. Uncover, spread with cilantro, and bake for 5 minutes. Top with tomatoes, green onions and avocado, place on serving plates and enjoy.

Beef Sausage Casserole

Ready in about: 60 minutes | Serves: 8
Per serving: Kcal 456, Fat 35g, Net Carbs 4g, Protein 32g

Ingredients

⅓ cup almond flour
2 eggs
2 pounds beef sausage, chopped
Salt and black pepper, to taste
1 tbsp dried parsley
¼ tsp red pepper flakes
¼ cup Parmesan cheese, grated
¼ tsp onion powder
½ tsp garlic powder
¼ tsp dried oregano
1 cup ricotta cheese
1 cup sugar-free marinara sauce
1 ½ cups cheddar cheese, shredded

Directions

In a bowl, combine the sausage, black pepper, pepper flakes, oregano, eggs, Parmesan cheese, onion powder, almond flour, salt, parsley, and garlic powder. Form balls, lay them on a greased baking sheet, place in the oven at 370ºF, and bake for 15 minutes.

Remove the balls from the oven and cover with half of the marinara sauce. Pour ricotta cheese all over followed by the rest of the marinara sauce. Scatter the cheddar cheese and bake in the oven for 10 minutes. Allow the meatballs casserole to cool before serving.

Jalapeno Beef Pot Roasted

Ready in about: 1 hour 25 minutes | Serves: 4
Per serving: Kcal 745, Fat 46g, Net Carbs 3.2g, Protein 87g

Ingredients

3½ pounds beef roast
4 ounces mushrooms, sliced
12 ounces beef stock
1 ounce onion soup mix
½ cup Italian dressing
2 jalapeño peppers, shredded

Directions

In a bowl, combine the stock with the Italian dressing and onion soup mixture. Place the beef roast in a pan, stir in the stock mixture, mushrooms, and jalapeños; cover with aluminum foil.

Set in the oven at 300ºF, and bake for 1 hour. Take out the foil and continue baking for 15 minutes. Allow the roast to cool, slice, and serve alongside a topping of the gravy.

Beef Cheeseburger Casserole

Ready in about: 30 minutes | Serves: 6
Per serving: Kcal 385, Fat 25g, Net Carbs 5g, Protein 20g

Ingredients

2 lb ground beef
Salt and black pepper to taste
1 cup cauli rice
2 cups chopped cabbage
14 oz can diced tomatoes
1 cup shredded colby jack cheese

Directions

Preheat oven to 370ºF and grease a baking dish with cooking spray. Put beef in a pot and season with salt and black pepper and cook over medium heat for 6 minutes until no longer pink. Drain the grease. Add cauli rice, cabbage, tomatoes, and ¼ cup water. Stir and bring to boil covered for 5 minutes to thicken the sauce. Adjust taste with salt and black pepper.
Spoon the beef mixture into the baking dish and spread evenly. Sprinkle with cheese and bake in the oven for 15 minutes until cheese has melted and it's golden brown. Remove and cool for 4 minutes and serve with low carb crusted bread.

Beef Stuffed Roasted Squash

Ready in about: 1 hour 15 minutes | Serves: 4
Per serving: Kcal 406, Fat 14.7g, Net Carbs 12.4g, Protein 34g

Ingredients

2 lb butternut squash, pricked with a fork
Salt and black pepper, to taste
3 garlic cloves, minced
1 onion, chopped
1 button mushroom, sliced
28 ounces canned diced tomatoes
1 tsp dried oregano
¼ tsp cayenne pepper
½ tsp dried thyme
1 pound ground beef
1 green bell pepper, chopped

Directions

Lay the butternut squash on a lined baking sheet, set in the oven at 400ºF, and bake for 40 minutes. After, cut in half, set aside to let cool, deseed, scoop out most of the flesh and let sit. Heat a greased pan over medium heat, add in the garlic, mushrooms, onion, and beef, and cook until the meat browns.
Stir in the green pepper, salt, thyme, tomatoes, oregano, black pepper, and cayenne, and cook for 10 minutes; stir in the flesh. Stuff the squash halves with the beef mixture, and bake in the oven for 10 minutes. Split into plates and enjoy.

Broccoli & Ground Beef Casserole

Ready in about: 4 hours 15 minutes | Serves: 6
Per serving: Kcal 434, Fat 21g, Net Carbs 5.6g, Protein 51g

Ingredients

1 tbsp olive oil
2 pounds ground beef
1 head broccoli, cut into florets
Salt and black pepper, to taste
2 tsp mustard
2 tsp Worcestershire sauce
28 ounces canned diced tomatoes
2 cups mozzarella cheese, grated
16 ounces tomato sauce
2 tbsp fresh parsley, chopped
1 tsp dried oregano

Directions

Apply black pepper and salt to the broccoli florets, set them into a bowl, drizzle over the olive oil, and toss well to coat completely. In a separate bowl, combine the beef with Worcestershire sauce, salt, mustard, and black pepper, and stir well. Press on the slow cooker's bottom.
Scatter in the broccoli, add the tomatoes, parsley, mozzarella, oregano, and tomato sauce. Cook for 4 hours on low; covered. Split the casserole among bowls and enjoy while hot.

Beef Meatballs

Ready in about: 45 minutes | Serves: 5
Per serving: Kcal 332, Fat 18g, Net Carbs 7g, Protein 25g

Ingredients

½ cup pork rinds, crushed
1 egg
Salt and black pepper, to taste
1½ pounds ground beef
10 ounces canned onion soup
1 tbsp almond flour
¼ cup free-sugar ketchup
3 tsp Worcestershire sauce
½ tsp dry mustard
¼ cup water

Directions

In a bowl, combine ⅓ cup of the onion soup with the beef, pepper, pork rinds, egg, and salt. Heat a pan over medium heat, shape the mixture into 12 meatballs. Brown in the pan for 12 minutes on both sides.
In a separate bowl, combine the rest of the soup with the almond flour, dry mustard, ketchup, Worcestershire sauce, and water. Pour this over the beef meatballs, cover the pan, and cook for 20 minutes as you stir occasionally. Split among serving bowls and serve.

Beef Meatballs with Onion Sauce

Ready in about: 35 minutes | Serves: 5
Per serving: Kcal 435, Fat 23g, Net Carbs 6g, Protein 32g

Ingredients

2 pounds ground beef
Salt and black pepper, to taste
½ tsp garlic powder
1 ¼ tbsp coconut aminos

1 cup beef stock
¾ cup almond flour
1 tbsp fresh parsley, chopped
1 tbsp dried onion flakes
1 onion, sliced
2 tbsp butter
¼ cup sour cream

Directions

In a bowl, combine the beef with salt, garlic powder, almond flour, onion flakes, parsley, 1 tablespoon coconut aminos, black pepper, ¼ cup of beef stock. Form 6 patties, place them on a baking sheet, put in the oven at 370ºF, and bake for 18 minutes.

Set a pan with the butter over medium heat, stir in the onion, and cook for 3 minutes. Stir in the remaining beef stock, sour cream, and remaining coconut aminos, and bring to a simmer. Remove from heat, adjust the seasonings. Serve the meatballs topped with onion sauce.

Roasted Spicy Beef

Ready in about: 70 minutes | Serves: 4
Per serving: Kcal 480, Fat 23.5g, Net Carbs 3.5g, Protein 55g

Ingredients

2 lb beef brisket
½ tsp celery salt
1 tsp chili powder
1 tbsp avocado oil
1 tbsp sweet paprika
A pinch of cayenne pepper
½ tsp garlic powder
½ cup beef stock
1 tbsp garlic, minced
¼ tsp dry mustard

Directions

Preheat oven to 340ºF. In a bowl, combine the paprika with dry mustard, chili powder, salt, garlic powder, cayenne pepper, and celery salt. Rub the meat with this mixture.

Set a pan over medium heat and warm avocado oil, place in the beef, and sear until brown. Remove to a baking dish. Pour in the stock, add garlic and bake for 60 minutes.

Set the beef to a cutting board, leave to cool before slicing and splitting in serving plates. Take the juices from the baking dish and strain, sprinkle over the meat, and enjoy.

Beef and Feta Salad

Ready in about: 35 minutes | Serves: 4
Per serving: Kcal 434, Fat 43g, Net Carbs 3.5g, Protein 17g

Ingredients

3 tbsp olive oil
½ pound beef rump steak, cut into strips
Salt and black pepper, to taste
1 tsp cumin
A pinch of dried thyme
2 garlic cloves, minced

4 ounces feta cheese, crumbled
½ cup pecans, toasted
2 cups spinach
1½ tbsp lemon juice
¼ cup fresh mint, chopped

Directions

Season the beef with salt, 1 tbsp of olive oil, garlic, thyme, pepper, and cumin. Place on a preheated to medium heat grill, and cook for 10 minutes, flip once. Remove the grilled beef to a cutting board, leave to cool, and slice into strips.

Sprinkle the pecans on a lined baking sheet, place in the oven at 350ºF, and toast for 10 minutes. In a salad bowl, combine the spinach with black pepper, mint, remaining olive oil, salt, lemon juice, feta cheese, and pecans, and toss well to coat. Top with the beef slices and enjoy.

Mexican Beef Chili

Ready in about: 45 minutes | Serves: 4
Per serving: Kcal 437, Fat 26g, Net Carbs 5g, Protein 17g

Ingredients

1 onion, chopped
2 tbsp olive oil
2 pounds ground beef
15 oz canned tomatoes with green chilies, chopped
3 ounces tomato paste
½ cup pickled jalapeños, chopped
1 tsp chipotle chili paste
4 tbsp garlic, minced
3 celery stalks, chopped
2 tbsp coconut aminos
Salt and black pepper, to taste
A pinch of cayenne pepper
2 tbsp cumin
1 tsp onion powder
1 tsp garlic powder
1 bay leaf
1 tsp chopped cilantro

Directions

Heat oil in a pan over medium heat, add in the onion, celery, garlic, beef, black pepper, and salt; cook until the meat browns. Stir in jalapeños, tomato paste, canned tomatoes with green chilies, salt, garlic powder, bay leaf, onion powder, cayenne, coconut aminos, chipotle chili paste, and cumin, and cook for 30 minutes while covered. Remove and discard bay leaf. Serve in bowls sprinkled with cilantro.

Russian Beef Gratin

Ready in about: 45 minutes | Serves: 5
Per serving: Kcal 584, Fat 48g, Net Carbs 5g, Protein 41g

Ingredients

2 tsp onion flakes
2 pounds ground beef
2 garlic cloves, minced
Salt and black pepper, to taste
1 cup mozzarella cheese, shredded

2 cups fontina cheese, shredded
1 cup Russian dressing
2 tbsp sesame seeds, toasted
20 dill pickle slices
1 iceberg lettuce head, torn

Set a pan over medium heat, place in beef, garlic, salt, onion flakes, and pepper, and cook for 5 minutes. Remove to a baking dish, stir in Russian dressing, mozzarella, and spread 1 cup of the fontina cheese.

Lay the pickle slices on top, spread over the remaining fontina cheese and sesame seeds, place in the oven at 350ºF, and bake for 20 minutes. Arrange the lettuce on a serving platter and top with the gratin.

Beef Bourguignon

Ready in about: 60 minutes + marinated time | Serves: 4
Per serving: Kcal 435, Fat 26g, Net Carbs 7g, Protein 45g

Ingredients

3 tbsp coconut oil
1 tbsp dried parsley flakes
1 cup red wine
1 tsp dried thyme
Salt and black pepper, to taste
1 bay leaf
⅓ cup coconut flour
2 lb beef, cubed
12 small white onions
4 pancetta slices, chopped
2 garlic cloves, minced
½ lb mushrooms, chopped

Directions

In a bowl, combine the wine with bay leaf, olive oil, thyme, pepper, parsley, salt, and the beef cubes; set aside for 3 hours. Drain the meat, and reserve the marinade. Toss the flour over the meat to coat.

Heat a pan over medium heat, stir in the pancetta, and cook until slightly browned. Place in the onions and garlic, and cook for 3 minutes. Stir-fry in the meat and mushrooms for 4-5 minutes.

Pour in the marinade and 1 cup of water; cover and cook for 50 minutes. Season to taste and serve.

Italian Sausage Stew

Ready in about: 35 minutes | Serves: 6
Per serving: Kcal 314, Fat 25g, Net Carbs 7g, Protein 16g

Ingredients

1 pound Italian sausage, sliced
1 red bell pepper, seeded and chopped
2 onions, chopped
Salt and black pepper, to taste
1 cup fresh parsley, chopped
6 green onions, chopped
¼ cup avocado oil
1 cup beef stock
4 garlic cloves

24 ounces canned diced tomatoes
16 ounces okra, trimmed and sliced
6 ounces tomato sauce
2 tbsp coconut aminos
1 tbsp hot sauce

Directions

Set a pot over medium heat and warm oil, place in the sausages, and cook for 2 minutes. Stir in the onions, green onions, garlic, black pepper, bell pepper, and salt, and cook for 5 minutes.

Add in the hot sauce, stock, tomatoes, coconut aminos, okra, and tomato sauce, bring to a simmer and cook for 15 minutes. Adjust the seasoning with salt and black pepper. Share into serving bowls and sprinkle with fresh parsley to serve.

Caribbean Beef

Ready in about: 1 hour 10 minutes | Serves: 8
Per serving: Kcal 305, Fat 14g, Net Carbs 8g, Protein 25g

Ingredients

2 onions, chopped
2 tbsp avocado oil
2 pounds beef stew meat, cubed
2 red bell peppers, seeded and chopped
1 habanero pepper, chopped
4 green chilies, chopped
14.5 ounces canned diced tomatoes
2 tbsp fresh cilantro, chopped
4 garlic cloves, minced
½ cup vegetable broth
Salt and black pepper, to taste
1 ½ tsp cumin
½ cup black olives, chopped
1 tsp dried oregano

Directions

Set a pan over medium heat and warm avocado oil. Brown the beef on all sides; remove and set aside. Stir-fry in the red bell peppers, green chilies, oregano, garlic, habanero pepper, onions, and cumin, for about 5-6 minutes. Pour in the tomatoes and broth, and cook for 1 hour. Stir in the olives, adjust the seasonings and serve in bowls sprinkled with fresh cilantro.

Beef Stew with Bacon

Ready in about: 1 hour 15 minutes | Serves: 6
Per serving: Kcal 592, Fat 36g, Net Carbs 5.7g, Protein 63g

Ingredients

8 ounces bacon, chopped
4 lb beef meat for stew, cubed
4 garlic cloves, minced
2 brown onions, chopped
2 tbsp olive oil
4 tbsp red vinegar
4 cups beef stock
2 tbsp tomato puree
2 cinnamon sticks
3 lemon peel strips

½ cup fresh parsley, chopped
4 thyme sprigs
2 tbsp butter
Salt and black pepper, to taste

Directions

Set a saucepan over medium heat and warm oil, add in the garlic, bacon, and onion, and cook for 5 minutes. Stir in the beef, and cook until slightly brown. Pour in the vinegar, black pepper, butter, lemon peel strips, stock, salt, tomato puree, cinnamon sticks and thyme; stir for 3 minutes.

Cook for 1 hour while covered. Get rid of the thyme, lemon peel, and cinnamon sticks. Split into serving bowls and sprinkle with parsley to serve.

Thai Beef with Shiitake Mushrooms

Ready in about: 30 minutes | Serves: 6
Per serving: Kcal 224, Fat 15g, Net Carbs 3g, Protein 19g

Ingredients

1 cup beef stock
4 tbsp butter
¼ tsp garlic powder
¼ tsp onion powder
1 tbsp coconut aminos
1½ tsp lemon pepper
1 pound beef steak, cut into strips
Salt and black pepper, to taste
1 cup shiitake mushrooms, sliced
3 green onions, chopped
1 tbsp thai red curry paste

Directions

Melt butter in a pan over medium heat, add in the beef, season with garlic powder, black pepper, salt, and onion powder and cook for 4 minutes. Mix in the mushrooms and stir-fry for 5 minutes.

Pour in the stock, coconut aminos, lemon pepper, and thai curry paste and cook for 15 minutes. Serve sprinkled with the green onions.

Beef and Butternut Squash Stew

Ready in about: 40 minutes | Serves: 4
Per serving: Kcal 343, Fat 17g, Net Carbs 7.3g, Protein 32g

Ingredients

3 tsp olive oil
1 pound ground beef
1 cup beef stock
14 ounces canned tomatoes with juice
1 tbsp stevia
1 pound butternut squash, chopped
1 tbsp Worcestershire sauce
2 bay leaves
Salt and black pepper, to taste
1 onion, chopped
1 tsp dried sage
1 tbsp garlic, minced

Directions

Set a pan over medium heat and heat olive oil, stir in the onion, garlic, and beef, and cook for 10 minutes.

Add in butternut squash, Worcestershire sauce, bay leaves, stevia, beef stock, canned tomatoes, and sage, and bring to a boil. Reduce heat, and simmer for 30 minutes.

Remove and discard the bay leaves and adjust the seasonings. Split into bowls and enjoy.

Herby Beef & Veggie Stew

Ready in about: 30 minutes | Serves: 4
Per serving: Kcal 253, Fat 13g, Net Carbs 5.2g, Protein 30g

Ingredients

1 pound ground beef
2 tbsp olive oil
1 onion, chopped
2 garlic cloves, minced
14 ounces canned diced tomatoes
1 tbsp dried rosemary
1 tbsp dried sage
1 tbsp dried oregano
1 tbsp dried basil
1 tbsp dried marjoram
Salt and black pepper, to taste
2 carrots, sliced
2 celery stalks, chopped
1 cup vegetable broth

Directions

Set a pan over medium heat, add in the olive oil, onion, celery, and garlic, and sauté for 5 minutes. Place in the beef, and cook for 6 minutes. Stir in the tomatoes, carrots, broth, black pepper, oregano, marjoram, basil, rosemary, salt, and sage, and simmer for 15 minutes. Serve and enjoy!

Beef Provençal

Ready in about: 50 minutes | Serves: 4
Per serving: Kcal 230, Fat 11.3g, Net Carbs 5.2g, Protein 19g

Ingredients

12 ounces beef steak racks
2 fennel bulbs, sliced
Salt and black pepper, to taste
3 tbsp olive oil
½ cup apple cider vinegar
1 tsp herbs de Provence
1 tbsp swerve

Directions

In a bowl, mix the fennel with 2 tbsp of oil, swerve, and vinegar, toss to coat well, and set to a baking dish. Season with herbs de Provence, pepper and salt, and cook in the oven at 400ºF for 15 minutes.

Sprinkle black pepper and salt to the beef, place into an oiled pan over medium heat, and cook for a couple of minutes. Place the beef to the baking dish with the fennel, and bake for 20 minutes. Split everything among plates and enjoy.

Parsley Beef Burgers

Ready in about: 25 minutes | Serves: 6
Per serving: Kcal 354, Fat: 28g, Net Carbs: 2.5g,
Protein: 27g

Ingredients
2 lb ground beef
1 tbsp onion flakes
¾ cup almond flour
¼ cup beef broth
1 tbsp chopped parsley
1 tbsp Worcestershire sauce

Directions
Combine all ingredients in a bowl. Mix well with your
hands and make 6 patties out of the mixture. Arrange
on a lined baking sheet. Bake at 370ºF, for about 18
minutes, until nice and crispy.

Pecorino Veal Cutlets

Ready in about: 1 hour 15 minutes | Serves: 6
Per serving: Kcal 362, Fat 21g, Net Carbs 6g, Protein
26g

Ingredients
6 veal cutlets
½ cup Pecorino cheese, grated
6 provolone cheese slices
Salt and black pepper, to taste
4 cups tomato sauce
A pinch of garlic salt
2 tbsp butter
2 tbsp coconut oil, melted
1 tsp Italian seasoning

Directions
Season the veal cutlets with garlic salt, black pepper,
and salt. Set a pan over medium heat and warm oil
and butter, place in the veal, and cook until browned
on all sides. Spread half of the tomato sauce on the
bottom of a baking dish that is coated with some
cooking spray.
Place in the veal cutlets then spread with Italian
seasoning and sprinkle over the remaining sauce. Set
in the oven at 360º F, and bake for 40 minutes.
Scatter with the provolone cheese, then sprinkle with
Pecorino cheese, and bake for another 5 minutes
until the cheese is golden and melted. Serve.

Chuck Roast Beef

Ready in about: 3 hours 15 minutes | Serves: 6
Per serving: Kcal 325, Fat 18g, Net Carbs 7g, Protein
28g

Ingredients
2 pounds beef chuck roast, cubed
2 tbsp olive oil
14.5 ounces canned diced tomatoes
2 carrots, chopped
Salt and black pepper, to taste
½ pound mushrooms, sliced
2 celery stalks, chopped
2 yellow onions, chopped
1 cup beef stock

1 tbsp fresh thyme, chopped
½ tsp dry mustard
3 tbsp almond flour

Directions
Set an ovenproof pot over medium heat, warm olive
oil and brown the beef on each side for a few minutes.
Stir in the tomatoes, onions, salt, pepper, mustard,
carrots, mushrooms, celery, and stock.
In a bowl, combine 1 cup water with flour. Place this
to the pot, stir then set in the oven, and bake for 3
hours at 325ºF stirring at intervals of 30 minutes.
Scatter the fresh thyme over and serve warm.

Rack of Lamb in Red Bell Pepper Butter Sauce

Ready in about: 65 minutes + cooling time | Serves: 4
Per serving: Kcal 415, Fat 25g, Carbs 2g, Protein 46g

Ingredients
1 lb rack of lamb
Salt to cure
3 cloves garlic, minced
⅓ cup olive oil
⅓ cup white wine
6 sprigs fresh rosemary
Sauce
2 tbsp olive oil
1 large red bell pepper, seeded, diced
2 cloves garlic, minced
1 cup chicken broth
2 oz butter
Salt and white pepper to taste

Directions
Fill a large bowl with water and soak in the lamb for
30 minutes. Drain the meat after and season with salt.
Let the lamb sit on a rack to drain completely and
then rinse it afterward. Put in a bowl.
Mix the olive oil with wine and garlic, and brush the
mixture all over the lamb. Drop the rosemary sprigs
on it, cover the bowl with plastic wrap, and place in
the refrigerator to marinate the meat.
The next day, preheat the grill to 450ºF and cook the
lamb for 6 minutes on both sides. Remove after and
let rest for 4 minutes.
Heat the olive oil in a frying pan and sauté the garlic
and bell pepper for 5 minutes. Pour in the chicken
broth and continue cooking the ingredients until the
liquid reduces by half, about 10 minutes. Add the
butter, salt, and white pepper. Stir to melt the butter
and turn the heat off.
Use the stick blender to puree the ingredients until
very smooth and strain the sauce through a fine
mesh into a bowl. Slice the lamb, serve with the sauce,
and your favorite red wine.

Veal Stew

Ready in about: 2 hours | Serves: 6
Per serving: Kcal 415, Fat 21g, Net Carbs 5.2g,
Protein 44g

Ingredients

2 tbsp olive oil
3 pounds veal shoulder, cubed
1 onion, chopped
1 garlic clove, minced
Salt and black pepper, to taste
1 cup water
1 ½ cups red wine
12 ounces canned tomato sauce
1 carrot, chopped
1 cup mushrooms, chopped
½ cup green beans
2 tsp dried oregano

Directions

Set a pot over medium heat and warm the oil. Brown the veal for 5-6 minutes. Stir in the onion, and garlic, and cook for 3 minutes. Place in the wine, oregano, carrot, black pepper, salt, tomato sauce, water, and mushrooms, bring to a boil, reduce the heat to low. Cook for 1 hour and 45 minutes, then add in the green beans and cook for 5 minutes. Adjust the seasoning and split among serving bowls to serve.

Venison Tenderloin with Cheese Stuffing

Ready in about: 30 minutes | Serves: 8
Per serving: Kcal 194, Fat: 12g, Net Carbs: 1.7g,
Protein: 25g

Ingredients

2 pounds venison tenderloin
2 garlic cloves, minced
2 tbsp chopped almonds
½ cup gorgonzola cheese
½ cup feta cheese
1 tsp chopped onion
½ tsp salt

Directions

Preheat your grill to medium. Slice the tenderloin lengthwise to make a pocket for the filling. Combine the rest of the ingredients in a bowl. Stuff the tenderloin with the filling. Shut the meat with skewers and grill for as long as it takes to reach your desired density.

Winter Veal and Sauerkraut

Ready in about: 60 minutes | Serves: 4
Per serving: Kcal 430, Fat 27g, Net Carbs 6g, Protein
29g

Ingredients

1 pound veal, cut into cubes
18 ounces sauerkraut, rinsed and drained
Salt and black pepper, to taste
½ cup ham, chopped
1 onion, chopped
2 garlic cloves, minced
1 tbsp butter
½ cup Parmesan cheese, grated
½ cup sour cream

Directions

Heat a pot with the butter over medium heat, add in the onion, and cook for 3 minutes. Stir in garlic, and cook for 1 minute. Place in the veal and ham, and cook until slightly browned. Place in the sauerkraut, and cook until the meat becomes tender, about 30 minutes. Stir in sour cream, pepper, and salt. Top with Parmesan cheese and bake for 20 minutes at 350ºF.

Lamb Shashlyk

Ready in about: 20 minutes | Serves: 4
Per serving: Kcal 467, Fat: 37g, Net Carbs: 3.2g,
Protein: 27g

Ingredients

1 pound ground lamb
¼ tsp cinnamon
1 egg
1 grated onion
Salt and ground black pepper, to taste

Directions

Place all ingredients in a bowl. Mix with your hands to combine well. Divide the meat into 4 pieces. Shape all meat portions around previously-soaked skewers. Preheat grill to medium and grill the kebabs for about 5 minutes per side.

North African Lamb

Ready in about: 25 minutes | Serves: 4
Per serving: Kcal 445, Fat 32g, Net Carbs 4g, Protein
34g

Ingredients

2 tsp paprika
2 garlic cloves, minced
2 tsp dried oregano
2 tbsp sumac
12 lamb cutlets
¼ cup sesame oil
2 tsp cumin
4 carrots, sliced
¼ cup fresh parsley, chopped
2 tsp harissa paste
1 tbsp red wine vinegar
Salt and black pepper, to taste
2 tbsp black olives, sliced
2 cucumbers, sliced

Directions

In a bowl, combine the cutlets with the paprika, oregano, black pepper, 2 tbsp water, half of the oil, sumac, garlic, and salt, and rub well. Add the carrots in a pot, cover with water, bring to a boil over medium heat, cook for 2 minutes then drain before placing them in a salad bowl.

Place the cucumbers and olives to the carrots. In another bowl, combine the harissa with the rest of the oil, a splash of water, parsley, vinegar, and cumin. Place this to the carrots mixture, season with pepper and salt, and toss well to coat.

Preheat the grill to medium heat and arrange the lamb cutlets on it, grill each side for 3 minutes, and split among separate plates. Serve alongside the carrot salad.

Lamb Stew with Veggies

Ready in about: 1 hour 50 minutes | Serves: 2
Per serving: Kcal 584, Fat 42g, Net Carbs 8.1g, Protein 38g

Ingredients

1 garlic clove, minced
1 parsnip, chopped
1 onion, chopped
1 tbsp olive oil
1 celery stalk, chopped
10 ounces lamb fillet, cut into pieces
Salt and black pepper, to taste
1 ¼ cups vegetable stock
1 carrot, chopped
½ tbsp fresh rosemary, chopped
1 leek, chopped
1 tbsp mint sauce
1 tsp stevia
1 tbsp tomato puree
½ head cauliflower, cut into florets
½ head celeriac, chopped
2 tbsp butter

Directions

Set a pot over medium heat and warm the oil, stir in the celery, onion, and garlic, and cook for 5 minutes. Stir in the lamb pieces, and cook for 3 minutes.

Add in the stevia, carrot, parsnip, rosemary, mint sauce, stock, leek, tomato puree, boil the mixture, and cook for 1 hour and 30 minutes.

Meanwhile, heat a pot with water over medium heat, place in the celeriac, cover, and simmer for 10 minutes. Place in the cauliflower florets, cook for 15 minutes, drain everything, and combine with butter, black pepper, and salt.

Mash using a potato masher, and split the mash between 2 plates. Top with vegetable mixture and lamb and enjoy.

Rolled Lamb Shoulder with Basil & Pine Nuts

Ready in about: 1 hour | Serves: 4
Per serving: Kcal 547, Fat 37.7g, Net Carbs 2.2g, Protein 42.7g

Ingredients

1 lb rolled lamb shoulder, boneless
1 ½ cups basil leaves, chopped
5 tbsp pine nuts, chopped
½ cup green olives, pitted and chopped
3 cloves garlic, minced
Salt and black pepper to taste

Directions

Preheat the oven to 450ºF.

In a bowl, combine the basil, pine nuts, olives, and garlic. Season with salt and pepper. Untie the lamb flat onto a chopping board, spread the basil mixture all over, and rub the spices onto the meat.

Roll the lamb over the spice mixture and tie it together using 3 to 4 strings of butcher's twine. Place the lamb onto a baking dish and cook in the oven for 10 minutes. Reduce the heat to 350ºF and continue cooking for 40 minutes. When ready, transfer the meat to a cleaned chopping board; let it rest for 10 minutes before slicing. Serve with roasted root vegetables.

Grilled Lamb on Lemony Sauce

Ready in about: 25 minutes | Serves: 4
Per serving: Kcal 392, Fat: 31g, Net Carbs: 1g, Protein: 29g

Ingredients

8 lamb chops
2 tbsp favorite spice mix
2 tbsp olive oil
Sauce:
¼ cup olive oil
1 tsp red pepper flakes
2 tbsp lemon juice
2 tbsp fresh mint
3 garlic cloves, pressed
2 tbsp lemon zest
¼ cup parsley
½ tsp smoked paprika

Directions

Rub lamb with olive oil and sprinkle with the seasoning. Preheat the grill to medium. Grill the lamb chops for about 3 minutes per side. Whisk together the sauce ingredients. Serve the lamb with sauce.

White Wine Lamb Chops

Ready in about: 1 hour 10 minutes | Serves: 6
Per serving: Kcal 397, Fat: 30g, Net Carbs: 4.3g, Protein: 16g

Ingredients

6 lamb chops
1 tbsp sage
1 tsp thyme
1 onion, sliced
3 garlic cloves, minced
2 tbsp olive oil
½ cup white wine
Salt and black pepper, to taste

Directions

Heat the olive oil in a pan. Add onion and garlic and cook for 3 minutes, until soft. Rub the sage and thyme over the lamb chops. Cook the lamb for about 3 minutes per side. Set aside.

Pour the white wine and 1 cup of water into the pan, bring the mixture to a boil. Cook until the liquid is reduced by half. Add the chops in the pan, reduce the heat, and let simmer for 1 hour.

SEAFOOD & FISH RECIPES

Trout and Fennel Parcels

Ready in about: 20 minutes | Serves: 4
Per serving: Kcal 234, Fat 9.3g, Net Carbs 2.8g,
Protein 17g

Ingredients

½ lb deboned trout, butterflied
Salt and black pepper to season
3 tbsp olive oil + extra for tossing
4 sprigs rosemary
4 sprigs thyme
4 butter cubes
1 cup thinly sliced fennel
1 medium red onion, sliced
8 lemon slices
3 tsp capers to garnish

Directions

Preheat the oven to 400ºF. Cut out parchment paper wide enough for each trout. In a bowl, toss the fennel and onion with a little bit of olive oil and share into the middle parts of the papers.

Place the fish on each veggie mound, top with a drizzle of olive oil each, a pinch of salt and black pepper, a sprig of rosemary and thyme, and 1 cube of butter. Also, lay the lemon slices on the fish. Wrap and close the fish packets securely, and place them on a baking sheet. Bake in the oven for 15 minutes, and remove once ready. Plate them and garnish the fish with capers and serve with a squash mash.

Shrimp Stuffed Zucchini

Ready in about: 56 minutes | Serves: 4
Per serving: Kcal 135, Fat 14.4g, Net Carbs 3.2g,
Protein 24.6g

Ingredients

4 medium zucchinis
1 lb small shrimp, peeled, deveined
1 tbsp minced onion
2 tsp butter
¼ cup chopped tomatoes
Salt and black pepper to taste
1 cup pork rinds, crushed
1 tbsp chopped basil leaves
2 tbsp melted butter

Directions

Preheat the oven to 350ºF and trim off the top and bottom ends of the zucchinis. Lay them flat on a chopping board, and cut a ¼ -inch off the top to create a boat for the stuffing. Scoop out the seeds with a spoon and set the zucchinis aside.

Melt the firm butter in a small skillet and sauté the onion and tomato for 6 minutes. Transfer the mixture to a bowl and add the shrimp, half of the pork rinds, basil leaves, salt, and black pepper.

Combine the ingredients and stuff the zucchini boats with the mixture. Sprinkle the top of the boats with the remaining pork rinds and drizzle the melted butter over them.

Place on a baking sheet and bake for 15 to 20 minutes. The shrimp should no longer be pink by this time. Remove the zucchinis after and serve with a tomato and mozzarella salad.

Spicy Sea Bass with Hazelnuts

Ready in about: 20 minutes | Serves: 2
Per serving: Kcal 467, Fat: 31g, Net Carbs: 2.8g,
Protein: 40g

Ingredients

2 sea bass fillets
2 tbsp butter
⅓ cup roasted hazelnuts
A pinch of cayenne pepper

Directions

Preheat your oven to 425ºF. Line a baking dish with waxed paper. Melt the butter and brush it over the fish. Process the cayenne pepper and hazelnuts in a food processor to achieve a smooth consistency. Coat the sea bass with the hazelnut mixture. Place in the oven and bake for about 15 minutes.

Creamy Hoki with Almond Bread Crust

Ready in about: 50 minutes | Serves: 4
Per serving: Kcal 386, Fat 27g, Net Carbs 3.5g,
Protein 28.5g

Ingredients

1 cup flaked smoked hoki, bones removed
1 cup cubed hoki fillets, cubed
4 eggs
1 cup water
3 tbsp almond flour
1 onion, sliced
2 cups sour cream
1 tbsp chopped parsley
1 cup pork rinds, crushed
1 cup grated cheddar cheese
Salt and black pepper to taste
2 tbsp butter

Directions

Preheat the oven to 360ºF and lightly grease a baking dish with cooking spray.

Then, boil the eggs in water in a pot over medium heat to be well done for 10 minutes, run the eggs under cold water and peel the shells. After, place on a cutting board and chop them.

Melt the butter in a saucepan over medium heat and sauté the onion for 4 minutes. Turn the heat off and stir in the almond flour to form a roux. Turn the heat back on and cook the roux to be golden brown and stir in the cream until the mixture is smooth. Season with salt and black pepper, and stir in the parsley.

Spread the smoked and cubed fish in the baking dish, sprinkle the eggs on top, and spoon the sauce over. In a bowl, mix the pork rinds with the cheddar cheese, and sprinkle it over the sauce.

Bake the casserole in the oven for 20 minutes until the top is golden and the sauce and cheese are bubbly. Remove the bake after and serve with a steamed green vegetable mix.

Tuna Steaks with Shirataki Noodles

Ready in about: 30 minutes | Serves: 4
Per serving: Kcal 310, Fat 18.2g, Net Carbs 2g, Protein 22g

Ingredients

1 pack (7 oz) miracle noodle angel hair
3 cups water
1 red bell pepper, seeded and halved
4 tuna steaks
Salt and black pepper to taste
Olive oil for brushing
2 tbsp pickled ginger
2 tbsp chopped cilantro

Directions

Cook the shirataki rice as per package instructions: In a colander, rinse the shirataki noodles with running cold water. Bring a pot of salted water to a boil; blanch the noodles for 2 minutes. Drain and transfer to a dry skillet over medium heat. Dry roast for a minute until opaque.

Grease a grill's grate with cooking spray and preheat on medium heat. Season the red bell pepper and tuna with salt and black pepper, brush with olive oil, and grill covered. Cook both for 3 minutes on each side. Transfer to a plate to cool. Dice bell pepper with a knife.

Assemble the noodles, tuna, and bell pepper in serving plate. Top with pickled ginger and garnish with cilantro. Serve with roasted sesame sauce.

Salmon Panzanella

Ready in about: 22 minutes | Serves: 4
Per serving: Kcal 338, Fat 21.7g, Net Carbs 3.1g, Protein 28.5g

Ingredients

1 lb skinned salmon, cut into 4 steaks each
1 cucumber, peeled, seeded, cubed
Salt and black pepper to taste
8 black olives, pitted and chopped
1 tbsp capers, rinsed
2 large tomatoes, diced
3 tbsp red wine vinegar
¼ cup thinly sliced red onion
3 tbsp olive oil
2 slices zero carb bread, cubed
¼ cup thinly sliced basil leaves

Directions

Preheat a grill to 350ºF and prepare the salad. In a bowl, mix the cucumbers, olives, pepper, capers, tomatoes, wine vinegar, onion, olive oil, bread, and basil leaves. Let sit for the flavors to incorporate.

Season the salmon steaks with salt and pepper; grill them on both sides for 8 minutes in total. Serve the salmon steaks warm on a bed of the veggies' salad.

Blackened Fish Tacos with Slaw

Ready in about: 20 minutes | Serves: 4
Per serving: Kcal 268, Fat: 20g, Net Carbs: 3.5g, Protein: 13.8g

Ingredients

1 tbsp olive oil
1 tsp chili powder
2 tilapia fillets
1 tsp paprika
4 low carb tortillas

Slaw:
½ cup red cabbage, shredded
1 tbsp lemon juice
1 tsp apple cider vinegar
1 tbsp olive oil
Salt and black pepper to taste

Directions

Season the tilapia with chili powder and paprika. Heat the olive oil in a skillet over medium heat.

Add tilapia and cook until blackened, about 3 minutes per side. Cut into strips. Divide the tilapia between the tortillas. Combine all slaw ingredients in a bowl and top the fish to serve.

Red Cabbage Tilapia Taco Bowl

Ready in about: 20 minutes | Serves: 4
Per serving: Kcal 269, Fat 23.4g, Net Carbs 4g, Protein 16.5g

Ingredients

2 cups cauli rice
2 tsp ghee
4 tilapia fillets, cut into cubes
¼ tsp taco seasoning
Salt and chili pepper to taste
¼ head red cabbage, shredded
1 ripe avocado, pitted and chopped

Directions

Sprinkle cauli rice in a bowl with a little water and microwave for 3 minutes. Fluff after with a fork and set aside. Melt ghee in a skillet over medium heat, rub the tilapia with the taco seasoning, salt, and chili pepper, and fry until brown on all sides, for about 8 minutes in total.

Transfer to a plate and set aside. In 4 serving bowls, share the cauli rice, cabbage, fish, and avocado. Serve with chipotle lime sour cream dressing.

Sicilian-Style Zoodle Spaghetti

Ready in about: 10 minutes | Serves: 2
Per serving: Kcal 355, Fat: 31g, Net Carbs: 6g, Protein: 20g

Ingredients

4 cups zoodles (spiralled zucchini)
2 ounces cubed bacon
4 ounces canned sardines, chopped
½ cup canned chopped tomatoes
1 tbsp capers
1 tbsp parsley
1 tsp minced garlic

Directions

Pour some of the sardine oil in a pan. Add garlic and cook for 1 minute. Add the bacon and cook for 2 more minutes. Stir in the tomatoes and let simmer for 5 minutes. Add zoodles and sardines and cook for 3 minutes.

Sour Cream Salmon with Parmesan

Ready in about: 25 minutes | Serves: 4
Per serving: Kcal 288, Fat 23.4g, Net Carbs 1.2g, Protein 16.2g

Ingredients

1 cup sour cream
½ tbsp minced dill
½ lemon, zested and juiced
Pink salt and black pepper to season
4 salmon steaks
½ cup grated Parmesan cheese

Directions

Preheat oven to 400ºF and line a baking sheet with parchment paper; set aside. In a bowl, mix the sour cream, dill, lemon zest, juice, salt and black pepper, and set aside.

Season the fish with salt and black pepper, drizzle lemon juice on both sides of the fish and arrange them in the baking sheet. Spread the sour cream mixture on each fish and sprinkle with Parmesan.

Bake the fish for 15 minutes and after broil the top for 2 minutes with a close watch for a nice a brown color. Plate the fish and serve with buttery green beans.

Sushi Shrimp Rolls

Ready in about: 10 minutes | Serves: 5
Per serving: Kcal 216, Fat: 10g, Net Carbs: 1g, Protein: 18.7g

Ingredients

2 cups cooked and chopped shrimp
1 tbsp sriracha sauce
¼ cucumber, julienned
5 hand roll nori sheets
¼ cup mayonnaise

Directions

Combine shrimp, mayonnaise, cucumber and sriracha sauce in a bowl. Lay out a single nori sheet on a flat surface and spread about 1/5 of the shrimp mixture. Roll the nori sheet as desired. Repeat with the other ingredients. Serve with sugar-free soy sauce.

Grilled Shrimp with Chimichurri Sauce

Ready in about: 55 minutes | Serves: 4
Per serving: Kcal 283, Fat: 20.3g, Net Carbs: 3.5g, Protein: 16g

Ingredients

1 pound shrimp, peeled and deveined
2 tbsp olive oil
Juice of 1 lime
Chimichurri
½ tsp salt
¼ cup olive oil
2 garlic cloves
¼ cup red onions, chopped
¼ cup red wine vinegar
½ tsp pepper
2 cups parsley
¼ tsp red pepper flakes

Directions

Process the chimichurri ingredients in a blender until smooth; set aside. Combine shrimp, olive oil, and lime juice, in a bowl, and let marinate in the fridge for 30 minutes. Preheat your grill to medium. Add shrimp and cook about 2 minutes per side. Serve shrimp drizzled with the chimichurri sauce.

Coconut Crab Patties

Ready in about: 15 minutes | Serves: 8
Per serving: Kcal 215, Fat: 11.5g, Net Carbs: 3.6g, Protein: 15.3g

Ingredients

2 tbsp coconut oil
1 tbsp lemon juice
1 cup lump crab meat
2 tsp Dijon mustard
1 egg, beaten
1 ½ tbsp coconut flour

Directions

In a bowl to the crabmeat, add all the ingredients, except for the oil; mix well to combine. Make patties out of the mixture. Melt the coconut oil in a skillet over medium heat. Add the crab patties and cook for about 2-3 minutes per side.

Shrimp in Curry Sauce

Ready in about: 15 minutes | Serves: 2
Per serving: Kcal 560, Fat: 41g, Net Carbs: 4.3g, Protein: 24.4g

Ingredients

½ ounce grated Parmesan cheese
1 egg, beaten
¼ tsp curry powder
2 tsp almond flour
12 shrimp, shelled
3 tbsp coconut oil
Sauce
2 tbsp curry leaves
2 tbsp butter
½ onion, diced
½ cup heavy cream
½ ounce cheddar cheese, shredded

Directions

Combine all dry ingredients for the batter. Melt the coconut oil in a skillet over medium heat. Dip the shrimp in the egg first, and then coat with the dry mixture. Fry until golden and crispy.

In another skillet, melt butter. Add onion and cook for 3 minutes. Add curry leaves and cook for 30 seconds. Stir in heavy cream and cheddar and cook until thickened. Add shrimp and coat well. Serve.

Tilapia with Olives & Tomato Sauce

Ready in about: 30 minutes | Serves: 4
Per serving: Kcal 282, Fat: 15g, Net Carbs: 6g, Protein: 23g

Ingredients

4 tilapia fillets
2 garlic cloves, minced
2 tsp oregano
14 ounces diced tomatoes
1 tbsp olive oil
½ red onion, chopped
2 tbsp parsley
¼ cup kalamata olives

Directions

Heat olive oil in a skillet over medium heat and cook the onion for 3 minutes. Add garlic and oregano and cook for 30 seconds. Stir in tomatoes and bring the mixture to a boil. Reduce the heat and simmer for 5 minutes. Add olives and tilapia, and cook for about 8 minutes. Serve the tilapia with tomato sauce.

Lemon Garlic Shrimp

Ready in about: 22 minutes | Serves: 6
Per serving: Kcal 258, Fat 22g, Net Carbs 2g, Protein 13g

Ingredients

½ cup butter, divided
2 lb shrimp, peeled and deveined
Salt and black pepper to taste
¼ tsp sweet paprika
1 tbsp minced garlic
3 tbsp water
1 lemon, zested and juiced
2 tbsp chopped parsley

Directions

Melt half of the butter in a large skillet over medium heat, season the shrimp with salt, black pepper, paprika, and add to the butter. Stir in the garlic and cook the shrimp for 4 minutes on both sides until pink. Remove to a bowl and set aside.
Put the remaining butter in the skillet; include the lemon zest, juice, and water. Add the shrimp, parsley, and adjust the taste with salt and pepper. Cook for 2 minutes. Serve shrimp and sauce with squash pasta.

Seared Scallops with Chorizo and Asiago Cheese

Ready in about: 15 minutes | Serves: 4
Per serving: Kcal 491, Fat 32g, Net Carbs 5g, Protein 36g

Ingredients

2 tbsp ghee
16 fresh scallops
8 ounces chorizo, chopped
1 red bell pepper, seeds removed, sliced
1 cup red onions, finely chopped
1 cup asiago cheese, grated
Salt and black pepper to taste

Directions

Melt half of the ghee in a skillet over medium heat, and cook the onion and bell pepper for 5 minutes until tender. Add the chorizo and stir-fry for another 3 minutes. Remove and set aside.
Pat dry the scallops with paper towels, and season with salt and pepper. Add the remaining ghee to the skillet and sear the scallops for 2 minutes on each side to have a golden brown color. Add the chorizo mixture back and warm through. Transfer to serving platter and top with asiago cheese.

Pistachio-Crusted Salmon

Ready in about: 35 minutes | Serves: 4
Per serving: Kcal 563, Fat: 47g, Net Carbs: 6g, Protein: 34g

Ingredients

4 salmon fillets
½ tsp pepper
1 tsp salt
¼ cup mayonnaise
½ cup chopped pistachios

Sauce

1 chopped shallot
2 tsp lemon zest
1 tbsp olive oil
A pinch of black pepper
1 cup heavy cream

Directions

Preheat the oven to 370ºF.
Brush the salmon with mayonnaise and season with salt and pepper. Coat with pistachios, place in a lined baking dish and bake for 15 minutes.
Heat olive oil in a saucepan and sauté the shallot for 3 minutes. Stir in the rest of the sauce ingredients. Bring the mixture to a boil and cook until thickened. Serve the fish with the sauce.

Coconut Curry Mussels

Ready in about: 25 minutes | Serves: 6
Per serving: Kcal 356, Fat 20.6g, Net Carbs 0.3g, Protein 21.1g

Ingredients

3 lb mussels, cleaned, de-bearded
1 cup minced shallots
3 tbsp minced garlic
1 ½ cups coconut milk
2 cups dry white wine
2 tsp red curry powder
⅓ cup coconut oil
⅓ cup chopped green onions
⅓ cup chopped parsley

Directions

Pour the wine into a large saucepan and cook the shallots and garlic over low heat. Stir in the coconut milk and red curry powder and cook for 3 minutes.
Add the mussels and steam for 7 minutes or until their shells are opened. Then, use a slotted spoon to remove to a bowl leaving the sauce in the pan. Discard any closed mussels at this point.

Stir the coconut oil into the sauce, turn the heat off, and stir in the parsley and green onions. Serve the sauce immediately with a butternut squash mash.

Cod in Garlic Butter Sauce

Ready in about: 20 minutes | Serves: 6
Per serving: Kcal 264, Fat 17.3g, Net Carbs 2.3g, Protein 20g

Ingredients

2 tsp olive oil
6 Alaska cod fillets
Salt and black pepper to taste
4 tbsp salted butter
4 cloves garlic, minced
⅓ cup lemon juice
3 tbsp white wine
2 tbsp chopped chives

Directions

Heat the oil in a skillet over medium heat and season the cod with salt and black pepper. Fry the fillets in the oil for 4 minutes on one side, flip and cook for 1 minute. Take out, plate, and set aside.

In another skillet over low heat, melt the butter and sauté the garlic for 3 minutes. Add the lemon juice, wine, and chives. Season with salt, black pepper, and cook for 3 minutes until the wine slightly reduces. Put the fish in the skillet, spoon sauce over, cook for 30 seconds and turn the heat off.

Divide fish into 6 plates, top with sauce, and serve with buttered green beans.

Dilled Salmon in Creamy Sauce

Ready in about: 15 minutes | Serves: 2
Per serving: Kcal 468, Fat: 40g, Net Carbs: 1.5g, Protein: 22g

Ingredients

2 salmon fillets
¾ tsp dried tarragon
2 tbsp olive oil
¾ tsp dried dill

Sauce

2 tbsp butter
½ tsp dill
½ tsp tarragon
¼ cup heavy cream
Salt and black pepper to taste

Directions

Season the salmon with dill and tarragon. Warm the olive oil in a pan over medium heat. Add salmon and cook for about 4 minutes on both sides. Set aside.

To make the sauce: melt the butter and add the dill and tarragon. Cook for 30 seconds to infuse the flavors. Whisk in the heavy cream, season with salt and black pepper, and cook for 2-3 minutes. Serve the salmon topped with the sauce.

Parmesan Fish Bake

Ready in about: 40 minutes | Serves: 4
Per serving: Kcal 354, Fat 17g, Net Carbs 4g, Protein 28g

Ingredients

2 salmon fillets, cubed
3 white fish, cubed
1 head broccoli, cut into florets
1 tbsp butter, melted
Salt and black pepper to taste
1 cup crème fraiche
¼ cup grated Parmesan cheese
Grated Parmesan cheese for topping

Directions

Preheat oven to 400ºF and grease an 8 x 8 inches casserole dish with cooking spray. Toss the fish cubes and broccoli in butter and season with salt and pepper to taste. Spread in the greased dish.

Mix the crème fraiche with Parmesan cheese, pour and smear the cream on the fish, and sprinkle with some more Parmesan cheese. Bake for 25 to 30 minutes until golden brown on top, take the dish out, sit for 5 minutes and spoon into plates. Serve with lemon-mustard asparagus.

MEATLESS MEALS

Vegetable Greek Mousaka

Ready in about: 50 minutes | Serves: 6
Per serving: Kcal 476, Fat 35g, Net Carbs 9.6g, Protein 33g

2 large eggplants, cut into strips
1 cup diced celery
1 cup diced carrots
1 small white onion, chopped
2 eggs
1 tsp olive oil
3 cups grated Parmesan
1 cup ricotta cheese
3 cloves garlic, minced
2 tsp Italian seasoning blend
Salt to taste

Sauce:

1 ½ cups heavy cream
¼ cup butter, melted
1 cup grated mozzarella cheese
2 tsp Italian seasoning
¾ cup almond flour

Directions

Preheat the oven to 350ºF. Lay the eggplant strips on a paper towel, sprinkle with salt and let sit there to exude liquid. Heat olive oil in a skillet over medium heat and sauté the onion, celery, and carrots for 5 minutes. Stir in the garlic and cook further for 30 seconds; set aside to cool.

Mix the eggs, 1 cup of Parmesan cheese, ricotta cheese, and salt in a bowl; set aside. Pour the heavy cream in a pot and bring to heat over a medium fire while continually stirring. Stir in the remaining Parmesan cheese, and 1 teaspoon of Italian seasoning. Turn the heat off and set aside.

To lay the mousaka, spread a small amount of the sauce at the bottom of the baking dish. Pat dry the eggplant strips and make a single layer on the sauce. Spread a layer of ricotta cheese on the eggplants, sprinkle some veggies on it, and repeat the layering process until all the ingredients are exhausted.

In a small bowl, evenly mix the melted butter, almond flour, and 1 teaspoon of Italian seasoning. Spread the top of the mousaka layers with it and sprinkle the top with mozzarella cheese. Cover the dish with foil and place it in the oven to bake for 25 minutes. Remove the foil and bake for 5 minutes until the cheese is slightly burned. Slice the mousaka and serve warm.

Vegetable Tempeh Kabobs

Ready in about: 2 hours 26 minutes | Serves: 4
Per serving: Kcal 228, Fat 15g, Net Carbs 3.6g, Protein 13.2g

Ingredients

10 oz tempeh, cut into chunks
1 ½ cups water
1 red onion, cut into chunks
1 red bell pepper, cut chunks
1 yellow bell pepper, cut into chunks
2 tbsp olive oil
1 cup sugar-free barbecue sauce

Directions

Bring the water to boil in a pot over medium heat and once it has boiled, turn the heat off, and add the tempeh. Cover the pot and let the tempeh steam for 5 minutes to remove its bitterness.

Drain the tempeh after. Pour the barbecue sauce in a bowl, add the tempeh to it, and coat with the sauce. Cover the bowl and marinate in the fridge for 2 hours. Preheat grill to 350ºF, and thread the tempeh, yellow bell pepper, red bell pepper, and onion.

Brush the grate of the grill with olive oil, place the skewers on it, and brush with barbecue sauce. Cook the kabobs for 3 minutes on each side while rotating and brushing with more barbecue sauce.

Once ready, transfer the kabobs to a plate and serve with lemon cauli couscous and a tomato sauce.

Cauliflower Gouda Casserole

Ready in about: 21 minutes | Serves: 4
Per serving: Kcal 215, Fat 15g, Net Carbs 4g, Protein 12g

Ingredients

2 heads cauliflower, cut into florets
⅓ cup butter, cubed
2 tbsp melted butter
1 white onion, chopped
Salt and black pepper to taste
¼ almond milk
½ cup almond flour
1 ½ cups grated gouda cheese

Directions

Preheat oven to 350ºF and put the cauli florets in a large microwave-safe bowl. Sprinkle with a bit of water, and steam in the microwave for 4 to 5 minutes. Melt the ⅓ cup of butter in a saucepan over medium heat and sauté the onion for 3 minutes. Add the cauliflower, season with salt and black pepper and mix in almond milk. Simmer for 3 minutes.

Mix the remaining melted butter with almond flour. Stir into the cauliflower as well as half of the cheese. Sprinkle the top with the remaining cheese and bake for 10 minutes until the cheese has melted and golden brown on the top. Plate the bake and serve with salad.

Creamy Vegetable Stew

Ready in about: 32 minutes | Serves: 4
Per serving: Kcal 310, Fat 26.4g, Net Carbs 6g,
Protein 8g

Ingredients

2 tbsp ghee
1 tbsp onion garlic puree
4 medium carrots, chopped
1 large head cauliflower, cut into florets
2 cups green beans, halved
Salt and black pepper to taste
1 cup water
1 ½ cups heavy cream

Directions

Melt ghee in a saucepan over medium heat and sauté onion-garlic puree to be fragrant, 2 minutes.
Stir in carrots, cauliflower, and green beans, salt, and black pepper, add the water, stir again, and cook the vegetables on low heat for 25 minutes to soften. Mix in the heavy cream to be incorporated, turn the heat off, and adjust the taste with salt and pepper. Serve the stew with almond flour bread.

Zucchini Lasagna with Ricotta and Spinach

Ready in about: 50 minutes | Serves: 4
Per serving: Kcal 390, Fat 39g, Net Carbs 2g, Protein 7g

Ingredients

2 zucchinis, sliced
Salt and black pepper to taste
2 cups ricotta cheese
2 cups shredded mozzarella cheese
3 cups tomato sauce
1 cup baby spinach

Directions

Preheat oven to 370ºF and grease a baking dish with cooking spray.
Put the zucchini slices in a colander and sprinkle with salt. Let sit and drain liquid for 5 minutes and pat dry with paper towels. Mix the ricotta, mozzarella cheese, salt, and black pepper to evenly combine and spread ¼ cup of the mixture in the bottom of the baking dish.
Layer ⅓ of the zucchini slices on top spread 1 cup of tomato sauce over, and scatter a ⅓ cup of spinach on top. Repeat the layering process two more times to exhaust the ingredients while making sure to layer with the last ¼ cup of cheese mixture finally.
Grease one end of foil with cooking spray and cover the baking dish with the foil. Bake for 35 minutes, remove foil, and bake further for 5 to 10 minutes or until the cheese has a nice golden brown color. Remove the dish, sit for 5 minutes, make slices of the lasagna, and serve warm.

Tofu Sandwich with Cabbage Slaw

Ready in about: 4 hours 10 minutes | Serves: 4

Per serving: Kcal 386, Fat 33g, Net Carbs 7.8g,
Protein 14g

Ingredients

½ lb firm tofu, sliced
4 low carb buns
1 tbsp olive oil

Marinade

Salt and black pepper to taste
2 tsp allspice
1 tbsp erythritol
2 tsp chopped thyme
1 habanero pepper, seeded and minced
3 green onions, thinly sliced
2 cloves garlic
¼ cup olive oil

Slaw

½ small cabbage, shredded
1 carrot, grated
½ red onion, grated
2 tsp swerve
2 tbsp white vinegar
1 pinch Italian seasoning
¼ cup olive oil
1 tsp Dijon mustard
Salt and black pepper to taste

Directions

In a food processor, make the marinade by blending the allspice, salt, black pepper, erythritol, thyme, habanero, green onions, garlic, and olive oil, for a minute. Pour the mixture in a bowl and put the tofu in it, coating it to be covered with marinade. Place in the fridge to marinate for 4 hours.
Make the slaw next: In a large bowl, evenly combine the white vinegar, swerve, olive oil, Dijon mustard, Italian seasoning, salt, and pepper. Stir in the cabbage, carrot, and onion, and place it in the refrigerator to chill while the tofu marinates.
Heat 1 teaspoon of oil in a skillet over medium heat, remove the tofu from the marinade, and cook it in the oil to brown on both sides for 6 minutes in total. Remove onto a plate after and toast the buns in the skillet. In the buns, add the tofu and top with the slaw. Close the bread and serve with a sweet chili sauce.

Creamy Cucumber Avocado Soup

Ready in about: 15 minutes | Serves: 4
Per serving: Kcal 170, Fat 7.4g, Net Carbs 4.1g,
Protein 3.7g

Ingredients

4 large cucumbers, seeded, chopped
1 large avocado, peeled and pitted
Salt and black pepper to taste
2 cups water
1 tbsp cilantro, chopped
3 tbsp olive oil
2 limes, juiced
2 tsp minced garlic
2 tomatoes, chopped
1 chopped avocado for garnish

Directions

Pour the cucumbers, avocado halves, salt, black pepper, olive oil, lime juice, cilantro, water, and garlic in the food processor. Puree the ingredients for 2 minutes or until smooth. Pour the mixture in a bowl and top with avocado and tomatoes. Serve chilled with zero-carb bread.

Lemon Cauliflower "Couscous" with Halloumi

Ready in about: 5 minutes | Serves: 4
Per serving: Kcal 185, Fat 15.6g, Net Carbs 2.1g, Protein 12g

Ingredients

4 oz halloumi, sliced
1 cauliflower head, cut into small florets
¼ cup chopped cilantro
¼ cup chopped parsley
¼ cup chopped mint
½ lemon juiced
Salt and black pepper to taste
Sliced avocado to garnish

Directions

Place a skillet over medium heat and lightly grease it with cooking spray.
Add the halloumi and fry for 2 minutes on each side until golden brown, set aside. Turn the heat off.
Next, pour the cauli florets in a food processor and pulse until it crumbles and resembles couscous. Transfer to a bowl and steam in the microwave for 2 minutes. They should be slightly cooked but crunchy. Remove the bowl from the microwave and let the cauli cool.
Stir in the cilantro, parsley, mint, lemon juice, salt, and black pepper. Garnish the couscous with avocado slices and serve with grilled halloumi and vegetable sauce.

Asparagus and Tarragon Flan

Ready in about: 65 minutes | Serves: 4
Per serving: Kcal 264, Fat 11.6g, Net Carbs 2.5g, Protein 12.5g

Ingredients

16 asparagus, stems trimmed
1 cup water
½ cup whipping cream
1 cup almond milk
2 eggs + 2 egg yolks, beaten in a bowl
2 tbsp chopped tarragon, fresh
Salt and black pepper to taste
A small pinch of nutmeg
2 tbsp grated Parmesan cheese
3 cups water
2 tbsp butter, melted
1 tbsp butter, softened

Directions

Pour the water and some salt in a pot, add the asparagus, and bring them to boil over medium heat on a stovetop for 6 minutes. Drain the asparagus; cut their tips and reserve for garnishing. Chop the remaining asparagus into small pieces.

In a blender, add the chopped asparagus, whipping cream, almond milk, tarragon, ½ teaspoon of salt, nutmeg, pepper, and Parmesan cheese. Process the ingredients on high speed until smooth. Pour the mixture through a sieve into a bowl and whisk the eggs into it.
Preheat the oven to 350ºF. Grease the ramekins with softened butter and share the asparagus mixture among the ramekins. Pour the melted butter over each mixture and top with 2-3 asparagus tips. Pour the remaining water into a baking dish, place in the ramekins, and insert in the oven.
Bake for 45 minutes until their middle parts are no longer watery. Remove the ramekins and let cool. Garnish the flan with the asparagus tips and serve with chilled white wine.

Parmesan Roasted Cabbage

Ready in about: 25 minutes | Serves: 4
Per serving: Kcal 268, Fat 19.3g, Net Carbs 4g, Protein 17.5g

Ingredients

1 large head green cabbage
4 tbsp melted butter
1 tsp garlic powder
Salt and black pepper to taste
1 cup grated Parmesan cheese
Grated Parmesan cheese for topping
1 tbsp chopped parsley to garnish

Directions

Preheat oven to 400ºF, line a baking sheet with foil, and grease with cooking spray.
Stand the cabbage and run a knife from the top to bottom to cut the cabbage into wedges. Remove stems and wilted leaves. Mix the butter, garlic, salt, and black pepper until evenly combined.
Brush the mixture on all sides of the cabbage wedges and sprinkle with Parmesan cheese.
Place on the baking sheet, and bake for 20 minutes to soften the cabbage and melt the cheese. Remove the cabbages when golden brown, plate and sprinkle with extra cheese and parsley. Serve warm with pan-glazed tofu.

Briam with Tomato Sauce

Ready in about: 70 minutes | Serves: 4
Per serving: Kcal 365, Fat 12g, Net Carbs 12.5g, Protein 11.3g

Ingredients

3 tbsp olive oil
1 large eggplant, halved and sliced
1 large onion, thinly sliced
3 cloves garlic, sliced
5 tomatoes, diced
3 rutabagas, diced
1 cup sugar-free tomato sauce
4 zucchinis, sliced
¼ cup water
Salt and black pepper to taste
1 tbsp dried oregano

2 tbsp chopped parsley

Directions

Preheat the oven to 400ºF. Heat the olive oil in a skillet over medium heat and cook the eggplant in for 6 minutes until on the edges. After, remove to a medium bowl. Sauté the onion and garlic in the oil for 3 minutes and add them to the eggplants. Turn the heat off.

In the eggplant bowl, mix in the tomatoes, rutabagas, tomato sauce, and zucchinis. Add the water and stir in the salt, black pepper, oregano, and parsley. Pour the mixture in the casserole dish. Place the dish in the oven and bake for 45 to 60 minutes. Serve the briam warm on a bed of cauli rice.

Spicy Cauliflower Steaks with Steamed Green Beans

Ready in about: 20 minutes | Serves: 4
Per serving: Kcal 118, Fat 9g, Net Carbs 4g, Protein 2g

Ingredients
2 heads cauliflower, sliced lengthwise into 'steaks'
¼ cup olive oil
¼ cup chili sauce
2 tsp erythritol
Salt and black pepper to taste
2 shallots, diced
1 bunch green beans, trimmed
2 tbsp fresh lemon juice
1 cup water
Dried parsley to garnish

Directions
In a bowl, mix the olive oil, chili sauce, and erythritol. Brush the cauliflower with the mixture. Place them on the grill, close the lid, and grill for 6 minutes. Flip the cauliflower, cook further for 6 minutes.

Bring the water to boil over high heat, place the green beans in a sieve and set over the steam from the boiling water. Cover with a clean napkin to keep the steam trapped in the sieve. Cook for 6 minutes. After, remove to a bowl and toss with lemon juice. Remove the grilled caulis to a plate; sprinkle with salt, pepper, shallots, and parsley. Serve with the steamed green beans.

Cheesy Cauliflower Falafel

Ready in about: 15 minutes | Serves: 4
Per serving: Kcal 315, Fat 26g, Net Carbs 2g, Protein 8g

Ingredients
1 head cauliflower, cut into florets
⅓ cup silvered ground almonds
2 tbsp cheddar cheese, shredded
½ tsp mixed spice
Salt and chili pepper to taste
3 tbsp coconut flour
3 fresh eggs
4 tbsp ghee

Directions

Blend the cauli florets in a food processor until a grain meal consistency is formed. Pour the rice in a bowl, add the ground almonds, mixed spice, salt, cheddar cheese, chili pepper, and coconut flour, and mix until evenly combined.

Beat the eggs in a bowl until creamy in color and mix with the cauli mixture. Shape ¼ cup each into patties. Melt ghee in a frying pan over medium heat and fry the patties for 5 minutes on each side to be firm and browned. Remove onto a wire rack to cool, share into serving plates, and top with tahini sauce.

Tofu Sesame Skewers with Warm Kale Salad

Ready in about: 2 hours 40 minutes | Serves: 4
Per serving: Kcal 263, Fat 12.9g, Net Carbs 6.1g, Protein 5.6g

Ingredients
14 oz Firm tofu
4 tsp sesame oil
1 lemon, juiced
5 tbsp sugar-free soy sauce
3 tsp garlic powder
4 tbsp coconut flour
½ cup sesame seeds
Warm Kale Salad:
4 cups chopped kale
2 tsp + 2 tsp olive oil
1 white onion, thinly sliced
3 cloves garlic, minced
1 cup sliced white mushrooms
1 tsp chopped rosemary
Salt and black pepper to season
1 tbsp balsamic vinegar

Directions
In a bowl, mix sesame oil, lemon juice, soy sauce, garlic powder, and coconut flour. Wrap the tofu in a paper towel, squeeze out as much liquid from it, and cut it into strips. Stick on the skewers, height wise. Place onto a plate, pour the soy sauce mixture over, and turn in the sauce to be adequately coated. Cover the dish with cling film and marinate in the fridge for 2 hours.

Heat the griddle pan over high heat. Pour the sesame seeds in a plate and roll the tofu skewers in the seeds for a generous coat. Grill the tofu in the griddle pan to be golden brown on both sides, about 12 minutes in total.

Heat 2 tablespoons of olive oil in a skillet over medium heat and sauté onion to begin browning for 10 minutes with continuous stirring. Add the remaining olive oil and mushrooms. Continue cooking for 10 minutes. Add garlic, rosemary, salt, pepper, and balsamic vinegar. Cook for 1 minute.

Put the kale in a salad bowl; when the onion mixture is ready, pour it on the kale and toss well. Serve the tofu skewers with the warm kale salad and a peanut butter dipping sauce.

Roasted Asparagus with Spicy Eggplant Dip

Ready in about: 35 minutes | Serves: 6
Per serving: Kcal 149; Fat: 12.1g, Net Carbs: 9g, Protein: 3.6g

Ingredients

1 ½ pounds asparagus spears, trimmed
¼ cup olive oil
Salt and black pepper, to taste
½ tsp paprika

For Eggplant Dip

¾ pound eggplants
2 tsp olive oil
½ cup scallions, chopped
2 cloves garlic, minced
1 tbsp fresh lemon juice
½ tsp chili pepper
Salt and black pepper, to taste
¼ cup fresh cilantro, chopped

Directions

Set the oven to 390ºF. Line a parchment paper to a baking sheet. Add in the asparagus spears. Toss with ¼ cup of olive, paprika, black pepper, and salt. Bake until cooked through for 9 minutes.

Set the oven to 425 ºF. Add eggplants on a lined cookie sheet. Place under the broiler for about 20 minutes; let the eggplants to cool. Peel them and discard the stems.

Place a frying pan over medium heat and warm olive 2 tsp olive oil. Add in garlic and scallions and sauté until tender.

In a food processor, pulse together black pepper, roasted eggplants, salt, lemon juice, scallion mixture, and chili pepper; mix evenly. Add in cilantro and serve alongside roasted asparagus spears.

Keto Pizza Margherita

Ready in about: 25 minutes | Serves: 2
Per serving: Kcal 510, Fat: 39g, Net Carbs: 3.7g, Protein: 31g

Ingredients

Crust

6 ounces mozzarella cheese
2 tbsp cream cheese
2 tbsp Parmesan cheese, grated
1 tsp dried oregano
½ cup almond flour
2 tbsp psyllium husk

Topping

4 ounces grated cheddar cheese
¼ cup Marinara sauce
1 bell pepper, sliced
1 tomato, sliced
2 tbsp chopped basil

Directions

Preheat the oven to 400ºF. Melt the mozzarella cheese in a microwave. Combine the remaining crust ingredients in a large bowl and add the mozzarella cheese. Mix with your hands to combine.

Divide the dough in two. Roll out the two crusts in circles and place on a lined baking sheet. Bake for about 10 minutes. Remove and spread the marinara sauce evenly.

Top with cheddar cheese, bell pepper, and tomato slices. Return to the oven and bake for 10 more minutes. Serve sprinkled with basil.

Sriracha Tofu with Yogurt Sauce

Ready in about: 40 minutes | Serves: 4
Per serving: Kcal 351; Fat: 25.9g, Net Carbs: 8.1g, Protein: 17.5g

Ingredients

12 ounces tofu, pressed and sliced
1 cup green onions, chopped
1 garlic clove, minced
2 tbsp vinegar
1 tbsp sriracha sauce
2 tbsp olive oil

For yogurt sauce

2 cloves garlic, pressed
2 tbsp fresh lemon juice
Sea salt and black pepper, to taste
1 tsp fresh dill weed
1 cup Greek yogurt
1 cucumber, shredded

Directions

Put tofu slices, garlic, sriracha sauce, vinegar, and green onions in a bowl; allow to settle for 30 minutes. Set a nonstick skillet to medium heat and add oil to warm. Cook tofu for 5 minutes until golden brown.

For the preparation of sauce, use a bowl to mix garlic, salt, yogurt, black pepper, lemon juice, and dill. Add in shredded cucumber as you stir to combine. Serve the tofu with a dollop of yogurt sauce.

Grilled Cheese the Keto Way

Ready in about: 15 minutes | Serves: 1
Per serving: Kcal 623, Fat: 51g, Net Carbs: 6.1g, Protein: 25g

Ingredients

2 eggs
½ tsp baking powder
2 tbsp butter
2 tbsp almond flour
1 ½ tbsp psyllium husk powder
2 ounces cheddar cheese, shredded

Directions

Whisk together all ingredients, except 1 tbsp butter and cheddar cheese. Place in a square oven-proof bowl, and microwave for 90 seconds. Flip the bun over and cut in half. Place the cheddar cheese on one half of the bun and top with the other. Melt the remaining butter in a skillet. Add the sandwich and grill until the cheese is melted and the bun is crispy.

Zesty Frittata with Roasted Chilies

Ready in about: 17 minutes | Serves: 4
Per serving: Kcal 153, Fat 10.3g, Net Carbs 2.3g, Protein 6.4g

Ingredients

2 large green bell peppers, seeded, chopped
4 red and yellow chilies, roasted
2 tbsp red wine vinegar
1 knob butter, melted
8 sprigs parsley, chopped
8 eggs, cracked into a bowl
4 tbsp olive oil
½ cup grated Parmesan cheese
¼ cup crumbled goat cheese
4 cloves garlic, minced
1 cup loosely filled salad leaves

Directions

Preheat the oven to 400ºF. With a knife, seed the chilies, cut into long strips, and pour into a bowl.

Mix in the vinegar, butter, half of the parsley, half of the olive oil, and garlic; set aside. In another bowl, whisk the eggs with salt, pepper, bell peppers, Parmesan cheese, and the remaining parsley.

Now, heat the remaining oil in the cast iron over medium heat and pour the egg mixture along with half of the goat cheese. Let cook for 3 minutes and when it is near done, sprinkle the remaining goat cheese on it, and transfer the cast iron to the oven.

Bake the frittata for 4 more minutes, remove and drizzle with the chili oil. Garnish the frittata with salad greens and serve for lunch.

Portobello Mushroom Burgers

Ready in about: 15 minutes | Serves: 4
Per serving: Kcal 190, Fat 8g, Net Carbs 3g, Protein 16g

Ingredients

4 low carb buns
4 portobello mushroom caps
1 clove garlic, minced
½ tsp salt
2 tbsp olive oil
½ cup sliced roasted red peppers
2 medium tomatoes, chopped
¼ cup crumbled feta cheese
1 tbsp red wine vinegar
2 tbsp pitted kalamata olives, chopped
½ tsp dried oregano
2 cups baby salad greens

Directions

Heat the grill pan over medium heat and while it heats, crush the garlic with salt in a bowl using the back of a spoon. Stir in 1 tablespoon of oil and brush the mushrooms and each inner side of the buns with the mixture. Place the mushrooms in the heated pan and grill them on both sides for 8 minutes until tender.Also, toast the buns in the pan until they are crisp, about 2 minutes. Set aside.

In a bowl, mix the red peppers, tomatoes, olives, feta cheese, vinegar, oregano, baby salad greens, and remaining oil; toss them. Assemble the burger: in a slice of bun, add a mushroom cap, a scoop of vegetables, and another slice of bread. Serve with cheese dip.

Avocado and Tomato Burritos

Ready in about: 5 minutes | Serves: 4
Per serving: Kcal 303, Fat 25g, Net Carbs 6g, Protein 8g

Ingredients

2 cups cauli rice
6 low carb tortillas
2 cups sour cream sauce
1 ½ cups tomato herb salsa
2 avocados, peeled, pitted, sliced

Directions

Pour the cauli rice in a bowl, sprinkle with a bit of water, and soften in the microwave for 2 minutes. On the tortillas, spread the sour cream all over and distribute the salsa on top. Top with cauli rice and scatter the avocado evenly on top. Fold and tuck the burritos and cut into two.

Vegan Mushroom Pizza

Ready in about: 35 minutes | Serves: 4
Per serving: Kcal 295, Fat 20g, Net Carbs 8g, Protein 15g

Ingredients

2 tsp olive oil
1 cup chopped button mushrooms
½ cup sliced mixed colored bell peppers
Salt and black pepper to taste
2 cauliflower pizza crusts
1 cup tomato sauce
1 tsp vegan Parmesan cheese
Vegan Parmesan cheese for garnish

Directions

Warm olive oil in a skillet over medium heat, sauté the mushrooms and bell peppers for 10 minutes to soften. Season with salt and black pepper. Turn the heat off.

Put the pizza crusts on a large pan and bake in the oven at 400ºF for 10 minutes. Remove and let sit for 5 minutes. Spread the tomato sauce all over the top and scatter vegetables evenly on top. Season with a little more salt and sprinkle with Parmesan cheese.

Return to the oven and bake for 5-10 minutes until the vegetables are soft and the cheese has melted and is bubbly. Garnish with extra Parmesan cheese. Serve with chilled berry juice.

Cremini Mushroom Stroganoff

Ready in about: 25 minutes | Serves: 4
Per serving: Kcal 284, Fat 28g, Net Carbs 1,5g, Protein 8g

Ingredients

3 tbsp butter
1 white onion, chopped
4 cups cremini mushrooms, cubed
2 cups water
½ cup heavy cream
½ cup grated Parmesan cheese
1 ½ tbsp dried mixed herbs
Salt and black pepper to taste

Directions

Melt the butter in a saucepan over medium heat and sauté the onion for 3 minutes until soft.

Stir in the mushrooms and cook until tender, about 5 minutes. Add the water, mix, and bring to boil for 10-15 minutes until the water reduces slightly.

Pour in the heavy cream and Parmesan cheese. Stir to melt the cheese. Also, mix in the dried herbs. Season with salt and black pepper, simmer for 5 minutes and turn the heat off. Ladle stroganoff over a bed of spaghetti squash and serve.

Stuffed Cremini Mushrooms

Ready in about: 35 minutes | Serves: 4
Per serving: Kcal 206; Fat: 13.4g, Net Carbs: 10g, Protein: 12.7g

Ingredients

½ head broccoli, cut into florets
1 pound cremini mushrooms, stems removed
2 tbsp coconut oil
1 onion, chopped
1 tsp garlic, minced
1 bell pepper, chopped
1 tsp cajun seasoning
Salt and black pepper, to taste
1 cup cheddar cheese, shredded

Directions

Use a food processor to pulse broccoli florets until become like small rice-like granules.

Set oven to 360ºF. Bake mushroom caps until tender for 8 to 12 minutes. In a heavy-bottomed skillet, melt the oil; stir in bell pepper, garlic, and onion and sauté until fragrant. Place in black pepper, salt, and cajun seasoning. Fold in broccoli rice.

Equally separate the filling mixture among mushroom caps. Cover with cheddar cheese and bake for 17 more minutes. Serve warm.

Vegetable Burritos

Ready in about: 10 minutes | Serves: 4
Per serving: Kcal 373, Fat 23.2g, Net Carbs 5.4g, Protein 17.9g

Ingredients

2 large low carb tortillas
2 tsp olive oil
1 small onion, sliced

1 bell pepper, seeded and sliced
1 large ripe avocado, pitted and sliced
1 cup lemon cauli couscous
Salt and black pepper to taste
⅓ cup sour cream
3 tbsp Mexican salsa

Directions

Heat the olive oil in a skillet and sauté the onion and bell pepper until they start to brown on the edges, about 4 minutes. Turn the heat off and set the skillet aside.

Lay the tortillas on a flat surface and top each with the bell pepper mixture, avocado, cauli couscous, season with salt and black pepper, sour cream, and Mexican salsa. Fold in the sides of each tortilla, and roll them in and over the filling to be completely enclosed. Wrap with foil, cut in halves, and serve warm.

Walnut Tofu Sauté

Ready in about: 15 minutes | Serves: 4
Per serving: Kcal 320, Fat 24g, Net Carbs 4g, Protein 18g

Ingredients

1 tbsp olive oil
1 (8 oz) block firm tofu, cubed
1 tbsp tomato paste with garlic and onion
1 tbsp balsamic vinegar
Salt and black pepper to taste
½ tsp mixed dried herbs
1 cup chopped raw walnuts

Directions

Heat the oil in a skillet over medium heat and cook the tofu for 3 minutes while stirring to brown.

Mix the tomato paste with the vinegar and add to the tofu. Stir, season with salt and black pepper, and cook for another 4 minutes.

Add the herbs and walnuts. Stir and cook on low heat for 3 minutes to be fragrant. Spoon to a side of squash mash and a sweet berry sauce to serve.

Wild Mushroom and Asparagus Stew

Ready in about: 25 minutes | Serves: 4
Per serving: Kcal 114; Fat: 7.3g, Net Carbs: 9.5g, Protein: 2.1g

Ingredients

2 tbsp olive oil
1 cup onions, chopped
2 garlic cloves, pressed
½ cup celery, chopped
2 carrots, chopped
1 cup wild mushrooms, sliced
2 tbsp dry white wine
2 rosemary sprigs, chopped
1 thyme sprig, chopped
4 cups vegetable stock
½ tsp chili pepper
1 tsp smoked paprika
2 tomatoes, chopped
1 tbsp flax seed meal

Set a pot over medium heat and warm oil. Add in onions and cook until tender, about 3 minutes.Place in carrots, celery, and garlic and cook until soft for 4 more minutes. Add in mushrooms and cook until the liquid evaporates; then set aside. Stir in wine to deglaze the pot's bottom.

Place in thyme and rosemary. Pour in tomatoes, vegetable stock, paprika, and chili pepper; add in reserved vegetables and allow to boil. On low heat, allow the mixture to simmer for 15 minutes. Stir in flax seed meal to thicken the stew. Plate into individual bowls and serve.

Vegetable Tempura

Ready in about: 17 minutes | Serves: 4
Per serving: Kcal 218, Fat 17g, Net Carbs 0.9g, Protein 3g

Ingredients

½ cup coconut flour + extra for dredging
Salt and black pepper to taste
3 egg yolks
2 red bell peppers, cut into strips
1 squash, peeled and cut into strips
1 broccoli, cut into florets
1 cup Chilled water
Olive oil for frying
Lemon wedges to serve
Sugar-free soy sauce to serve

Directions

In a deep frying pan or wok, heat the olive oil over medium heat. Beat the eggs lightly with ½ cup of coconut flour and water. The mixture should be lumpy. Dredge the vegetables lightly in some flour, shake off the excess flour, dip it in the batter, and then into the hot oil.

Fry in batches for 1 minute each, not more, and remove with a perforated spoon onto a wire rack. Sprinkle with salt and pepper and serve with the lemon wedges and soy sauce.

Classic Tangy Ratatouille

Ready in about: 47 minutes | Serves: 6
Per serving: Kcal 154, Fat 12.1g, Net Carbs 5.6g, Protein 1.7g

Ingredients

2 eggplants, chopped
3 zucchinis, chopped
2 red onions, diced
1 (28 oz) can tomatoes
2 red bell peppers, cut in chunks
1 yellow bell pepper, cut in chunks
3 cloves garlic, sliced
½ cup basil leaves, chop half
4 sprigs thyme
1 tbsp balsamic vinegar
2 tbsp olive oil
½ lemon, zested

Directions

In a casserole pot, heat the olive oil and sauté the eggplants, zucchinis, and bell peppers over medium heat for 5 minutes. Spoon the veggies into a large bowl.

In the same pan, sauté garlic, onions, and thyme leaves for 5 minutes and return the cooked veggies to the pan along with the canned tomatoes, balsamic vinegar, chopped basil, salt, and black pepper to taste. Stir and cover the pot, and cook the ingredients on low heat for 30 minutes.

Open the lid and stir in the remaining basil leaves, lemon zest, and adjust the seasoning. Turn the heat off. Plate the ratatouille and serve with some low carb crusted bread.

Vegetarian Burgers

Ready in about: 20 minutes | Serves: 2
Per serving: Kcal 637, Fat: 55g, Net Carbs: 8.5g, Protein: 23g

Ingredients

1 garlic clove, minced
2 portobello mushrooms, sliced
1 tbsp coconut oil, melted
1 tbsp chopped basil
1 tbsp oregano
2 eggs, fried
2 low carb buns
2 tbsp mayonnaise
2 lettuce leaves
Salt to taste

Directions

Combine the melted coconut oil, garlic, herbs, and salt, in a bowl. Place the mushrooms in the bowl and coat well. Form into burger patties. Preheat the grill to medium heat. Grill the mushroom patties for 2 minutes per side.

Cut the low carb buns in half. Add the lettuce leaves, grilled mushrooms, eggs, and mayonnaise. Top with the other bun half.

Pumpkin Bake

Ready in about: 45 minutes | Serves: 6
Per serving: Kcal 125, Fat 4.8g, Net Carbs 5.7g, Protein 2.7g

Ingredients

3 large pumpkins, peeled and sliced
1 cup almond flour
1 cup grated mozzarella cheese
3 tbsp olive oil
½ cup chopped parsley

Directions

Preheat oven to 350ºF. Arrange the pumpkin slices in a baking dish, drizzle with olive oil; bake for 35 minutes. Mix almond flour, mozzarella, and parsley and when the pumpkin is ready, remove it from the oven, and sprinkle the cheese mixture all over. Place back in the oven and bake the top for 5 minutes.

Bianca Pizza

Ready in about: 17 minutes | Serves: 1
Per serving: Kcal 591, Fat: 55g, Net Carbs: 2g, Protein: 22g

Ingredients

2 large eggs
1 tbsp water
½ jalapeño pepper, diced
1 ounce Monterey Jack cheese, shredded
1 chopped green onion
1 cup egg Alfredo sauce
¼ tsp cumin
2 tbsp olive oil

Directions

Preheat the oven to 350ºF.
Heat the olive oil in a skillet. Whisk the eggs along with water and cumin. Pour the eggs into the skillet. Cook until set. Top with the alfredo sauce and jalapeno pepper. Sprinkle the green onion and cheese over. Place in the oven and bake for 5 minutes.

Stuffed Portobello Mushrooms

Ready in about: 30 minutes | Serves: 2
Per serving: Kcal 334, Fat: 29g, Net Carbs: 5.5g, Protein: 14g

Ingredients

4 portobello mushrooms, stems removed
2 tbsp olive oil
2 cups lettuce
1 cup crumbled blue cheese

Directions

Preheat the oven to 350ºF. Fill the mushrooms with blue cheese and place on a lined baking sheet; bake for 20 minutes. Serve with lettuce drizzled with olive oil.

Spaghetti Squash with Eggplant & Parmesan

Ready in about: 15 minutes | Serves: 4
Per serving: Kcal 139, Fat: 8.2g, Net Carbs: 6.8g, Protein: 6.9g

Ingredients

1 tbsp butter
1 cup cherry tomatoes
2 tbsp parsley
1 eggplant, cubed
¼ cup Parmesan cheese, shredded
3 tbsp scallions, chopped
1 cup snap peas
1 tsp lemon zest
2 cups cooked spaghetti squash
Salt and black pepper to taste

Directions

Melt butter in a saucepan and cook eggplant for 5 minutes until tender. Add tomatoes and peas, and cook for 5 minutes. Stir in parsley, zest, scallions, salt, and pepper; remove the pan from heat. Stir in spaghetti squash and Parmesan cheese to serve.

Cauliflower & Mushrooms Stuffed Peppers

Ready in about: 40 minutes | Serves: 4
Per serving: Kcal: 77; Fat 4.8g, Net Carbs 8.4g, Protein 1.6g,

Ingredients

1 head cauliflower
4 bell peppers
1 cup mushrooms, sliced
1 ½ tbsp oil
1 onion, chopped
1 cup celery, chopped
1 garlic clove, minced
1 tsp chili powder
2 tomatoes, pureed
Sea salt and pepper, to taste

Directions

To prepare cauliflower rice, grate the cauliflower into rice-size. Set in a kitchen towel to attract and remove any excess moisture. Set oven to 360ºF.
Lightly oil a casserole dish. Chop off bell pepper tops, do away with the seeds and core. Line a baking pan with a parchment paper and roast the peppers for 18 minutes until the skin starts to brown.
Warm the oil over medium heat. Add in garlic, celery, and onion and sauté until soft and translucent.Stir in chili powder, mushrooms, and cauliflower rice. Cook for 6 minutes until the cauliflower rice becomes tender. Split the cauliflower mixture among the bell peppers. Set in the casserole dish.Combine pepper, salt, and tomatoes. Top the peppers with the tomato mixture. Bake for 10 minutes.

Cauliflower Risotto with Mushrooms

Ready in about: 15 minutes | Serves: 4
Per serving: Kcal 264, Fat: 18g, Net Carbs: 8.4g, Protein: 11g

Ingredients

2 shallots, diced
3 tbsp olive oil
¼ cup veggie broth
⅓ cup Parmesan cheese, shredded
2 tbsp butter
3 tbsp chopped chives
2 pounds mushrooms, sliced
4 cups cauliflower rice
Salt and black pepper to taste
2 tbsp parsley, chopped

Directions

Heat olive oil in a saucepan over medium heat. Add the mushrooms and shallots and cook for about 5 minutes until tender. Remove from the pan and set aside.
Add in the cauliflower, broth, salt, and black pepper, and cook until the liquid is absorbed, about 4-5 minutes. Stir in butter and Parmesan cheese until the cheese is melted. Sprinkle with parsley to serve.

Onion & Nuts Stuffed Mushrooms

Ready in about: 30 minutes | Serves: 4
Per serving: Kcal 139; Fat: 11.2g, Net Carbs: 7.4g,
Protein: 4.8g

Ingredients

1 tbsp sesame oil
1 onion, chopped
1 garlic clove, minced
1 pound mushrooms, stems removed
Salt and black pepper, to taste
¼ cup raw pine nuts
2 tbsp parsley, chopped

Directions

Set oven to 360ºF. Use a nonstick cooking spray to grease a large baking sheet. Into a frying pan, add sesame oil and warm. Place in garlic and onion and cook until soft.

Chop mushroom stems and cook until tender. Sprinkle with pepper and salt; add in pine nuts. Take the nut/mushroom mixture and stuff them to the mushroom caps and set on the baking sheet.

Bake the stuffed mushrooms for 30 minutes and remove to a wire rack to cool slightly. Add fresh parsley for garnish and serve.

Colorful Vegan Soup

Ready in about: 25 minutes | Serves: 6
Per serving: Kcal 142; Fat: 11.4g, Net Carbs: 9g,
Protein: 2.9g

Ingredients

2 tsp olive oil
1 red onion, chopped
2 cloves garlic, minced
1 celery stalk, chopped
1 head broccoli, chopped
1 carrot, sliced
1 cup spinach, torn into pieces
1 cup collard greens, chopped
Salt and black pepper, to taste
2 thyme sprigs, chopped
1 rosemary sprig, chopped
2 bay leaves
6 cups vegetable stock
2 tomatoes, chopped
1 cup almond milk
1 tbsp white miso paste
½ cup arugula

Directions

Place a large pot over medium heat and warm oil. Add in carrot, celery, onion, broccoli, garlic, and sauté until soft, about 5 minutes.

Place in spinach, salt, rosemary, tomatoes, bay leaves, black pepper, collard greens, thyme, and vegetable stock. On low heat, simmer the mixture for 15 minutes while the lid is slightly open. Stir in white miso paste, arugula, and almond milk and cook for 5 more minutes.

Sautéed Celeriac with Tomato Sauce

Ready in about: 20 minutes | Serves: 4
Per serving: Kcal 135; Fat: 13.6g, Net Carbs: 3g,
Protein: 0.9g

Ingredients

2 tbsp olive oil
1 garlic clove, crushed
1 celeriac, sliced
¼ cup vegetable stock
Salt and black pepper, to taste
For the sauce
2 tomatoes, halved
2 tbsp olive oil
½ cup onions, chopped
2 cloves garlic, minced
1 chili, minced
1 bunch fresh basil, chopped
1 tbsp fresh cilantro, chopped
Salt and black pepper, to taste

Directions

Set a pan over medium heat and warm olive oil. Add in garlic and sauté for 1 minute. Stir in celeriac slices, stock and cook until softened. Sprinkle with black pepper and salt; kill the heat. Brush olive oil to the tomato halves. Microwave for 15 minutes; get rid of any excess liquid.

Remove the cooked tomatoes to a food processor; add the rest of the ingredients for the sauce and puree to obtain the desired consistency. Serve the celeriac topped with tomato sauce.

Cauliflower Mac and Cheese

Ready in about: 45 minutes | Serves: 4
Per serving: Kcal 160, Fat: 12g, Net Carbs: 2g, Protein:
8.6g

Ingredients

1 cauliflower head, riced
1 ½ cups shredded mozzarella cheese
2 tsp paprika
¾ tsp rosemary
2 tsp turmeric
Salt and black pepper to taste

Directions

Microwave the cauliflower for 5 minutes. Place it in cheesecloth and squeeze the extra juices out. Place the cauli in a pot over medium heat. Add paprika, turmeric, salt, pepper, and rosemary. Stir in mozzarella cheese and cook until the cheese is melted and thoroughly combined. Serve topped with rosemary.

Vegan Cheesy Chips with Tomatoes

Ready in about: 15 minutes | Serves: 6
Per serving: Kcal 161; Fat: 14g, Net Carbs: 7.2g, Protein: 4.6g

Ingredients

5 tomatoes, sliced
¼ cup olive oil
1 tbsp chili seasoning mix

For vegan cheese

½ cup pepitas seeds
1 tbsp nutritional yeast
Salt and black pepper, to taste
1 tsp garlic puree

Directions

Over the sliced tomatoes, drizzle olive oil. Set oven to 400ºF.

In a food processor, add all vegan cheese ingredients and pulse until the desired consistency is attained. Transfer to a bowl and stir in chili seasoning mix. Toss in the tomato slices to coat. Set the tomato slices on the prepared baking pan and bake for 10 minutes.

Smoked Tofu with Rosemary Sauce

Ready in about: 20 minutes | Serves: 4
Per serving: Kcal 336; Fat: 22.2g, Net Carbs: 9.3g, Protein: 27.6g

Ingredients

10 ounces smoked tofu
2 tbsp sesame oil
1 onion, chopped
1 tsp garlic, minced
½ cup vegetable broth
½ tsp turmeric powder
Salt and black pepper, to taste

For the sauce

½ tbsp olive oil
1 cup tomato sauce
2 tbsp white wine
1 tsp fresh rosemary, chopped
1 tsp chili garlic sauce

Directions

Pat dry the tofu using a paper towel and chop into 1-inch cubes. Set a frying pan over medium heat and warm sesame oil. Add in the tofu cubes and fry until browned. Stir in salt, broth, black pepper, garlic, turmeric powder, and onions. Cook until all liquid evaporates.

As the process goes on, you can prepare the sauce. Set a pan over medium heat and warm olive oil. Place in tomato sauce and heat until cooked through. Place in the rest of the ingredients and simmer for 10 minutes over medium heat. Serve with prepared tofu cubes!

Cream of Zucchini and Avocado

Ready in about: 35 minutes | Serves: 4
Per serving: Kcal 165 Fat: 13.4g, Net Carbs: 9g, Protein: 2.2g

Ingredients

3 tsp vegetable oil
1 onion, chopped
1 carrot, sliced
1 turnip, sliced
3 cups zucchinis, chopped
1 avocado, peeled and diced
¼ tsp ground black pepper
4 cups vegetable broth
1 tomato, pureed

Directions

In a pot, warm the oil and sauté onion until translucent, about 3 minutes. Add in turnip, zucchini, and carrot and cook for 7 minutes; add black pepper for seasoning.

Mix in pureed tomato, and broth; boil. Change heat to low and allow the mixture to simmer for 20 minutes. Lift from the heat. Add the soup and avocado to a blender. Blend until creamy and smooth.

Greek Salad with Poppy Seed Dressing

Ready in about: 3 hours 15 minutes | Serves: 4
Per serving: Kcal 208; Fat: 15.6g, Net Carbs: 6.7g, Protein: 7.6g

Ingredients

For the dressing

1 cup poppy seeds
2 cups water
2 tbsp green onions, chopped
1 garlic clove, minced
1 lime, freshly squeezed
Salt and black pepper, to taste
¼ tsp dill, minced
2 tbsp almond milk

For the salad

1 head lettuce, separated into leaves
3 tomatoes, diced
3 cucumbers, sliced
2 tbsp kalamata olives, pitted

Directions

Put all dressing ingredients, except for the poppy seeds, in a food processor and pulse until well incorporated. Add in poppy seeds and mix well with a fork. Mix and divide salad ingredients between 4 plates. Add the dressing to each and shake to serve.

Spicy Tofu with Worcestershire Sauce

Ready in about: 25 minutes | Serves: 4
Per serving: Kcal 182; Fat: 10.3g, Net Carbs: 8.3g, Protein: 8.1g

Ingredients

2 tbsp olive oil
14 ounces block tofu, pressed and cubed
1 celery stalk, chopped
1 bunch scallions, chopped
1 tsp cayenne pepper
1 tsp garlic powder
2 tbsp Worcestershire sauce
Salt and black pepper, to taste
1 pound green cabbage, shredded
½ tsp turmeric powder

¼ tsp dried basil

Directions

Set a large skillet over medium heat and warm 1 tablespoon of olive oil. Stir in tofu cubes and cook for 8 minutes. Place in scallions and celery; cook for 5 minutes until soft.

Stir in cayenne, Worcestershire sauce, pepper, salt, and garlic; cook for 3 more minutes; set aside.

In the same pan, warm the remaining 1 tablespoon of oil. Add in shredded cabbage and the remaining seasonings and cook for 4 minutes. Mix in tofu mixture and serve warm.

Cauliflower & Hazelnut Salad

Ready in about: 15 minutes + chilling time | Serves: 4
Per serving: Kcal 221; Fat: 18g, Net Carbs: 6.6g, Protein: 4.2g

Ingredients

1 head cauliflower, cut into florets
1 cup green onions, chopped
4 ounces bottled roasted peppers, chopped
¼ cup extra-virgin olive oil
1 tbsp wine vinegar
1 tsp yellow mustard
Salt and black pepper, to taste
½ cup black olives, pitted and chopped
½ cup hazelnuts, chopped

Directions

Place the cauliflower florets in a steamer basket over boiling water. Cover and steam for 5 minutes; let cool and set aside. Add roasted peppers and green onions in a salad bowl.

Using a mixing dish, combine salt, olive oil, mustard, black pepper, and vinegar. Sprinkle the mixture over the veggies. Place in the reserved cauliflower and shake to mix well.

Top with hazelnuts and black olives and serve.

Parsnip Chips with Avocado Dip

Ready in about: 20 minutes | Serves: 6
Per serving: Kcal 269; Fat: 26.7g, Net Carbs: 9.4g, Protein: 2.3g

Ingredients

2 avocados, pitted
2 tsp lime juice
Salt and black pepper, to taste
2 garlic cloves, minced
2 tbsp olive oil
For parsnip chips
3 cups parsnips, sliced
1 tbsp olive oil
Salt and garlic powder, to taste

Directions

Use a fork to mash avocado pulp. Stir in fresh lime juice, pepper, 2 tbsp of olive oil, garlic, and salt until well combined. Remove to a bowl and set the oven to 300ºF. Grease a baking sheet with spray.

Set parsnip slices on the baking sheet; toss with garlic powder, 1 tbsp of olive oil, and salt. Bake for 15 minutes until slices become dry. Serve alongside the well-chilled avocado dip.

Tomato Stuffed Avocado

Ready in about: 10 minutes | Serves: 4
Per serving: Kcal 263; Fat: 24.8g, Net Carbs: 5.5g, Protein: 3.5g

Ingredients

2 avocados
1 tomato, chopped
¼ cup walnuts, ground
2 carrots, chopped
1 garlic clove
1 tsp lemon juice
1 tbsp soy sauce
Salt and black pepper, to taste

Directions

Halve and pit the avocados. Spoon out some of the pulp of each avocado.

In a bowl, mix soy sauce, carrots, avocado pulp, tomato, lemon juice, and garlic. Add black pepper and salt. Fill the avocado halves with the mixture and scatter walnuts over to serve.

Zoodles with Avocado & Olives

Ready in about: 15 minutes | Serves: 4
Per serving: Kcal 449, Fat: 42g, Net Carbs: 8.4g, Protein: 6.3g

Ingredients

4 zucchinis, julienned or spiralized
½ cup pesto
2 avocados, sliced
1 cup kalamata olives, chopped
¼ cup chopped basil
2 tbsp olive oil
¼ cup chopped sun-dried tomatoes
Salt and black pepper to taste

Directions

Heat half of the olive oil in a pan over medium heat. Add zoodles and cook for 4 minutes. Transfer to a plate. Stir in pesto, basil, salt, black pepper, tomatoes, and olives. Top with avocado slices to serve.

Fried Tofu with Mushrooms

Ready in about: 40 minutes | Serves: 2
Per serving: Kcal 223; Fat: 15.9g, Net Carbs: 8.1g, Protein: 15.6g

Ingredients

12 ounces extra firm tofu, pressed and cubed
1 ½ tbsp flax seed meal
Salt and black pepper, to taste
1 tsp garlic clove, minced
½ tsp paprika
1 tsp onion powder
½ tsp ground bay leaf
1 tbsp olive oil
1 cup mushrooms, sliced
1 jalapeño pepper, deveined, sliced

Directions

In a container, add onion powder, tofu, salt, paprika, black pepper, jalapeño pepper, flaxseed, garlic, and bay leaf. While the container is closed, toss the mixture to coat, and allow to marinate for 30 minutes. In a pan, warm oil over medium heat. Cook mushrooms and tofu for 6 minutes, stirring continuously.

Bell Pepper Stuffed Avocado
Ready in about: 10 minutes | Serves: 8
Per serving: Kcal 255; Fat: 23.2g, Net Carbs: 7.4g, Protein: 2.4g
Ingredients
4 avocados, pitted and halved
2 tbsp olive oil
3 cups green bell peppers, chopped
1 onion, chopped
1 tsp garlic puree
Salt and black pepper, to taste
1 tsp deli mustard
1 tomato, chopped
Directions
From each half of the avocados, scoop out 2 teaspoons of flesh; set aside.
Use a sauté pan to warm oil over medium heat. Cook the garlic, onion, and bell peppers until tender. Mix in the reserved avocado. Add in tomato, salt, mustard, and black pepper. Separate the mixture and mix equally among the avocado halves and serve.

Brussels Sprouts with Tofu
Ready in about: 20 minutes | Serves: 4
Per serving: Kcal 179; Fat: 11.7g, Net Carbs: 9.1g, Protein: 10.5g
Ingredients
2 tbsp olive oil
2 garlic cloves, minced
½ cup onion, chopped
10 ounces tofu, crumbled
2 tbsp water
2 tbsp soy sauce
1 tbsp tomato puree
½ pound Brussels sprouts, quartered
Sea salt and black pepper, to taste
Directions
Set a saucepan over medium heat and warm the oil. Add onion and garlic and cook until tender, 3 minutes. Place in the soy sauce, water, and tofu. Cook for 5 minutes until the tofu starts to brown.
Add in brussels sprouts; adjust the seasonings; reduce heat to low and cook for 13 minutes while stirring frequently. Serve warm.

Carrot Noodles with Cashew Sauce
Ready in about: 15 minutes | Serves: 4
Per serving: Kcal 145; Fat: 10.6g, Net Carbs: 7,9g, Protein: 5.5g
Ingredients
4 carrots, peeled
2 tbsp olive oil
½ cup water
Salt and pepper to taste
For cashew sauce

½ cup raw cashews
3 tbsp nutritional yeast
Sea salt and black pepper, to taste
¼ tsp onion powder
½ tsp garlic powder
¼ cup olive oil
Directions
Cut the carrots into long strips. Set a pan over medium heat and warm oil; cook the carrots for 1 minute as you stir. Add in water and cook for an additional 6 minutes. Sprinkle with salt.
Place all dip ingredients in a food processor and pulse until you attain the required "cheese" consistency. Serve cooked noodles with a topping of cashew sauce.

Morning Coconut Smoothie
Ready in about: 5 minutes | Serves: 4
Per serving: Kcal 247; Fat: 21.7g, Net Carbs: 6.9g, Protein: 2.6g
Ingredients
½ cup water
1 ½ cups coconut milk
1 cup frozen strawberries
2 cups fresh blueberries
¼ tsp vanilla extract
1 tbsp protein powder
Directions
Using a blender, combine all the ingredients and blend well until you attain a uniform and creamy consistency. Divide in glasses and serve!

Chard Swiss Dip
Ready in about: 25 minutes | Serves: 6
Per serving: Kcal 105; Fat: 7.3g, Net Carbs: 7.9g, Protein: 2.9g
Ingredients
2 cups Swiss chard
1 cup tofu, pressed, drained, crumbled
½ cup almond milk
2 tsp nutritional yeast
2 garlic cloves, minced
2 tbsp olive oil
Salt and pepper to taste
½ tsp paprika
½ tsp chopped fresh mint leaves
Directions
In a pot over medium heat, boil Swiss chard until wilted. Drain and set aside. Using a blender, puree the remaining ingredients. Season with salt and black pepper. Stir in the Swiss chard to get a homogeneous mixture. Serve alongside baked vegetables.

Greek-Style Zucchini Pasta

Ready in about: 15 minutes | Serves: 4
Per serving: Kcal 231, Fat: 19.5g, Net Carbs: 6.5g, Protein: 6.5g

Ingredients

¼ cup sun-dried tomatoes
2 garlic cloves, minced
2 tbsp butter
1 cup spinach
2 large zucchinis, spiralized
¼ cup crumbled feta
¼ cup Parmesan cheese, shredded
10 kalamata olives, halved
2 tbsp olive oil
2 tbsp chopped parsley

Directions

Heat the olive oil and butter in a pan over medium heat. Add zoodles, garlic, and spinach and cook for about 5 minutes. Stir in the olives, tomatoes, feta cheese, and parsley. Cook for 2 more minutes, top with Parmesan cheese and serve.

Garlicky Bok Choy

Ready in about: 25 minutes | Serves: 4
Per serving: Kcal 118; Fat: 7g, Net Carbs: 13.4g, Protein: 2.9g

Ingredients

2 pounds bok choy, chopped
2 tbsp almond oil
1 tsp garlic, minced
½ tsp thyme
½ tsp red pepper flakes, crushed
Salt and black pepper, to the taste

Directions

Add bok choy in a pot with salted water and cook for 10 minutes over medium heat. Drain and set aside. Place a sauté pan over medium heat and warm oil. Add in garlic and cook until soft. Stir in the bok choy, red pepper, black pepper, salt, and thyme. Add more seasonings if needed and serve with cauli rice.

Tofu Stir Fry with Asparagus

Ready in about: 30 minutes | Serves: 4
Per serving: Kcal 138; Fat: 8.9g, Net Carbs: 5.9g, Protein: 6.4g

Ingredients

1 pound asparagus, cut off stems
2 tbsp olive oil
2 blocks tofu, pressed and cubed
2 garlic cloves, minced
1 tsp cajun spice mix
1 tsp mustard
1 bell pepper, chopped
¼ cup vegetable broth
Salt and black pepper, to taste

Directions

In a large saucepan with lightly salted water, place in asparagus and cook until tender for 10 minutes; drain. Set a wok over high heat and warm olive oil; stir in tofu cubes and cook for 6 minutes.
Place in garlic and cook for 30 seconds until soft. Stir in the rest of the ingredients, including reserved asparagus, and cook for an additional 4 minutes. Divide among plates and serve.

Zucchini Boats

Ready in about: 50 minutes | Serves: 4
Per serving: Kcal 148; Fat: 10g, Net Carbs: 9.8g, Protein: 7.5g

Ingredients

1 tbsp olive oil
12 ounces firm tofu, drained and crumbled
2 garlic cloves, pressed
½ cup onions, chopped
2 cups tomato paste
¼ tsp turmeric
Sea salt and chili pepper, to taste
3 zucchinis, cut into halves, scoop out the insides
1 tbsp nutritional yeast
¼ cup almonds, chopped

Directions

Set pan over medium heat and warm oil; add in onion, garlic, and tofu and cook for 5 minutes. Place in scooped zucchini flesh, turmeric and 1 cup of tomato paste; cook for 6 more minutes.
Preheat oven to 360ºF. Grease a baking dish with a cooking spray. Divide the tofu mixture among the zucchini shells. Arrange the stuffed zucchini shells in the baking dish. Stir in the remaining 1 cup of tomato paste. Bake for about 30 minutes. Sprinkle with almonds and nutritional yeast and continue baking for 5 to 6 more minutes.

Mushroom & Jalapeño Stew

Ready in about: 50 minutes | Serves: 4
Per serving: Kcal 65; Fat: 2.7g, Net Carbs: 9g, Protein: 2.7g

Ingredients

2 tsp olive oil
1 cup leeks, chopped
1 garlic clove, minced
½ cup celery stalks, chopped
½ cup carrots, chopped
1 green bell pepper, chopped
1 jalapeño pepper, chopped
2 ½ cups mushrooms, sliced
1 ½ cups vegetable stock
2 tomatoes, chopped
2 thyme sprigs, chopped
1 rosemary sprig, chopped
2 bay leaves
½ tsp salt
¼ tsp ground black pepper
2 tbsp vinegar

Directions

Set a pot over medium heat and warm oil. Add in garlic and leeks and sauté until soft and translucent.

Add in the black pepper, celery, mushrooms, and carrots.

Cook as you stir for 12 minutes; stir in a splash of vegetable stock to ensure there is no sticking. Stir in the rest of the ingredients. Set heat to medium; allow to simmer for 25 to 35 minutes or until cooked through. Divide into individual bowls and serve warm.

Easy Cauliflower Soup

Ready in about: 15 minutes | Serves: 4
Per serving: Kcal 172; Fat: 10.3g, Net Carbs: 11.8g, Protein: 8.1g

Ingredients

2 tbsp olive oil
2 onions, finely chopped
1 tsp garlic, minced
1 pound cauliflower, cut into florets
1 cup kale, chopped
4 cups vegetable broth
½ cup almond milk
½ tsp salt
½ tsp red pepper flakes
1 tbsp fresh chopped parsley

Directions

Set a pot over medium heat and warm the oil. Add garlic and onions and sauté until browned and softened. Place in vegetable broth, kale, and cauliflower; cook for 10 minutes until the mixture boils. Stir in the pepper flakes, salt, and almond milk; reduce the heat and simmer the soup for 5 minutes. Transfer the soup to an immersion blender and blend to achieve the desired consistency; top with parsley and serve immediately.

Crispy-Topped Baked Vegetables

Ready in about: 40 minutes | Serves: 4
Per serving: Kcal 242; Fat: 16.3g, Net Carbs: 8.6g, Protein: 16.3g

Ingredients

2 tbsp olive oil
1 onion, chopped
1 celery stalk, chopped
2 carrots, grated
½ pound turnips, sliced
1 cup vegetable broth
1 tsp turmeric
Sea salt and black pepper, to taste
½ tsp liquid smoke
1 cup Parmesan cheese, shredded
2 tbsp fresh chives, chopped

Directions

Set oven to 360ºF and grease a baking dish with olive oil. Set a skillet over medium heat and warm olive oil. Sweat the onion until soft, and place in the turnips, carrots and celery; and cook for 4 minutes. Remove the vegetable mixture to the baking dish.

Combine vegetable broth with turmeric, pepper, liquid smoke, and salt. Spread this mixture over the vegetables. Sprinkle with Parmesan cheese and bake for about 30 minutes. Garnish with chives to serve.

Morning Granola

Ready in about: 1 hour | Serves: 8
Per serving: Kcal 262; Fat: 24.3g, Net Carbs: 9.2g, Protein: 5.1g

Ingredients

1 tbsp coconut oil
⅓ cup almond flakes
½ cup almond milk
½ tbsp liquid stevia
1/8 tsp salt
1 tsp lime zest
1/8 tsp nutmeg, grated
½ tsp ground cinnamon
½ cup pecans, chopped
½ cup almonds, slivered
2 tbsp pepitas
3 tbsp sunflower seeds
¼ cup flax seed

Directions

Set a deep pan over medium heat and warm the coconut oil. Add almond flakes and toast for about 2 minutes. Stir in the remaining ingredients.

Set the oven to 300ºF. Lay the mixture in an even layer onto a baking sheet lined with a parchment paper. Bake for 1 hour, making sure that you shake gently in intervals of 15 minutes. Serve alongside additional almond milk.

Tasty Cauliflower Dip

Ready in about: 10 minutes | Serves: 4
Per serving: Kcal 100; Fat: 8.2g, Net Carbs: 4.7g, Protein: 3.7g

Ingredients

¾ pound cauliflower, cut into florets
¼ cup olive oil
Salt and black pepper, to taste
1 garlic clove, smashed
1 tbsp sesame paste
1 tbsp fresh lime juice
½ tsp garam masala

Directions

Boil cauliflower until tender for 7 minutes in salted water, in a large pot. Transfer to a blender and pulse until you attain a rice-like consistency. Place in garam masala, oil, black paper, lime juice, garlic, salt, and sesame paste. Blend the mixture until well combined. Decorate with some olive oil and serve.

Spiced Cauliflower & Peppers

Ready in about: 35 minutes | Serves: 4
Per serving: Kcal 166; Fat: 13.9g, Net Carbs: 7.4g,
Protein: 3g

Ingredients

1 pound cauliflower, cut into florets
2 bell peppers, halved
¼ cup olive oil
Salt and black pepper, to taste
½ tsp cayenne pepper
1 tsp curry powder

Directions

Set oven to 425ºF. Line a parchment paper to a large baking sheet. Sprinkle olive oil to the peppers and cauliflower alongside curry powder, black pepper, salt, and cayenne pepper.

Set the vegetables on the baking sheet. Roast for 30 minutes as you toss in intervals until they start to brown. Serve alongside mushroom pate or homemade tomato dip!

Coconut Cauliflower & Parsnip Soup

Ready in about: 20 minutes | Serves: 4
Per serving: Kcal 94; Fat: 7.2g, Net Carbs: 7g, Protein: 2.7g

Ingredients

4 cups vegetable broth
2 heads cauliflower, cut into florets
1 cup parsnips, chopped
1 tbsp coconut oil
1 cup coconut milk
½ tsp red pepper flakes

Directions

Add broth in a pot set over medium heat and bring to a boil. Add in cauliflower florets and parsnips, and cook for about 10 minutes. Add in coconut oil, set to low heat, and cook for an additional 5 minutes. Puree the mixture in an immersion blender. After, stir in the coconut milk.

Plate into four separate soup bowls; decorate each with red pepper flakes. Serve warm.

Roasted Brussels Sprouts with Sunflower Seeds

Ready in about: 45 minutes | Serves: 6
Per serving: Kcal: 186; Fat 17g, Net Carbs 8g, Protein 2.1g

Ingredients

¼ cup olive oil
3 pounds brussels sprouts, halved
Salt and black pepper, to taste
1 tsp sunflower seeds
2 tbsp fresh chives, chopped

Directions

Set oven to 390ºF. Arrange sprout halves on a greased baking sheet. Shake in pepper, salt, sunflower seeds, and olive oil. Roast for 40 minutes,

until the cabbage becomes soft. Top with chives to serve.

Fall Roasted Vegetables

Ready in about: 45 minutes | Serves: 4
Per serving: Kcal 165; Fat: 14.3g, Net Carbs: 8.2g,
Protein: 2.1g

Ingredients

3 mixed bell peppers, sliced
½ head broccoli, cut into florets
2 zucchinis, sliced
2 leeks, chopped
4 garlic cloves, halved
2 thyme sprigs, chopped
1 tsp dried sage, crushed
4 tbsp olive oil
2 tbsp vinegar
4 tbsp tomato puree
Salt and cayenne pepper, to taste

Directions

Set oven to 425ºF. Apply nonstick cooking spray to a rimmed baking sheet. Mix all vegetables with oil, seasonings, and vinegar; shake well. Roast for 40 minutes, flipping once halfway through.

Walnuts with Tofu

Ready in about: 13 minutes | Serves: 4
Per serving: Kcal 232; Fat: 21.6g, Net Carbs: 5.3g,
Protein: 8.3g

Ingredients

3 tsp olive oil
1 cup extra firm tofu, cubed
¼ cup walnuts, chopped
1 ½ tbsp coconut aminos
3 tbsp vegetable broth
½ tsp smashed garlic
1 tsp cayenne pepper
½ tsp turmeric powder
Salt and black pepper, to taste
2 tsp sunflower seeds

Directions

Set a frying pan over medium heat and warm the oil. Add in tofu and fry as you stir until browned. Pour in the walnuts; turn temperature to higher and cook for 2 minutes. Stir in the remaining ingredients, set heat to medium-low and cook for 5 more minutes. Drizzle with hot sauce and serve!

Creamy Almond and Turnip Soup

Ready in about: 25 minutes | Serves: 4
Per serving: Kcal 114; Fat: 6.5g, Net Carbs: 9.2g,
Protein: 3.8g

Ingredients

1 tbsp olive oil
1 cup onion, chopped
1 celery, chopped
2 cloves garlic, minced
2 turnips, peeled and chopped
4 cups vegetable broth
Salt and white pepper, to taste
¼ cup ground almonds

1 cup almond milk
1 tbsp fresh cilantro, chopped

Set a pot over medium heat and warm oil. Add in celery, garlic, and onion and sauté for 6 minutes. Stir in white pepper, broth, salt, and almonds. Boil the mixture. Set heat to low and simmer for 17 minutes. Transfer the soup to an immersion blender and puree. Decorate with fresh cilantro before serving.

Mushroom & Cauliflower Bake

Ready in about: 30 minutes | Serves: 4
Per serving: Kcal 113; Fat: 6.7g, Net Carbs: 11.6g, Protein: 5g

Ingredients
Cooking spray
1 head cauliflower, cut into florets
8 ounces mushrooms, halved
2 garlic cloves, smashed
2 tomatoes, pureed
¼ cup coconut oil, melted
1 tsp chili paprika paste
¼ tsp marjoram
½ tsp curry powder
Salt and black pepper, to taste

Directions
Set oven to 390ºF. Apply a cooking spray to a baking dish. Lay mushrooms and cauliflower in the baking dish. Around the vegetables, scatter smashed garlic. Place in the pureed tomatoes. Sprinkle over melted coconut oil and place in chili paprika paste, curry, black pepper, salt, and marjoram. Roast for 25 minutes, turning once. Place in a serving plate and serve with green salad.

Bell Pepper & Pumpkin with Avocado Sauce

Ready in about: 15 minutes | Serves: 4
Per serving: Kcal 233; Fat: 20.2g, Net Carbs: 11g, Protein: 1.9g

Ingredients
½ pound pumpkin, peeled
½ pound bell peppers
1 tbsp olive oil
1 avocado, peeled and pitted
1 lemon, juiced and zested
2 tbsp sesame oil
2 tbsp cilantro, chopped
1 onion, chopped
1 jalapeño pepper, deveined and minced
Salt and black pepper, to taste

Directions
Use a spiralizer to spiralize bell peppers and pumpkin. Using a large nonstick skillet, warm olive oil. Add in bell peppers and pumpkin and sauté for 8 minutes. Combine the remaining ingredients to obtain a creamy mixture. Top the vegetable noodles with the avocado sauce and serve.

Easy Vanilla Granola

Ready in about: 1 hour | Serves: 6
Per serving: Kcal 449; Fat: 44.9g, Net Carbs: 5.1g, Protein: 9.3g

Ingredients
½ cup hazelnuts, chopped
1 cup walnuts, chopped
⅓ cup flax meal
⅓ cup coconut milk
⅓ cup poppy seeds
⅓ cup pumpkin seeds
8 drops stevia
⅓ cup coconut oil, melted
1 ½ tsp vanilla paste
1 tsp ground cloves
1 tsp grated nutmeg
1 tsp lemon zest
⅓ cup water

Directions
Set oven to 300ºF. Line a parchment paper to a baking sheet. Combine all ingredients. Spread the mixture onto the baking sheet in an even layer. Bake for 55 minutes, as you stir at intervals of 15 minutes. Let cool at room temperature.

Kale Cheese Waffles

Ready in about: 45 minutes | Serves: 4
Per serving: Kcal 283, Fat: 20.2g, Net Carbs: 3.6g, Protein: 16g

Ingredients
2 green onions, chopped
1 tbsp olive oil
2 eggs
⅓ cup Parmesan cheese
1 cup kale, chopped
1 cup mozzarella cheese
½ cauliflower head, chopped
1 tsp garlic powder
1 tbsp sesame seeds
2 tsp chopped thyme

Directions
Place the chopped cauliflower in the food processor and process until rice is formed. Add kale, spring onions, and thyme to the food processor. Pulse until smooth. Transfer to a bowl. Stir in the rest of the ingredients and mix to combine.
Heat waffle iron and spread in ¼ cup of the mixture, evenly. Cook following the manufacturer's instructions until golden, about 10 minutes in total. Repeat with the remaining batter.

SOUPS, STEW & SALADS

Homemade Cold Gazpacho Soup

Ready in about: 15 minutes + chilling time | Serves: 6
Per serving: Kcal 528, Fat: 45.8g, Net Carbs: 6.5g,
Protein: 7.5g

Ingredients

2 small green peppers, roasted
2 large red peppers, roasted
2 medium avocados, flesh scoped out
2 garlic cloves
2 spring onions, chopped
1 cucumber, chopped
1 cup olive oil
2 tbsp lemon juice
4 tomatoes, chopped
7 ounces goat cheese
1 small red onion, chopped
2 tbsp apple cider vinegar
Salt to taste

Directions

Place the peppers, tomatoes, avocados, red onion,
garlic, lemon juice, olive oil, vinegar, and salt, in a
food processor. Pulse until your desired consistency
is reached. Taste and adjust the seasoning.

Transfer the mixture to a pot. Stir in cucumber and
spring onions. Cover and chill in the fridge at least 2
hours. Divide the soup between 6 bowls. Serve
topped with goat cheese and an extra drizzle of olive
oil.

Tip: For more protein, add cooked and chopped
shrimp to this refreshing delight.

Cream of Thyme Tomato Soup

Ready in about: 20 minutes | Serves: 6
Per serving: Kcal 310, Fat 27g, Net Carbs 3g, Protein
11g

Ingredients

2 tbsp ghee
2 large red onions, diced
½ cup raw cashew nuts, diced
2 (28 oz) cans tomatoes
1 tsp fresh thyme leaves + extra to garnish
1 ½ cups water
Salt and black pepper to taste
1 cup heavy cream

Directions

Melt ghee in a pot over medium heat and sauté the
onions for 4 minutes until softened.

Stir in the tomatoes, thyme, water, cashews, and
season with salt and black pepper. Cover and bring to
simmer for 10 minutes until thoroughly cooked.

Open, turn the heat off, and puree the ingredients
with an immersion blender. Adjust to taste and stir in
the heavy cream. Spoon into soup bowls and serve.

Green Minestrone Soup

Ready in about: 25 minutes | Serves: 4
Per serving: Kcal 227, Fat 20.3g, Net Carbs 2g,
Protein 8g

Ingredients

2 tbsp ghee
2 tbsp onion-garlic puree
2 heads broccoli, cut in florets
2 stalks celery, chopped
5 cups vegetable broth
1 cup baby spinach
Salt and black pepper to taste
2 tbsp Gruyere cheese, grated

Directions

Melt the ghee in a saucepan over medium heat and
sauté the onion-garlic puree for 3 minutes until
softened. Mix in the broccoli and celery, and cook for
4 minutes until slightly tender. Pour in the broth,
bring to a boil, then reduce the heat to medium-low
and simmer covered for about 5 minutes.

Drop in the spinach to wilt, adjust the seasonings,
and cook for 4 minutes. Ladle soup into serving
bowls. Serve with a sprinkle of grated Gruyere
cheese.

Creamy Cauliflower Soup with Bacon Chips

Ready in about: 25 minutes | Serves: 4
Per serving: Kcal 402, Fat 37g, Net Carbs 6g, Protein
8g

Ingredients

2 tbsp ghee
1 onion, chopped
2 head cauliflower, cut into florets
2 cups water
Salt and black pepper to taste
3 cups almond milk
1 cup shredded white cheddar cheese
3 bacon strips

Directions

Melt the ghee in a saucepan over medium heat and
sauté the onion for 3 minutes until fragrant.

Include the cauli florets, sauté for 3 minutes to
slightly soften, add the water, and season with salt
and black pepper. Bring to a boil, and then reduce the
heat to low. Cover and cook for 10 minutes. Puree
cauliflower with an immersion blender until the
ingredients are evenly combined and stir in the
almond milk and cheese until the cheese melts.
Adjust taste with salt and black pepper.

In a non-stick skillet over high heat, fry the bacon,
until crispy. Divide soup between serving bowls, top
with crispy bacon, and serve hot.

Power Green Soup

Ready in about: 30 minutes | Serves: 6
Per serving: Kcal 392, Fat: 37.6g, Net Carbs: 5.8g, Protein: 4.9g

Ingredients

1 broccoli head, chopped
1 cup spinach
1 onion, chopped
2 garlic cloves, minced
½ cup watercress
5 cups veggie stock
1 cup coconut milk
1 tbsp ghee
1 bay leaf
Salt and black pepper, to taste

Directions

Melt the ghee in a large pot over medium heat. Add onion and garlic, and cook for 3 minutes. Add broccoli and cook for an additional 5 minutes. Pour the stock over and add the bay leaf. Close the lid, bring to a boil, and reduce the heat. Simmer for about 3 minutes.

At the end, add spinach and watercress, and cook for 3 more minutes. Stir in the coconut cream, salt and black pepper. Discard the bay leaf, and blend the soup with a hand blender.

Slow Cooker Beer Soup with Cheddar & Sausage

Ready in about: 8 hr | Serves: 8
Per serving: Kcal 244, Fat: 17g, Net Carbs: 4g, Protein: 5g

Ingredients

1 cup heavy cream
10 ounces sausages, sliced
1 cup celery, chopped
1 cup carrots, chopped
4 garlic cloves, minced
8 ounces cream cheese
1 tsp red pepper flakes
6 ounces beer
16 ounces beef stock
1 onion, diced
1 cup cheddar cheese, grated
Salt and black pepper, to taste
Fresh cilantro, chopped, to garnish

Directions

Turn on the slow cooker. Add beef stock, beer, sausages, carrots, onion, garlic, celery, salt, red pepper flakes, and black pepper, and stir to combine. Pour in enough water to cover all the ingredients by roughly 2 inches. Close the lid and cook for 6 hours on Low.

Open the lid and stir in the heavy cream, cheddar, and cream cheese, and cook for 2 more hours. Ladle the soup into bowls and garnish with cilantro before serving. Yummy!

Beef Reuben Soup

Ready in about: 20 minutes | Serves: 6
Per serving: Kcal 450, Fat: 37g, Net Carbs: 8g, Protein: 23g

Ingredients

1 onion, diced
6 cups beef stock
1 tsp caraway seeds
2 celery stalks, diced
2 garlic cloves, minced
2 cups heavy cream
1 cup sauerkraut, shredded
1 pound corned beef, chopped
3 tbsp butter
1 ½ cup swiss cheese, shredded
Salt and black pepper, to taste

Directions

Melt the butter in a large pot. Add onion and celery, and fry for 3 minutes until tender. Add garlic and cook for another minute.

Pour the beef stock over and stir in sauerkraut, salt, caraway seeds, and add a pinch of black pepper. Bring to a boil. Reduce the heat to low, and add the corned beef. Cook for about 15 minutes, adjust the seasoning. Stir in heavy cream and cheese and cook for 1 minute.

Coconut, Green Beans & Shrimp Curry Soup

Ready in about: 20 minutes | Serves: 4
Per serving: Kcal 375, Fat 35.4g, Net Carbs 2g, Protein 9g

Ingredients

2 tbsp ghee
1 lb jumbo shrimp, peeled and deveined
2 tsp ginger-garlic puree
2 tbsp red curry paste
6 oz coconut milk
Salt and chili pepper to taste
1 bunch green beans, halved

Directions

Melt ghee in a medium saucepan over medium heat. Add the shrimp, season with salt and black pepper, and cook until they are opaque, 2 to 3 minutes. Remove shrimp to a plate. Add the ginger-garlic puree and red curry paste to the ghee and sauté for 2 minutes until fragrant.

Stir in the coconut milk; add the shrimp, salt, chili pepper, and green beans. Cook for 4 minutes. Reduce the heat to a simmer and cook an additional 3 minutes, occasionally stirring. Adjust taste with salt, fetch soup into serving bowls, and serve with cauli rice.

Brazilian Moqueca (Shrimp Stew)

Ready in about: 25 minutes | Serves: 6
Per serving: Kcal 324, Fat: 21g, Net Carbs: 5g, Protein: 23.1g

Ingredients

1 cup coconut milk
2 tbsp lime juice
¼ cup diced roasted peppers
1 ½ pounds shrimp, peeled and deveined
¼ cup olive oil
1 garlic clove, minced
14 ounces diced tomatoes
2 tbsp sriracha sauce
1 chopped onion
¼ cup chopped cilantro
Fresh dill, chopped to garnish
Salt and black pepper, to taste

Directions

Heat the olive oil in a pot over medium heat. Add onion and cook for 3 minutes or until translucent. Add the garlic and cook for another minute, until soft. Add tomatoes, shrimp, and cilantro. Cook until the shrimp becomes opaque, about 3-4 minutes.

Stir in sriracha sauce and coconut milk, and cook for 2 minutes. Do not bring to a boil. Stir in the lime juice and season with salt and pepper. Spoon the stew in bowls, garnish with fresh dill to serve.

Broccoli Cheese Soup

Ready in about: 20 minutes | Serves: 4
Per serving: Kcal 561, Fat: 52.3g, Net Carbs: 7g, Protein: 23.8g

Ingredients

¾ cup heavy cream
1 onion, diced
1 tsp minced garlic
4 cups chopped broccoli
4 cups veggie broth
2 tbsp butter
3 cups grated cheddar cheese
Salt and black pepper, to taste
½ bunch fresh mint, chopped

Directions

Melt the butter in a large pot over medium heat. Sauté onion and garlic for 3 minutes or until tender, stirring occasionally. Season with salt and black pepper. Add the broth, broccoli and bring to a boil.

Reduce the heat and simmer for 10 minutes. Puree the soup with a hand blender until smooth. Add in 2 ¾ cups of the cheddar cheese and cook about 1 minute. Taste and adjust the seasoning. Stir in the heavy cream. Serve in bowls with the remaining cheddar cheese and sprinkled with fresh mint.

Salsa Verde Chicken Soup

Ready in about: 15 minutes | Serves: 4
Per serving: Kcal 346, Fat: 23g, Net Carbs: 3g, Protein: 25g

Ingredients

½ cup salsa verde
2 cups cooked and shredded chicken
2 cups chicken broth
1 cup shredded cheddar cheese
4 ounces cream cheese
½ tsp chili powder
½ tsp ground cumin
½ tsp fresh cilantro, chopped
Salt and black pepper, to taste

Directions

Combine the cream cheese, salsa verde, and broth, in a food processor; pulse until smooth. Transfer the mixture to a pot and place over medium heat. Cook until hot, but do not bring to a boil. Add chicken, chili powder, and cumin and cook for about 3-5 minutes, or until it is heated through.

Stir in cheddar cheese and season with salt and pepper to taste. If it is very thick, add a few tablespoons of water and boil for 1-3 more minutes. Serve hot in bowls sprinkled with fresh cilantro.

Pumpkin & Meat Peanut Stew

Ready in about: 45 minutes | Serves: 6
Per serving: Kcal 451, Fat: 33g, Net Carbs: 4g, Protein: 27.5g

Ingredients

1 cup pumpkin puree
2 pounds chopped pork stew meat
1 tbsp peanut butter
4 tbsp chopped peanuts
1 garlic clove, minced
½ cup chopped onion
½ cup white wine
1 tbsp olive oil
1 tsp lemon juice
¼ cup granulated sweetener
¼ tsp cardamom powder
¼ tsp allspice
2 cups water
2 cups chicken stock

Directions

Heat the olive oil in a large pot and sauté onion for 3 minutes, until translucent. Add garlic and cook for 30 more seconds. Add the pork and cook until browned, about 5-6 minutes, stirring occasionally. Pour in the wine and cook for one minute.

Add in the remaining ingredients, except for the lemon juice and peanuts. Bring the mixture to a boil, and cook for 5 minutes. Reduce the heat to low, cover the pot, and let cook for about 30 minutes. Adjust seasonings and stir in the lemon juice before serving. Ladle into bowls and serve topped with peanuts.

Creamy Cauliflower Soup with Chorizo Sausage

Ready in about: 40 minutes | Serves: 4
Per serving: Kcal 251, Fat: 19.1g, Net Carbs: 5.7g, Protein: 10g

Ingredients

1 cauliflower head, chopped
1 turnip, chopped
3 tbsp butter
1 chorizo sausage, sliced
2 cups chicken broth
1 small onion, chopped
2 cups water
Salt and black pepper, to taste

Directions

Melt 2 tbsp of the butter in a large pot over medium heat. Stir in onion and cook until soft and golden, about 3-4 minutes. Add cauliflower and turnip, and cook for another 5 minutes.

Pour the broth and water over. Bring to a boil, simmer covered, and cook for about 20 minutes until the vegetables are tender. Remove from heat. Melt the remaining butter in a skillet. Add the chorizo sausage and cook for 5 minutes until crispy. Puree the soup with a hand blender until smooth. Taste and adjust the seasonings. Serve the soup in deep bowls topped with the chorizo sausage.

Thyme & Wild Mushroom Soup

Ready in about: 25 minutes | Serves: 4
Per serving: Kcal 281, Fat: 25g, Net Carbs: 5.8g, Protein: 6.1g

Ingredients

¼ cup butter
½ cup crème fraiche
12 oz wild mushrooms, chopped
2 tsp thyme leaves
2 garlic cloves, minced
4 cups chicken broth
Salt and black pepper, to taste

Directions

Melt the butter in a large pot over medium heat. Add garlic and cook for one minute until tender. Add mushrooms, salt and pepper, and cook for 10 minutes. Pour the broth over and bring to a boil.

Reduce the heat and simmer for 10 minutes. Puree the soup with a hand blender until smooth. Stir in crème fraiche. Garnish with thyme leaves before serving.

Chicken Creamy Soup

Ready in about: 15 minutes | Serves: 4
Per serving: Kcal 406, Fat: 29.5g, Net Carbs: 5g, Protein: 26.5g

Ingredients

2 cups cooked and shredded chicken
3 tbsp butter, melted
4 cups chicken broth

4 tbsp chopped cilantro
⅓ cup buffalo sauce
½ cup cream cheese
Salt and black pepper, to taste

Directions

Blend the butter, buffalo sauce, and cream cheese, in a food processor, until smooth. Transfer to a pot, add chicken broth and heat until hot but do not bring to a boil. Stir in chicken, salt, black pepper and cook until heated through. When ready, remove to soup bowls and serve garnished with cilantro.

Mediterranean Salad

Ready in about: 10 minutes | Serves: 4
Per serving: Kcal 290, Fat: 25g, Net Carbs: 4.3g, Protein: 9g

Ingredients

3 tomatoes, sliced
1 large avocado, sliced
8 kalamata olives
¼ lb buffalo mozzarella cheese, sliced
2 tbsp pesto sauce
2 tbsp olive oil

Directions

Arrange the tomato slices on a serving platter and place the avocado slices in the middle. Arrange the olives around the avocado slices and drop pieces of mozzarella on the platter. Drizzle the pesto sauce all over, and drizzle olive oil as well.

Cobb Egg Salad in Lettuce Cups

Ready in about: 25 minutes | Serves: 4
Per serving: Kcal 325, Fat 24.5g, Net Carbs 4g, Protein 21g

Ingredients

2 chicken breasts, cut into pieces
1 tbsp olive oil
Salt and black pepper to season
6 large eggs
1 ½ cups water
2 tomatoes, seeded, chopped
6 tbsp Greek yogurt
1 head green lettuce, firm leaves removed for cups

Directions

Preheat oven to 400ºF. Put the chicken pieces in a bowl, drizzle with olive oil, and sprinkle with salt and black pepper. Mix the ingredients until the chicken is well coated with the seasoning.

Put the chicken on a prepared baking sheet and spread out evenly. Slide the baking sheet in the oven and bake the chicken until cooked through and golden brown for 8 minutes, turning once.

Bring the eggs to boil in salted water in a pot over medium heat for 10 minutes. Run the eggs in cold water, peel, and chop into small pieces. Transfer to a salad bowl.

Remove the chicken from the oven when ready and add to the salad bowl. Include the tomatoes and Greek yogurt; mix evenly with a spoon. Layer two lettuce leaves each as cups and fill with two tablespoons of egg salad each. Serve with chilled blueberry juice.

Tuna Caprese Salad

Ready in about: 10 minutes | Serves: 4
Per serving: Kcal 360, Fat 31g, Net Carbs 1g, Protein 21g

Ingredients

2 (10 oz) cans tuna chunks in water, drained
2 tomatoes, sliced
8 oz fresh mozzarella cheese, sliced
6 basil leaves
½ cup black olives, pitted and sliced
2 tbsp extra virgin olive oil
½ lemon, juiced

Directions

Place the tuna in the center of a serving platter. Arrange the cheese and tomato slices around the tuna. Alternate a slice of tomato, cheese, and a basil leaf.
To finish, scatter the black olives over the top, drizzle with olive oil and lemon juice and serve.

Tuna Salad with Lettuce & Olives

Ready in about: 5 minutes | Serves: 2
Per serving: Kcal 248, Fat: 20g, Net Carbs: 2g, Protein: 18.5g

Ingredients

1 cup canned tuna, drained
1 tsp onion flakes
3 tbsp mayonnaise
1 cup shredded romaine lettuce
1 tbsp lime juice
Sea salt, to taste
6 black olives, pitted and sliced

Directions

Combine the tuna, mayonnaise, lime juice, and salt in a small bowl; mix to combine well. In a salad platter, arrange the shredded lettuce and onion flakes. Spread the tuna mixture over; top with black olives to serve.

Arugula Prawn Salad with Mayo Dressing

Ready in about: 15 minutes | Serves: 4
Per serving: Kcal 215, Fat 20.3g, Net Carbs 2g, Protein 8g

Ingredients

4 cups baby arugula
½ cup garlic mayonnaise
3 tbsp olive oil
1 lb tiger prawns, peeled and deveined
1 tsp Dijon mustard
Salt and chili pepper to season
2 tbsp lemon juice

Directions

First, make the dressing: add the mayonnaise, lemon juice and mustard in a small bowl. Mix until smooth and creamy. Set aside until ready to use.

Heat 2 tbsp of olive oil in a skillet over medium heat, add the prawns, season with salt, and chili pepper, and fry for 3 minutes on each side until prawns are pink. Set aside to a plate.
Place the arugula in a serving bowl and pour half of the dressing on the salad. Toss with 2 spoons until mixed, and add the remaining dressing. Divide salad onto 4 plates and top with prawns.

Lobster Salad with Mayo Dressing

Ready in about: 1 hour 10 minutes | Serves: 4
Per serving: Kcal 182, Fat: 15g, Net Carbs: 2g, Protein: 12g

Ingredients

1 small head cauliflower, cut into florets
⅓ cup diced celery
½ cup sliced black olives
2 cups cooked large shrimp
1 tbsp dill, chopped

Dressing:

½ cup mayonnaise
1 tsp apple cider vinegar
¼ tsp celery seeds
A pinch of black pepper
2 tbsp lemon juice
2 tsp swerve
Salt to taste

Directions

Combine the cauliflower, celery, shrimp, and dill in a large bowl.
Whisk together the mayonnaise, vinegar, celery seeds, black pepper, sweetener, and lemon juice in another bowl. Season with salt to taste. Pour the dressing over and gently toss to combine; refrigerate for 1 hour. Top with olives to serve.

Caesar Salad with Smoked Salmon and Poached Eggs

Ready in about: 15 minutes | Serves: 4
Per serving: Kcal 260, Fat 21g, Net Carbs 5g, Protein 8g

Ingredients

3 cups water
8 eggs
2 cups torn romaine lettuce
½ cup smoked salmon, chopped
6 slices bacon
2 tbsp Heinz low carb Caesar dressing

Directions

Boil the water in a pot over medium heat for 5 minutes and bring to simmer. Crack each egg into a small bowl and gently slide into the water. Poach for 2 to 3 minutes, remove with a perforated spoon, transfer to a paper towel to dry, and plate. Poach the remaining 7 eggs.
Put the bacon in a skillet and fry over medium heat until browned and crispy, about 6 minutes, turning once. Remove, allow cooling, and chop in small pieces. Toss the lettuce, smoked salmon, bacon, and Caesar dressing in a salad bowl. Divide the salad into 4

plates, top with two eggs each, and serve immediately or chilled.

Green Mackerel Salad
Ready in about: 25 minutes | Serves: 2
Per serving: Kcal 525, Fat: 41.9g, Net Carbs: 7.6g, Protein: 27.3g
Ingredients
2 mackerel fillets
2 hard-boiled eggs, sliced
1 tbsp coconut oil
2 cups green beans
1 avocado, sliced
4 cups mixed salad greens
2 tbsp olive oil
2 tbsp lemon juice
1 tsp Dijon mustard
Salt and black pepper, to taste
Directions
Fill a saucepan with water and add the green beans and salt. Cook over medium heat for about 3 minutes. Drain and set aside.
Melt the coconut oil in a pan over medium heat. Add the mackerel fillets and cook for about 4 minutes per side, or until opaque and crispy. Divide the green beans between two salad bowls. Top with mackerel, eggs, and avocado slices.
In a bowl, whisk together the lemon juice, olive oil, mustard, salt, and pepper, and drizzle over the salad.

Brussels Sprouts Salad with Pecorino Romano
Ready in about: 35 minutes | Serves: 6
Per serving: Kcal 210, Fat 18g, Net Carbs 6g, Protein 4g
Ingredients
2 lb Brussels sprouts, halved
3 tbsp olive oil
Salt and black pepper to taste
2 ½ tbsp balsamic vinegar
¼ head red cabbage, shredded
1 tbsp Dijon mustard
1 cup pecorino romano cheese, grated
Directions
Preheat oven to 400ºF and line a baking sheet with foil. Toss the brussels sprouts with olive oil, a little salt, black pepper, and balsamic vinegar, in a bowl, and spread on the baking sheet in an even layer. Bake until tender on the inside and crispy on the outside, about 20 to 25 minutes.
Transfer to a salad bowl and add the red cabbage, Dijon mustard and half of the cheese. Mix until well combined. Sprinkle with the remaining cheese, share the salad onto serving plates, and serve with syrup-grilled salmon.

Pork Burger Salad with Yellow Cheddar
Ready in about: 25 minutes | Serves: 4
Per serving: Kcal 310, Fat 23g, Net Carbs 2g, Protein 22g
Ingredients
1 lb ground pork
Salt and black pepper to season
1 tbsp olive oil
2 hearts romaine lettuce, torn into pieces
2 firm tomatoes, sliced
¼ red onion, sliced
3 oz yellow cheddar cheese, shredded
Directions
Season the pork with salt and black pepper, mix and make medium-sized patties out of them.
Heat the oil in a skillet over medium heat and fry the patties on both sides for 10 minutes until browned and cook within. Transfer to a wire rack to drain oil. When cooled, cut into quarters.
Mix the lettuce, tomatoes, and red onion in a salad bowl, season with a little oil, salt, and black pepper. Toss and add the pork on top.
Melt the cheese in the microwave for about 90 seconds. Drizzle the cheese over the salad and serve.

Bacon and Spinach Salad
Ready in about: 20 minutes | Serves: 4
Per serving: Kcal 350, Fat: 33g, Net Carbs: 3.4g, Protein: 7g
Ingredients
2 large avocados, 1 chopped and 1 sliced
1 spring onion, sliced
4 cooked bacon slices, crumbled
2 cups spinach
2 small lettuce heads, chopped
2 hard-boiled eggs, chopped
Vinaigrette:
3 tbsp olive oil
1 tsp Dijon mustard
1 tbsp apple cider vinegar
Directions
Combine the spinach, lettuce, eggs, chopped avocado, and spring onion, in a large bowl. Whisk together the vinaigrette ingredients in another bowl. Pour the dressing over, toss to combine and top with the sliced avocado and bacon.

Traditional Greek Salad
Ready in about: 10 minutes | Serves: 4
Per serving: Kcal 323, Fat: 28g, Net Carbs: 8g, Protein: 9.3g
Ingredients
5 tomatoes, chopped
1 large cucumber, chopped
1 green bell pepper, chopped
1 small red onion, chopped
16 kalamata olives, chopped
4 tbsp capers
1 cup feta cheese, chopped
1 tsp oregano, dried
4 tbsp olive oil
Salt to taste
Directions

Place tomatoes, bell pepper, cucumber, onion, feta cheese and olives in a bowl; mix to combine well. Season with salt. Combine capers, olive oil, and oregano, in a bowl. Drizzle with the dressing to serve.

Garlic Chicken Salad
Ready in about: 15 minutes | Serves: 4
Per serving: Kcal 286, Fat 23g, Net Carbs 4g, Protein 14g
Ingredients
2 chicken breasts, boneless, skinless, flattened
Salt and black pepper to taste
2 tbsp garlic powder
1 tsp olive oil
1 ½ cups mixed salad greens
1 tbsp red wine vinegar
1 cup crumbled blue cheese
Directions
Season the chicken with salt, black pepper, and garlic powder. Heat oil in a pan over high heat and fry the chicken for 4 minutes on both sides until golden brown. Remove chicken to a cutting board and let cool before slicing.
Toss salad greens with red wine vinegar and share the salads into 4 plates. Divide chicken slices on top and sprinkle with blue cheese. Serve salad with carrots fries.

Strawberry Salad with Spinach, Cheese & Almonds
Ready in about: 20 minutes | Serves: 2
Per serving: Kcal 445, Fat: 34.2g, Net Carbs: 5.3g, Protein: 33g
Ingredients
4 cups spinach
4 strawberries, sliced
½ cup flaked almonds
1 ½ cup grated hard goat cheese
4 tbsp raspberry vinaigrette
Salt and black pepper, to taste
Directions
Preheat your oven to 400ºF. Arrange the grated goat cheese in two circles on two pieces of parchment paper. Place in the oven and bake for 10 minutes.
Find two same bowls, place them upside down, and carefully put the parchment paper on top to give the cheese a bowl-like shape. Let cool that way for 15 minutes. Divide spinach among the bowls stir in salt, pepper and drizzle with vinaigrette. Top with almonds and strawberries.

Green Salad with Bacon and Blue Cheese
Ready in about: 15 minutes | Serves: 4
Per serving: Kcal 205, Fat 20g, Net Carbs 2g, Protein 4g
Ingredients
2 (8 oz) pack mixed salad greens
8 strips bacon
1 ½ cups crumbled blue cheese

1 tbsp white wine vinegar
3 tbsp extra virgin olive oil
Salt and black pepper to taste
Directions
Pour the salad greens in a salad bowl; set aside. Fry bacon strips in a skillet over medium heat for 6 minutes, until browned and crispy. Chop the bacon and scatter over the salad. Add in half of the cheese, toss and set aside.
In a small bowl, whisk the white wine vinegar, olive oil, salt, and black pepper until dressing is well combined. Drizzle half of the dressing over the salad, toss, and top with remaining cheese. Divide salad into four plates and serve with crusted chicken fries along with the remaining dressing.

Crispy Bacon Salad with Mozzarella & Tomato
Ready in about: 10 minutes | Serves: 2
Per serving: Kcal 279, Fat: 26g, Net Carbs: 1.5g, Protein: 21g
Ingredients
1 large tomato, sliced
4 basil leaves
8 mozzarella cheese slices
2 tsp olive oil
4 bacon slices, chopped
1 tsp balsamic vinegar
Salt, to taste
Directions
Place the bacon in a skillet over medium heat and cook until crispy, about 5 minutes. Divide the tomato slices between two serving plates. Arrange the mozzarella slices over and top with the basil leaves. Add the crispy bacon on top, drizzle with olive oil and vinegar. Sprinkle with salt and serve.

Warm Baby Artichoke Salad
Ready in about: 30 minutes | Serves: 4
Per serving: Kcal 170, Fat: 13g, Net Carbs: 5g, Protein: 1g
Ingredients
6 baby artichokes
6 cups water
1 tbsp lemon juice
¼ cup cherry peppers, halved
¼ cup pitted olives, sliced
¼ cup olive oil
¼ tsp lemon zest
2 tsp balsamic vinegar, sugar-free
1 tbsp chopped dill
Salt and black pepper to taste
1 tbsp capers
¼ tsp caper brine
Directions
Combine the water and salt in a pot over medium heat. Trim and halve the artichokes; add to the pot. Bring to a boil, lower the heat, and let simmer for 20 minutes until tender. Combine the rest of the ingredients, except for the olives in a bowl. Drain and

place the artichokes in a serving plate. Pour the prepared mixture over; toss to combine well. Serve topped with the olives.

Spring Salad with Cheese Balls

Ready in about: 20 minutes | Serves: 6
Per serving: Kcal: 234; Fat 16.7g, Net Carbs 7.9g, Protein 12.4g

Ingredients

Cheese balls:

3 eggs
1 cup feta cheese, crumbled
½ cup pecorino cheese, shredded
1 cup almond flour
1 tbsp flax meal
1 tsp baking powder
Salt and black pepper, to taste

Salad:

1 head iceberg lettuce, leaves separated
½ cup cucumber, thinly sliced
2 tomatoes, seeded and chopped
½ cup red onion, thinly sliced
½ cup radishes, thinly sliced
⅓ cup mayonnaise
1 tsp mustard
1 tsp paprika
1 tsp oregano
Salt, to taste

Directions

Set oven to 390ºF. Line a piece of parchment paper to a baking sheet.
In a mixing dish, mix all ingredients for the cheese balls; form balls out of the mixture. Set the balls on the prepared baking sheet. Bake for 10 minutes until crisp. Arrange lettuce leaves on a large salad platter; add in radishes, tomatoes, cucumbers, and red onion. In a small mixing bowl, mix the mayonnaise, paprika, salt, oregano, and mustard. Sprinkle this mixture over the vegetables. Add cheese balls on top and serve.

Squid Salad with Mint, Cucumber & Chili Dressing

Ready in about: 30 minutes | Serves: 4
Per serving: Kcal 318, Fat 22.5g, Net Carbs 2.1g, Protein 24.6g

Ingredients

4 medium squid tubes, cut into strips
½ cup mint leaves
2 medium cucumbers, halved and cut in strips
½ cup coriander leaves, reserve the stems
½ red onion, finely sliced
Salt and black pepper to taste
1 tsp fish sauce
1 red chili, roughly chopped
1 clove garlic
2 limes, juiced
1 tbsp chopped coriander
1 tsp olive oil

Directions

In a salad bowl, mix mint leaves, cucumber strips, coriander leaves, and red onion. Season with salt, black pepper and some olive oil; set aside. In the mortar, pound the coriander stems, and red chili to form a paste using the pestle. Add the fish sauce and lime juice, and mix with the pestle.
Heat a skillet over high heat on a stovetop and sear the squid on both sides to lightly brown, about 5 minutes. Pour the squid on the salad and drizzle with the chili dressing. Toss the ingredients with two spoons, garnish with coriander, and serve the salad as a single dish or with some more seafood.

Sriracha Egg Salad with Mustard Dressing

Ready in about: 15 minutes | Serves: 8
Per serving: Kcal 174; Fat 13g, Net Carbs 7.7g, Protein 7.4g

Ingredients

10 eggs
¾ cup mayonnaise
1 tsp sriracha sauce
1 tbsp mustard
½ cup scallions
½ stalk celery, minced
½ tsp fresh lemon juice
½ tsp sea salt
½ tsp black pepper
1 head romaine lettuce, torn into pieces

Directions

Add the eggs in a pan and cover with enough water and boil. Get them from the heat and allow to set for 10 minutes while covered. Chop the eggs and add to a salad bowl. Stir in the remaining ingredients until everything is well combined. Refrigerate until ready to serve.

Cobb Salad with Blue Cheese Dressing

Ready in about: 30 minutes | Serves: 6
Per serving: Kcal 122, Fat 14g, Net Carbs 2g, Protein 23g

Ingredients

Dressing:

½ cup buttermilk
1 cup mayonnaise
2 tbsp Worcestershire sauce
½ cup sour cream
1 ½ cup crumbled blue cheese
Salt and black pepper to taste
2 tbsp chopped chives

Salad:

6 eggs
2 chicken breasts, boneless and skinless
5 strips bacon
1 iceberg lettuce, cut into chunks
1 romaine lettuce, chopped
1 bibb lettuce, cored and leaves removed
2 avocado, pitted and diced
2 large tomatoes, chopped
½ cup crumbled blue cheese

2 scallions, chopped

Directions

In a bowl, whisk the buttermilk, mayonnaise, Worcestershire sauce, and sour cream. Stir in the blue cheese, salt, black pepper, and chives. Place in the refrigerator to chill until ready to use.

Bring the eggs to boil in salted water over medium heat for 10 minutes. Once ready, drain the eggs and transfer to the ice bath. Peel and chop the eggs. Set aside.

Preheat the grill pan over high heat. Season the chicken with salt and pepper. Grill for 3 minutes on each side. Remove to a plate to cool for 3 minutes, and cut into bite-size chunks. Fry the bacon in another pan set over medium heat until crispy, about 6 minutes. Remove, let cool for 2 minutes, and chop.

Arrange the lettuce leaves in a salad bowl and in single piles, add the avocado, tomatoes, eggs, bacon, and chicken. Sprinkle the blue cheese over the salad as well as the scallions and black pepper. Drizzle the blue cheese dressing on the salad and serve with low carb bread.

Spinach Turnip Salad with Bacon

Ready in about: 40 minutes | Serves: 4
Per serving: Kcal 193, Fat 18.3g, Net Carbs 3.1g, Protein 9.5g

Ingredients

2 turnips, cut into wedges
1 tsp olive oil
1 cup baby spinach, chopped
3 radishes, sliced
3 bacon slices
4 tbsp sour cream
2 tsp mustard seeds
1 tsp Dijon mustard
1 tbsp red wine vinegar
Salt and black pepper to taste
1 tbsp chopped chives

Directions

Preheat the oven to 400ºF. Line a baking sheet with parchment paper, toss the turnips with salt and black pepper, drizzle with the olive oil, and bake for 25 minutes, turning halfway. Let cool.

Spread the baby spinach in the bottom of a salad bowl and top with the radishes. Remove the turnips to the salad bowl. Fry the bacon in a skillet over medium heat until crispy, about 5 minutes.

Mix sour cream, mustard seeds, mustard, vinegar, and salt with the bacon. Add a little water to deglaze the bottom of the skillet. Pour the bacon mixture over the vegetables, scatter the chives over it. Serve.

Caesar Salad with Chicken and Parmesan

Ready in about: 1 hour and 30 minutes | Serves: 4
Per serving: Kcal 529, Fat: 39g, Net Carbs: 5g, Protein: 33g

Ingredients

4 boneless, skinless chicken thighs

¼ cup lemon juice
2 garlic cloves, minced
4 tbsp olive oil
½ cup Caesar salad dressing, sugar-free
12 bok choy leaves
3 Parmesan crisps
Parmesan cheese, grated for garnishing

Directions

Mix chicken, lemon juice, 2 tbsp olive oil and garlic in a ziploc bag. Seal the bag, shake well, and refrigerate for 1 hour. Preheat the grill to medium and grill the chicken for 4 minutes per side. Cut bok choy lengthwise, and brush with the remaining oil. Grill the bok choy for about 3 minutes. Place on a bowl. Top with chicken and Parmesan; drizzle the dressing over. Top with Parmesan crisps to serve.

Shrimp with Avocado & Cauliflower Salad

Ready in about: 30 minutes | Serves: 6
Per serving: Kcal 214, Fat: 17g, Net Carbs: 5g, Protein: 15g

Ingredients

1 cauliflower head, florets only
1 pound medium shrimp
¼ cup + 1 tbsp olive oil
1 avocado, chopped
3 tbsp chopped dill
¼ cup lemon juice
2 tbsp lemon zest
Salt and black pepper to taste

Directions

Heat 1 tbsp olive oil in a skillet and cook shrimp for 8 minutes. Microwave cauliflower for 5 minutes. Place shrimp, cauliflower, and avocado in a bowl. Whisk the remaining olive oil, lemon zest, juice, dill, and salt, and pepper, in another bowl. Pour the dressing over, toss to combine and serve immediately.

Grilled Steak Salad with Pickled Peppers

Ready in about: 15 minutes | Serves: 4
Per serving: Kcal 315, Fat 26g, Net Carbs 2g, Protein 18g

Ingredients

1 lb skirt steak, sliced
Salt and black pepper to season
1 tsp olive oil
1 ½ cups mixed salad greens
3 chopped pickled peppers
2 tbsp red wine vinaigrette
½ cup crumbled queso fresco

Directions

Brush the steak slices with olive oil and season with salt and black pepper on both sides. Heat pan over high heat and cook the steaks on each side for about 5-6 minutes. Remove to a bow. Mix the salad greens, pickled peppers, and vinaigrette in a salad bowl. Add the beef and sprinkle with queso fresco.

Broccoli Slaw Salad with Mustard-Mayo Dressing

Ready in about: 10 minutes | Serves: 6
Per serving: Kcal 110, Fat: 10g, Net Carbs: 2g, Protein: 3g

Ingredients

2 tbsp granulated swerve
1 tbsp Dijon mustard
1 tbsp olive oil
4 cups broccoli slaw
⅓ cup mayonnaise, sugar-free
1 tsp celery seeds
1 ½ tbsp apple cider vinegar
Salt and black pepper, to taste

Directions

Whisk together all ingredients except the broccoli slaw. Place broccoli slaw in a large salad bowl. Pour the dressing over. Mix with your hands to combine well.

SIDE DISHES & SNACKS

Roasted Cauliflower with Serrano Ham & Pine Nuts

Ready in about: 30 minutes | Serves: 6
Per serving: Kcal 141, Fat 10g, Net Carbs 2.5g, Protein 10g

Ingredients

2 heads cauliflower, cut into 1-inch slices
2 tbsp olive oil
Salt and chili pepper to taste
1 tsp garlic powder
10 slices Serrano ham, chopped
¼ cup pine nuts, chopped
1 tsp capers
1 tsp parsley

Directions

Preheat oven to 450ºF and line a baking sheet with foil. Brush the cauli steaks with olive oil and season with chili pepper, garlic, and salt. Spread the cauli slices on the baking sheet.

Roast in the oven for 10 minutes until tender and lightly browned. Remove the sheet and sprinkle the ham and pine nuts all over the cauli. Bake for another 10 minutes until the ham is crispy and a nutty aroma is perceived. Take out, sprinkle with capers and parsley and serve.

Mascarpone Snapped Amaretti Biscuits

Ready in about: 25 minutes | Serves: 6
Per serving: Kcal 165, Fat 13g, Net Carbs 3g, Protein 9g

Ingredients

6 egg whites
1 egg yolk, beaten
1 tsp vanilla bean paste
8 oz swerve confectioner's sugar
A pinch of salt
¼ cup ground fragrant almonds
1 lemon juice
7 tbsp sugar-free amaretto liquor
¼ cup mascarpone cheese
¼ cup butter, room temperature
¾ cup swerve confectioner's sugar, for topping

Directions

Preheat an oven to 300ºF and line a baking sheet with parchment paper. Set aside.

In a bowl, beat eggs whites, salt, and vanilla paste with the hand mixer while you gradually spoon in 8 oz of swerve confectioner's sugar until a stiff mixture. Add almonds and fold in the egg yolk, lemon juice, and amaretto liquor. Spoon mixture into the piping bag and press out 50 mounds on the baking sheet.

Bake the biscuits for 15 minutes by which time they should be golden brown. Whisk the mascarpone cheese, butter, and swerve confectioner's sugar with the cleaned electric mixer; set aside.

When the biscuits are ready, transfer to a bowl and let cool. Spread a scoop of mascarpone cream onto one biscuit and snap with another biscuit. Sift some swerve confectioner's sugar on top to serve.

Balsamic Brussels Sprouts with Prosciutto

Ready in about: 40 minutes | Serves: 4
Per serving: Kcal 166, Fat 14g, Net Carbs 0g, Protein 8g

Ingredients

3 tbsp balsamic vinegar
1 tbsp erythritol
½ tbsp olive oil
Salt and black pepper to taste
1 lb Brussels sprouts, halved
5 slices prosciutto, chopped

Directions

Preheat oven to 400ºF and line a baking sheet with parchment paper. Mix balsamic vinegar, erythritol, olive oil, salt, and black pepper and combine with the brussels sprouts in a bowl. Spread the mixture on the baking sheet and roast for 30 minutes until tender on the inside and crispy on the outside. Toss with prosciutto, share among 4 plates, and serve with chicken breasts.

Parmesan Crackers with Guacamole

Ready in about: 10 minutes | Serves: 4
Per serving: Kcal 229, Fat 20g, Net Carbs 2g, Protein 10g

Ingredients

1 cup finely grated Parmesan cheese
¼ tsp sweet paprika
¼ tsp garlic powder
2 soft avocados, pitted and scooped
1 tomato, chopped
Salt to taste

Directions

Preheat oven to 350ºF and line a baking sheet with parchment paper. Mix Parmesan cheese, paprika, and garlic powder. Spoon 8 teaspoons on the baking sheet creating spaces between each mound. Flatten mounds. Bake for 5 minutes, cool, and remove to a plate.

To make the guacamole, mash avocado, with a fork in a bowl, add in tomato and continue to mash until mostly smooth. Season with salt. Serve crackers with guacamole.

Cheesy Chicken Fritters with Dill Dip

Ready in about: 40 minutes + cooling time | Serves: 4
Per serving: Kcal 151, Fat 7g, Net Carbs 0.8g, Protein 12g

Ingredients

1 lb chicken breasts, thinly sliced
1 ¼ cup mayonnaise
¼ cup coconut flour
2 eggs
Salt and black pepper to taste
1 cup mozzarella cheese, grated
4 tbsp dill, chopped

3 tbsp olive oil
1 cup sour cream
1 tsp garlic powder
1 tbsp parsley, chopped
1 onion, finely chopped

Directions

In a bowl, mix 1 cup of the mayonnaise, 3 tbsp of dill, sour cream, garlic powder, onion, and salt. Cover the bowl with plastic wrap and refrigerate for 30 minutes.

Mix the chicken, remaining mayonnaise, coconut flour, eggs, salt, black pepper, mozzarella, and remaining dill, in a bowl. Cover the bowl with plastic wrap and refrigerate it for 2 hours. After the marinating time is over, remove from the fridge.

Place a skillet over medium fire and heat the olive oil. Fetch 2 tablespoons of chicken mixture into the skillet, use the back of a spatula to flatten the top. Cook for 4 minutes, flip, and fry for 4 more.

Remove onto a wire rack and repeat the cooking process until the batter is finished, adding more oil as needed. Garnish the fritters with parsley and serve with dill dip.

Devilled Eggs with Sriracha Mayo

Ready in about: 15 minutes | Serves: 4
Per serving: Kcal 195, Fat 19g, Net Carbs 1g, Protein 4g

Ingredients

8 large eggs
3 cups water
Ice water bath
3 tbsp sriracha sauce
4 tbsp mayonnaise
Salt to taste
¼ tsp smoked paprika

Directions

Bring eggs to boil in salted water in a pot over high heat, and then reduce the heat to simmer for 10 minutes. Transfer eggs to an ice water bath, let cool completely and peel the shells.

Slice the eggs in half height wise and empty the yolks into a bowl. Smash with a fork and mix in sriracha sauce, mayonnaise, and half of the paprika until smooth. Spoon filling into a piping bag with a round nozzle and fill the egg whites to be slightly above the brim. Garnish with remaining paprika and serve.

Bacon Mashed Cauliflower

Ready in about: 40 minutes | Serves: 6
Per serving: Kcal 312, Fat 25g, Net Carbs 6g, Protein 14g

Ingredients

6 slices bacon
3 heads cauliflower, leaves removed
2 cups water
2 tbsp melted butter
½ cup buttermilk
Salt and black pepper to taste
¼ cup grated yellow cheddar cheese

2 tbsp chopped chives

Directions

Preheat oven to 350ºF. Fry bacon in a heated skillet over medium heat for 5 minutes until crispy. Remove to a paper towel-lined plate, allow to cool, and crumble. Set aside and keep bacon fat. Boil cauli heads in water in a pot over high heat for 7 minutes, until tender. Drain and put in a bowl.

Include butter, buttermilk, salt, black pepper, and puree using a hand blender until smooth and creamy. Lightly grease a casserole dish with the bacon fat and spread the mash on it.

Sprinkle with cheddar cheese and place under the broiler for 4 minutes on high until the cheese melts. Remove and top with bacon and chopped chives. Serve with pan-seared scallops.

Crunchy Pork Rind and Zucchini Sticks

Ready in about: 20 minutes | Serves: 4
Per serving: Kcal 180, Fat 14g, Net Carbs 2g, Protein 6g

Ingredients

¼ cup pork rind crumbs
1 tsp sweet paprika
¼ cup shredded Parmesan cheese
Salt and chili pepper to taste
3 fresh eggs
2 zucchinis, cut into strips

Aioli:

½ cup mayonnaise
1 garlic clove, minced
Juice and zest from ½ lemon

Directions

Preheat oven to 425ºF and line a baking sheet with foil. Grease with cooking spray and set aside. Mix the pork rinds, paprika, Parmesan cheese, salt, and chili pepper in a bowl. Beat the eggs in another bowl. Coat zucchini strips in eggs, then in Parmesan mixture, and arrange on the baking sheet. Grease lightly with cooking spray and bake for 15 minutes to be crispy.

To make the aioli, combine in a bowl mayonnaise, lemon juice, and garlic, and gently stir until everything is well incorporated. Add the lemon zest, adjust the seasoning and stir again. Cover and place in the refrigerator until ready to serve. Serve the zucchini strips with garlic aioli for dipping.

Baked Cheese & Spinach Balls

Ready in about: 30 minutes | Serves: 8
Per serving: Kcal 160, Fat: 15g, Net Carbs: 0.8g, Protein: 8g

Ingredients

⅓ cup crumbled ricotta cheese
¼ tsp nutmeg
¼ tsp pepper
3 tbsp heavy cream
1 tsp garlic powder
1 tbsp onion powder
2 tbsp butter, melted
⅓ cup Parmesan cheese, shredded

2 eggs
1 cup spinach
1 cup almond flour

Directions
Place all ingredients in a food processor. Process until smooth. Place in the freezer for about 10 minutes. Make balls out of the mixture and arrange them on a lined baking sheet. Bake in the oven at 350ºF for about 10-12 minutes.

Duo-Cheese Chicken Bake

Ready in about: 30 minutes | Serves: 6
Per serving: Kcal 216, Fat 16g, Net Carbs 3g, Protein 14g

Ingredients
2 tbsp olive oil
8 oz cream cheese
1 lb ground chicken
1 cup buffalo sauce
1 cup ranch dressing
3 cups grated yellow cheddar cheese

Directions
Preheat oven to 350ºF. Lightly grease a baking sheet with a cooking spray. Warm the oil in a skillet over medium heat and brown the chicken for a couple of minutes, take off the heat, and set aside.

Spread cream cheese at the bottom of the baking sheet, top with chicken, pour buffalo sauce over, add ranch dressing, and sprinkle with cheddar cheese. Bake for 23 minutes until cheese has melted and golden brown on top. Remove and serve with veggie sticks or low carb crackers.

Spicy Chicken Cucumber Bites

Ready in about: 5 minutes | Serves: 6
Per serving: Kcal 170, Fat 14g, Net Carbs 0g, Protein 10g

Ingredients
2 cucumbers, sliced with a 3-inch thickness
2 cups small dices leftover chicken
¼ jalapeño pepper, seeded and minced
1 tbsp Dijon mustard
⅓ cup mayonnaise
Salt and black pepper to taste

Directions
Cut mid-level holes in cucumber slices with a knife and set aside. Combine chicken, jalapeno pepper, mustard, mayonnaise, salt, and black pepper to be evenly mixed. Fill cucumber holes with chicken mixture and serve.

Cheesy Cauliflower Bake with Mayo Sauce

Ready in about: 27 minutes | Serves: 6
Per serving: Kcal 363, Fat 35g, Net Carbs 2g, Protein 6g

Ingredients
2 heads cauliflower, cut into florets
¼ cup melted butter
Salt and black pepper to taste

1 pinch red pepper flakes
½ cup mayonnaise
¼ tsp Dijon mustard
3 tbsp grated pecorino cheese

Directions
Preheat oven to 400ºF and grease a baking dish with cooking spray.

Combine the cauli florets, butter, salt, black pepper, and red pepper flakes in a bowl until well mixed. Mix the mayonnaise and Dijon mustard in a bowl, and set aside until ready to serve.

Arrange cauliflower florets on the prepared baking dish. Sprinkle with grated pecorino cheese and bake for 25 minutes until the cheese has melted and golden brown on the top. Remove, let sit for 3 minutes to cool, and serve with the mayo sauce.

Zucchini Gratin with Feta Cheese

Ready in about: 65 minutes | Serves: 6
Per serving: Kcal 264, Fat 21g, Net Carbs 4g, Protein 14g

Ingredients
2 lb zucchinis, sliced
2 red bell peppers, seeded and sliced
Salt and black pepper to taste
1 ½ cups crumbled feta cheese
2 tbsp butter, melted
¼ tsp xanthan gum
½ cup heavy whipping cream

Directions
Preheat oven to 370ºF. Place the sliced zucchinis in a colander over the sink, sprinkle with salt and let sit for 20 minutes. Transfer to paper towels to drain the excess liquid.

Grease a baking dish with cooking spray and make a layer of zucchini and bell peppers overlapping one another. Season with pepper, and sprinkle with feta cheese. Repeat the layering process a second time.

Combine the butter, xanthan gum, and whipping cream in a bowl, stir to mix completely, and pour over the vegetables. Bake for 30-40 minutes or until golden brown on top.

Coconut Ginger Macaroons

Ready in about: 20 minutes | Serves: 6
Per serving: Kcal 97, Fat 3.5g, Net Carbs 0.3g, Protein 6.8g

Ingredients
2 fingers ginger root, pureed
6 egg whites
1 cup finely shredded coconut
¼ cup swerve
A pinch of chili powder
1 cup water
Angel hair chili to garnish

Directions
Preheat the oven to 350ºF and line a baking sheet with parchment paper. Set aside.

In a heatproof bowl, whisk ginger, egg whites, coconut, swerve, and chili powder. Bring the water to boil in a pot over medium heat and place the heatproof bowl on the pot. Continue whisking the mixture until it is glossy, about 4 minutes. Do not let the bowl touch the water or be too hot so that the eggs don't cook.

Spoon the mixture into the piping bag after and pipe out 40 to 50 little mounds on the lined baking sheet. Bake the macaroons in the middle part of the oven for 15 minutes. Once they are ready, transfer them to a wire rack, garnish them with the angel hair chili, and serve.

Cheesy Green Bean Crisps

Ready in about: 30 minutes | Serves: 6
Per serving: Kcal 210, Fat 19g, Net Carbs 3g, Protein 5g

Ingredients

¼ cup pecorino romano cheese, shredded
¼ cup pork rind crumbs
1 tsp garlic powder
Salt and black pepper to taste
2 eggs
1 lb green beans, thread removed

Directions

Preheat oven to 425ºF and line two baking sheets with foil. Grease with cooking spray and set aside.
Mix the pecorino, pork rinds, garlic powder, salt, and black pepper in a bowl. Beat the eggs in another bowl. Coat green beans in eggs, then cheese mixture and arrange evenly on the baking sheets.
Grease lightly with cooking spray and bake for 15 minutes to be crispy. Transfer to a wire rack to cool before serving. Serve with sugar-free tomato dip.

Crispy Chorizo with Cheesy Topping

Ready in about: 30 minutes | Serves: 6
Per serving: Kcal 172, Fat: 13g, Net Carbs: 0g, Protein: 5g

Ingredients

7 ounces Spanish chorizo, sliced
4 ounces cream cheese
¼ cup chopped parsley

Directions

Preheat oven to 325ºF. Line a baking dish with waxed paper. Bake chorizo for 15 minutes until crispy. Remove and let cool. Arrange on a serving platter. Top with cream cheese. Serve sprinkled with parsley.

Mixed Roast Vegetables

Ready in about: 40 minutes | Serves: 4
Per serving: Kcal 65, Fat 3g, Net Carbs 8g, Protein 3g

Ingredients

1 large butternut squash, cut into chunks
¼ lb shallots, peeled
2 rutabagas, cut into chunks
¼ lb Brussels sprouts
1 sprig rosemary, chopped
1 sprig thyme, chopped
4 cloves garlic, peeled only
3 tbsp olive oil

Salt and black pepper to taste

Directions

Preheat the oven to 450ºF.
Pour the butternut squash, shallots, rutabagas, garlic cloves, and Brussels sprouts in a bowl. Season with salt, black pepper, olive oil, and toss. Pour the mixture on a baking sheet and sprinkle with the chopped thyme and rosemary. Roast the vegetables for 15–20 minutes. Once ready, remove and spoon into a serving bowl. Serve with oven roasted chicken thighs.

Buttery Herb Roasted Radishes

Ready in about: 25 minutes | Serves: 6
Per serving: Kcal 160, Fat 14g, Net Carbs 2g, Protein 5g

Ingredients

2 lb small radishes, greens removed
3 tbsp olive oil
Salt and black pepper to season
3 tbsp unsalted butter
1 tbsp chopped parsley
1 tbsp chopped tarragon

Directions

Preheat oven to 400ºF and line a baking sheet with parchment paper. Toss radishes with oil, salt, and black pepper. Spread on baking sheet and roast for 20 minutes until browned.
Heat butter in a large skillet over medium heat to brown and attain a nutty aroma, 2 to 3 minutes.
Take out the radishes from the oven and transfer to a serving plate. Pour over the browned butter atop and sprinkle with parsley and tarragon. Serve with roasted rosemary chicken.

Bacon-Wrapped Jalapeño Peppers

Ready in about: 30 minutes | Serves: 6
Per serving: Kcal 206, Fat 17g, Net Carbs 0g, Protein 14g

Ingredients

12 jalapeno peppers
¼ cup shredded colby cheese
6 oz cream cheese, softened
6 slices bacon, halved

Directions

Cut the jalapeno peppers in half, and then remove the membrane and seeds. Combine cheeses and stuff into the pepper halves. Wrap each pepper with a bacon strip and secure with toothpicks.
Place the filled peppers on a baking sheet lined with a piece of foil. Bake at 350ºF for 25 minutes until bacon has browned, and crispy and cheese is golden brown on the top. Remove to a paper towel lined plate to absorb grease, arrange on a serving plate, and serve warm.

Turkey Pastrami & Mascarpone Cheese Pinwheels

Ready in about: 40 minutes | Serves: 4
Per serving: Kcal 266, Fat 24g, Net Carbs 0g, Protein 13g

Ingredients

Cooking spray
8 oz mascarpone cheese
10 oz turkey pastrami, sliced
10 canned pepperoncini peppers, sliced and drained

Directions

Lay a 12 x 12 plastic wrap on a flat surface and arrange the pastrami all over slightly overlapping each other. Spread the cheese on top of the salami layers and arrange the pepperoncini on top.

Hold two opposite ends of the plastic wrap and roll the pastrami. Twist both ends to tighten and refrigerate for 2 hours. Unwrap the salami roll and slice into 2-inch pinwheels. Serve.

Garlicky Cheddar Biscuits

Ready in about: 20 minutes | Serves: 4
Per serving: Kcal 153, Fat 14.2g, Net Carbs 1.4g, Protein 5.4g

Ingredients

⅓ cup almond flour
2 tsp garlic powder
Salt to taste
1 tsp baking powder
5 eggs
⅓ cup butter, melted
1 ¼ cups grated sharp cheddar cheese
⅓ cup Greek yogurt

Directions

Preheat the oven to 350ºF.

Mix the flour, garlic powder, salt, baking powder, and cheddar cheese, in a bowl.

In a separate bowl, whisk the eggs, butter, and Greek yogurt, and then pour the resulting mixture into the dry ingredients. Stir well until a dough-like consistency has formed. Fetch half tbsp of the mixture onto a baking sheet with 2-inch intervals between each batter. Bake for 12 minutes golden brown.

Roasted Stuffed Piquillo Peppers

Ready in about: 20 minutes | Serves: 8
Per serving: Kcal 132, Fat: 11g, Net Carbs: 2.5g, Protein: 6g

Ingredients

8 canned roasted piquillo peppers
1 tbsp olive oil
3 slices prosciutto, cut into thin slices
1 tbsp balsamic vinegar
Filling:
8 ounces goat cheese
3 tbsp heavy cream
3 tbsp chopped parsley

½ tsp minced garlic
1 tbsp olive oil
1 tbsp chopped mint

Directions

Mix all filling ingredients in a bowl. Place in a freezer bag, press down and squeeze, and cut off the bottom. Drain and deseed the peppers. Squeeze about 2 tbsp of the filling into each pepper.

Wrap a prosciutto slice onto each pepper. Secure with toothpicks. Arrange them on a serving platter. Sprinkle the olive oil and vinegar over.

Herb Cheese Sticks

Ready in about: 15 minutes | Serves: 4
Per serving: Kcal 188, Fat 17.3g, Net Carbs 0g, Protein 8g

Ingredients

1 cup pork rinds, crushed
1 tbsp Italian herb mix
1 egg
1 lb swiss cheese, cut into sticks

Directions

Preheat oven to 350ºF and line a baking sheet with parchment paper. Combine pork rinds and herb mix in a bowl to be evenly mixed and beat the egg in another bowl. Coat the cheese sticks in the egg and then generously dredge in pork rind mixture. Arrange on the baking sheet. Bake for 4 to 5 minutes, take out after, let cool for 2 minutes, and serve with marinara sauce.

Buttered Broccoli

Ready in about: 10 minutes | Serves: 6
Per serving: Kcal 114, Fat: 7.8g, Net Carbs: 5.5g, Protein: 3.9g

Ingredients

1 broccoli head, florets only
Kosher salt and black pepper to taste
¼ cup butter

Directions

Place the broccoli in a pot filled with salted water and bring to a boil. Cook for about 3 minutes until crisp-tender. Drain the broccoli and transfer to a plate. Melt the butter in a microwave. Drizzle the butter over and season with some salt and black pepper.

Cheesy Cauliflower Fritters

Ready in about: 35 minutes | Serves: 4
Per serving: Kcal 69, Fat: 4.5g, Net Carbs: 3g, Protein: 4.5g

Ingredients

1 pound grated cauliflower
½ cup Parmesan cheese, grated
3 ounces chopped onion
½ tsp baking powder
½ cup almond flour
2 eggs
½ tsp lemon juice
2 tbsp olive oil
⅓ tsp salt

Directions

Sprinkle the salt over the cauliflower in a bowl, and let it stand for 10 minutes. Add in the other ingredients. Mix with your hands to combine. Place a skillet over medium heat, and heat olive oil.

Shape fritters out of the cauliflower mixture. Fry in batches, for about 3 minutes per side.

Italian-Style Chicken Wraps

Ready in about: 20 minutes | Serves: 8
Per serving: Kcal 174, Fat: 10g, Net Carbs: 0.7g, Protein: 17g

Ingredients

¼ tsp garlic powder
8 ounces provolone cheese
8 raw chicken tenders
Salt and black pepper to taste
8 prosciutto slices

Directions

Pound the chicken until half an inch thick. Season with salt, black pepper, and garlic powder. Cut the provolone cheese into 8 strips. Place a slice of prosciutto on a flat surface. Place one chicken tender on top. Top with a provolone strip.

Roll the chicken and secure with previously soaked skewers. Grill the wraps for 3 minutes per side.

Boiled Stuffed Eggs

Ready in about: 30 minutes | Serves: 6
Per serving: Kcal 178, Fat: 17g, Net Carbs: 5g, Protein: 6g

Ingredients

6 eggs
1 tbsp green tabasco
⅓ cup mayonnaise
Salt to taste

Directions

Place the eggs in a saucepan and cover with salted water. Bring to a boil over medium heat. Boil for 10 minutes. Place the eggs in an ice bath and let cool for 10 minutes.

Peel and slice in half lengthwise. Scoop out the yolks to a bowl; mash with a fork. Whisk together the tabasco, mayonnaise, mashed yolks, and salt, in a bowl. Spoon this mixture into egg whites.

Nutty Avocado Crostini with Nori

Ready in about: 12 minutes | Serves: 4
Per serving: Kcal 195, Fat 12.2g, Net Carbs 2.8g, Protein 13.7g

Ingredients

8 slices low carb bread (baguette)
4 nori sheets
1 cup mashed avocado
⅓ tsp salt
1 tsp lemon juice
1 ½ tbsp coconut oil
⅓ cup chopped raw walnuts
1 tbsp chia seeds

Directions

In a bowl, flake the nori sheets into the smallest possible pieces.

In another bowl, mix the avocado, salt, and lemon juice, and stir in half of the nori flakes. Set aside.

Place the bread slices on a baking sheet and toast in a broiler on medium heat for 2 minutes, making sure not to burn. Remove the crostini after and brush with coconut oil on both sides. Top each crostini with the avocado mixture and garnish with the chia seeds, chopped walnuts, Serve.

Parmesan Crackers

Ready in about: 25 minutes | Serves: 6
Per serving: Kcal 115, Fat 3g, Net Carbs 0.7g, Protein 5g

Ingredients

1 ⅓ cups coconut flour
1 ¼ cup grated Parmesan cheese
Salt and black pepper to taste
1 tsp garlic powder
⅓ cup butter, softened
⅓ tsp sweet paprika
⅓ cup heavy cream

Directions

Preheat the oven to 350ºF.

Mix the coconut flour, Parmesan cheese, salt, pepper, garlic powder, and paprika in a bowl. Add in the butter and mix well. Top with the heavy cream and mix again until a smooth, thick mixture has formed. Add 1 to 2 tablespoon of water at this point, if it is too thick.

Place the dough on a cutting board and cover with plastic wrap. Use a rolling pin to spread out the dough into a light rectangle. Cut cracker squares out of the dough and arrange them on a baking sheet without overlapping. Bake for 20 minutes and transfer to a serving bowl after.

Parsnip and Carrot Fries with Aioli

Ready in about: 40 minutes + chilling time | Serves: 4
Per serving: Kcal 155, Fat 7.4g, Net Carbs 7.4g, Protein 2.1g

Ingredients

Aioli:
4 tbsp mayonnaise
2 garlic cloves, minced
Salt and black pepper to taste
3 tbsp lemon juice
Parsnip and carrots fries:
4 medium parsnips, julienned
3 large carrots, julienned
2 tbsp olive oil
2 tbsp chopped parsley
Salt and black pepper to taste

Directions

Preheat the oven to 400ºF. Make the aioli by mixing the mayonnaise with garlic, salt, black pepper, and lemon juice; then refrigerate for 30 minutes.

Spread parsnips and carrots on a baking sheet. Drizzle with olive oil, sprinkle with salt and pepper, and rub the seasoning into the veggies. Bake for 35 minutes. Garnish with parsley and serve.

Spicy Devilled Eggs with Herbs
Ready in about: 30 minutes | Serves: 4
Per serving: Kcal 112, Fat 9.3g, Net Carbs 0.4g, Protein 6.7g

Ingredients

12 large eggs
1 ½ cups water
6 tbsp mayonnaise
Salt and chili pepper to taste
1 tsp mixed dried herbs
½ tsp sugar-free Worcestershire sauce
¼ tsp Dijon mustard
A pinch of sweet paprika
Chopped parsley to garnish

Directions

Pour the water into a saucepan, add the eggs, and bring to boil on high heat for 10 minutes. Cut the eggs in half lengthways and remove the yolks into a medium bowl. Use a fork to crush the yolks.

Add the mayonnaise, salt, chili pepper, dried herbs, Worcestershire sauce, mustard, and paprika. Mix together until a smooth paste has formed. Then, spoon the mixture into the piping bag and fill the egg white holes with it. Garnish with the chopped parsley and serve immediately.

Cocoa Nuts Goji Bars
Ready in about: 5 minutes | Serves: 6
Per serving: Kcal 170, Fat 11g, Net Carbs 6g, Protein 2g

Ingredients

1 cup raw almonds
1 cup raw walnuts
¼ tsp cinnamon powder
¼ cup dried goji berries
1 ½ tsp vanilla extract
2 tbsp unsweetened chocolate chips
2 tbsp coconut oil
1 tbsp golden flax meal
1 tsp erythritol

Directions

Combine the walnuts and almonds in the food processor and process until smooth. Add the cinnamon powder, goji berries, vanilla extract, chocolate chips, coconut oil, golden flax meal, and erythritol. Process further until the mixture begins to stick to each other, about 2 minutes.

Spread out a large piece of plastic wrap on a flat surface and place the dough on it. Wrap the dough and use a rolling pin to spread it out into a thick rectangle. Unwrap the dough after and use an oiled knife to cut the dough into bars.

Dill Pickles with Tuna-Mayo Topping
Ready in about: 40 minutes | Serves: 12
Per serving: Kcal 118, Fat: 10g, Net Carbs: 1.5g, Protein: 11g

Ingredients

18 ounces canned and drained tuna
6 large dill pickles
¼ tsp garlic powder
⅓ cup sugar-free mayonnaise
1 tbsp onion flakes

Directions

Combine the mayonnaise, tuna, onion flakes, and garlic powder in a bowl. Cut the pickles in half lengthwise. Top each half with tuna mixture. Place in the fridge for 30 minutes before serving.

Mozzarella & Prosciutto Wraps
Ready in about: 15 minutes | Serves: 6
Per serving: Kcal 163, Fat: 12g, Net Carbs: 0.1g, Protein: 13g

Ingredients

6 thin prosciutto slices
18 basil leaves
18 ciliegine mozzarella balls
2 tbsp extra virgin olive oil

Directions

Cut the prosciutto slices into three strips each. Place basil leaves at the end of each strip. Top with a ciliegine mozzarella ball. Wrap the mozzarella in prosciutto. Secure with toothpicks. Arrange on a platter, drizzle with olive oil, and serve.

Pecorino-Mushroom Balls
Ready in about: 20 minutes | Serves: 4
Per serving: Kcal 370; Fat: 30g, Net Carbs: 7.7g, Protein: 16.8g

Ingredients

2 tbsp butter, softened
2 tbsp olive oil
2 garlic cloves, minced
2 cups portobello mushrooms, chopped
4 tbsp blanched almond flour
4 tbsp ground flax seeds
4 tbsp hemp seeds
4 tbsp sunflower seeds
1 tbsp cajun seasoning
1 tsp mustard
2 eggs, whisked
½ cup Pecorino cheese, shredded

Directions

Set a pan over medium heat and warm the olive oil. Add in mushrooms and garlic and sauté until there is no more water in mushrooms. Remove to a plate and let cool for a few minutes.

In a bowl, place Pecorino cheese, almond flour, hemp seeds, mustard, eggs, sunflower seeds, flax seeds, mushrooms, and cajun seasoning. Create 4 burgers from the mixture.

To the same pan, add and warm the butter; fry the burgers for 7 minutes. Flip them over with a wide spatula and cook for 6 more minutes. Serve with guacamole.

Garlic and Basil Mashed Celeriac

Ready in about: 30 minutes | Serves: 4
Per serving: Kcal 94, Fat 0.5g, Net Carbs 6g, Protein 2.4g

Ingredients

2 lb celeriac, chopped
4 cups water
2 oz cream cheese
2 tbsp butter
⅓ cup sour cream
½ tsp garlic powder
2 tsp dried basil
Salt and black pepper to taste

Directions

Bring the celeriac and water to boil over high heat on a stovetop for 5 minutes and then reduce the heat to low to simmer for 15 minutes. Drain the celeriac through a colander after.
Then, pour the celeriac in a large bowl, add the cream cheese, butter, sour cream, garlic powder, dried basil, salt, and black pepper. Mix with a hand mixer on medium speed until well combined.Serve.

Cheesy Lettuce Rolls

Ready in about: 10 minutes | Serves: 6
Per serving: Kcal 370; Fat: 30g, Net Carbs: 4.9g, Protein: 19.5g

Ingredients

½ pound gouda cheese, grated
½ pound feta cheese, crumbled
1 tsp taco seasoning mix
2 tbsp olive oil
1 ½ cups guacamole
1 cup buttermilk
A head lettuce

Directions

Mix both types of cheese with taco seasoning mix. Set a pan over medium heat and warm the olive oil. Spread the shredded cheese mixture all over the pan. Fry for 5 minutes, turning once. Arrange some of the cheese mixture on each lettuce leaf, top with buttermilk and guacamole, then roll up folding in the ends to secure and serve.

Party Bacon and Pistachio Balls

Ready in about: 45 minutes | Serves: 8
Per serving: Kcal 145, Fat: 12g, Net Carbs: 1.5g, Protein: 7g

Ingredients

8 bacon slices, cooked and chopped
8 ounces Liverwurst
¼ cup chopped pistachios
1 tsp Dijon mustard
6 ounces cream cheese

Directions

Combine the liverwurst and pistachios in the bowl of food the processor. Pulse until smooth. Whisk the cream cheese and mustard in another bowl. Make 12 balls out of the liverwurst mixture.

Make a thin cream cheese layer over. Coat with bacon, arrange on a plate and chill for 30 minutes.

Spiced Gruyere Crisps

Ready in about: 10 minutes | Serves: 4
Per serving: Kcal 205; Fat: 15g, Net Carbs: 2.9g, Protein: 14.5g

Ingredients

2 cups Gruyere cheese, shredded
½ tsp garlic powder
¼ tsp onion powder
1 rosemary sprig, minced
½ tsp chili powder

Directions

Set oven to 400ºF. Coat two baking sheets with parchment paper.
Mix Gruyere cheese with the seasonings. Take 1 tablespoon of cheese mixture and form small mounds on the baking sheets. Bake for 6 minutes. Leave to cool. Serve.

Roasted String Beans, Mushrooms & Tomato Plate

Ready in about: 32 minutes | Serves: 4
Per serving: Kcal 121, Fat 2g, Net Carbs 6g, Protein 6g

Ingredients

2 cups string beans, cut in halves
1 lb cremini mushrooms, quartered
3 tomatoes, quartered
2 cloves garlic, minced
3 tbsp olive oil
3 shallots, julienned
½ tsp dried thyme
Salt and black pepper to season

Directions

Preheat oven to 450ºF. In a bowl, mix the strings beans, mushrooms, tomatoes, garlic, olive oil, shallots, thyme, salt, and pepper. Pour the vegetables in a baking sheet and spread them all around.
Place the baking sheet in the oven and bake the veggies for 20 to 25 minutes.

Lemony Fried Artichokes

Ready in about: 20 minutes | Serves: 4
Per serving: Kcal 35, Fat: 2.4g, Net Carbs: 2.9g, Protein: 2g

Ingredients

12 fresh baby artichokes
2 tbsp lemon juice
2 tbsp olive oil
Salt to taste

Directions

Slice the artichokes vertically into narrow wedges. Drain on paper towels before frying.
Heat olive oil in a skillet over high heat. Fry the artichokes until browned and crispy. Drain excess oil on paper towels. Sprinkle with salt and lemon juice.

Spinach and Ricotta Gnocchi

Ready in about: 13 minutes | Serves: 4
Per serving: Kcal 125, Fat 8.3g, Net Carbs 4.1g, Protein 6.5g

Ingredients

3 cups chopped spinach
1 cup ricotta cheese
1 cup Parmesan cheese , grated
¼ tsp nutmeg powder
1 egg, cracked into a bowl
Salt and black pepper
1 ½ cups almond flour
2 ½ cups water
2 tbsp butter

Directions

To a bowl, add the ricotta cheese, half of the Parmesan cheese, egg, nutmeg powder, salt, spinach, almond flour, and black pepper. Mix well. Make gnocchi of the mixture using 2 tbsp and set aside.

Bring the water to a boil over high heat on a stovetop, about 5 minutes. Place one gnocchi onto the water, if it breaks apart; add some more flour to the other gnocchi to firm it up.

Put the remaining gnocchi in the water to poach and rise to the top, about 2 minutes. Remove the gnocchi with a perforated spoon to a serving plate. Melt the butter in a microwave and pour over the gnocchi. Sprinkle with the remaining Parmesan cheese and serve with green salad.

Smoked Mackerel Patties

Ready in about: 30 minutes | Serves: 6
Per serving: Kcal 324, Fat 27.1g, Net Carbs 2.2g, Protein 16g

INGREDIENTS

1 turnip, diced
1 ½ cup water
Salt and chili pepper to taste
3 tbsp olive oil + for rubbing
4 smoked mackerel steaks, bones removed, flaked
3 eggs, beaten
2 tbsp mayonnaise
1 tbsp pork rinds, crushed

DIRECTIONS

Bring the turnip to boil in salted water in a saucepan over medium heat for 8 minutes or until tender. Drain the turnip through a colander, transfer to a mixing bowl, and mash the lumps.

Add the mackerel, eggs, mayonnaise, pork rinds, salt, and chili pepper; mix and make 6 compact patties. Heat olive oil in a skillet over medium heat and fry the patties for 3 minutes on each side until golden brown. Remove onto a wire rack to cool. Serve with sesame lime dipping sauce.

Swiss Chard Pesto Scrambled Eggs

Ready in about: 15 minutes | Serves: 4
Per serving: Kcal 495; Fat: 45g, Net Carbs: 6.3g, Protein: 19.5g

Ingredients

3 tbsp butter
8 eggs, beaten
¼ cup almond milk
Salt and black pepper, to taste

Swiss chard pesto

2 cups swiss chard
1 cup Parmesan cheese, grated
2 garlic cloves, minced
½ cup olive oil
2 tbsp lime juice
½ cup walnuts, chopped

Directions

Set a pan over medium heat and warm butter. Mix eggs, black pepper, salt, and almond milk. Cook the egg mixture while stirring gently, until eggs are set but still tender and moist.

In your blender, place all the ingredients for the pesto, excluding the olive oil. Pulse until roughly blended. While the machine is still running, slowly add in the olive oil until the desired consistency is attained. Serve alongside warm scrambled eggs.

BRUNCH & DINNER

Homemade Pizza Crust

Ready in about: 8 minutes | Serves: 8
Per serving: Kcal: 234; Fat 16.7g, Net Carbs 7.9g, Protein 12.4g

Ingredients

3 cups almond flour
3 tbsp butter, then melted
⅓ tsp salt
3 large eggs

Directions

Preheat the oven to 350ºF and in a bowl, mix the almond flour, butter, salt, and eggs until a dough forms. Mold the dough into a ball and place in between two wide parchment papers on a flat surface.

Use a rolling pin to roll it out into a circle of a quarter-inch thickness. Slide the pizza dough into the pizza pan and remove the parchment papers. Bake the dough for 20 minutes.

Salami & Prawn Pizza

Ready in about: 35 minutes | Serves: 6
Per serving: Kcal 267, Fat 13.3g, Net Carbs 4.3g, Protein 9.5g

Ingredients

1 low carb pizza crust (see "Homemade Pizza Crust")
1 cup sugar-free pizza sauce
2 ¼ cups grated mozzarella cheese
4 oz Hot Salami, thinly sliced
3 tomatoes, thinly sliced
16 green prawns, peeled, deveined, and halved
2 cloves garlic, finely sliced
2 cups baby arugula
2 tbsp toasted pine nuts
1 tbsp olive oil
Salt and black pepper to taste
10 basil leaves

Directions

Preheat the oven to 450ºF. With the pizza bread on the pizza pan, spread the pizza sauce on it and sprinkle with half of the mozzarella cheese. Top with the salami, tomatoes, prawns, and garlic, then sprinkle the remaining cheese over it. Place the pizza in the oven to bake for 15 minutes.

Once the cheese has melted, top with the basil leaves. In a bowl, toss the arugula and pine nuts with olive oil and adjust its seasoning to taste. Section the pizza with a slicer and serve with the arugula mixture.

Broccoli Rabe Pizza with Parmesan

Ready in about: 40 minutes | Serves: 2
Per serving: Kcal 673, Fat 47g, Net Carbs 10.7g, Protein 32.6g

Ingredients

1 cauliflower pizza crust
2 tbsp olive oil
2 parsnips, chopped
Salt and black pepper to taste
2 cups broccoli rabe
2 hard-boiled eggs, chopped
½ cup largely diced bacon
1 cup grated Parmesan cheese
2 tbsp chopped basil leaves

Directions

Preheat the oven to 400ºF. Drizzle the parsnips with 1 teaspoon of olive oil and sprinkle with salt and pepper. Rub the seasoning on them and place on a baking sheet. Bake for 20 minutes; set aside.

Toss the broccoli rabe with 2 tablespoons of olive oil in a bowl, season with salt and black pepper, and drain any liquid from the bowl.

Bake the pizza crust for 7 minutes in the oven. Then, let cool for a few minutes and brush with the remaining olive oil. Scatter the parsnips all over, top with the broccoli rabe, bacon and eggs and sprinkle with Parmesan cheese. Bake the pizza for 6-8 minutes until the cheese is melted. Garnish with basil and section with a pizza cutter. Serve the slices with sundried tomato salad.

Chipotle Pizza with Cotija & Cilantro

Ready in about: 15 minutes | Serves: 2
Per serving: Kcal 397, Fat: 31g, Net Carbs: 8.1g, Protein: 22g

Ingredients

Pizza crust:

4 eggs, beaten
¼ cup sour cream
2 tbsp flax seed meal
1 tsp chipotle pepper
¼ tsp cumin seeds, ground
½ tsp dried coriander leaves
Salt to taste
1 tbsp olive oil

Topping:

2 tbsp tomato paste
2 ounces Cotija cheese, shredded
Fresh chopped cilantro for garnish

Directions

Mix all crust ingredients, except for the oil.

Set a pan over medium heat and warm ½ tablespoon oil. Ladle ½ of crust mixture into the pan and evenly spread out. Cook until the edges are set; then, flip the crust and cook on the second side. Do the same process with the remaining crust mixture.

Warm the remaining ½ tablespoon of oil in the pan. Spread each pizza crust with tomato paste, then scatter over the cotija cheese. In batches, bake in the oven for 8-10 minutes at 425ºF until all the cheese melts. Garnish with cilantro and serve.

Roasted Vegetable and Goat Cheese Pizza

Ready in about: 45 minutes | Serves: 6 2
Per serving: Kcal 315, Fat 16g, Net Carbs 7.3g, Protein 12g

Ingredients

1 cauliflower pizza crust
1 sweet onion, cut into chunks
1 eggplant, cut into chunks
1 red bell pepper, cut into pieces
1 medium zucchini, cut into pieces
2 tbsp olive oil
Salt and black pepper to taste
1 tsp chopped thyme, fresh
½ cup pesto sauce
½ cup crumbled goat cheese

Directions

Preheat the oven to 425ºF. Bake the pizza crust in a greased baking sheet for 7 minutes. Let cool.
In a bowl, mix the onion, eggplant, red bell pepper, and zucchinis with olive oil, salt, black pepper, and thyme. Pour the mixture into a baking sheet and spread it well around. Bake for 30 minutes, stirring at 10 minutes intervals.
Remove the veggies and set aside. Spread the pesto on the pizza crust. Arrange the roasted veggies on top and sprinkle with goat cheese. Bake the pizza for 5-6 minutes until the cheese is melted.

Cheesy Basil Omelet

Ready in about: 10 minutes | Serves: 2
Per serving: Kcal 431; Fat: 33.1g, Net Carbs: 2.7g, Protein: 30.3g

Ingredients

4 slices cooked bacon, crumbled
4 eggs, beaten
1 tsp basil, chopped
1 tsp parsley, chopped
Sea salt and black pepper
½ cup cheddar cheese, grated

Directions

In a frying pan, cook the bacon until sizzling. Add in eggs, parsley, black pepper, salt, and basil.Scatter the cheese over the half of omelet; using a spatula fold in half over the filling. Cook for 1 extra minute or until cooked through and serve immediately.

Cheese Sticks with Mustard-Yogurt Dipping Sauce

Ready in about: 40 minutes | Serves: 8
Per serving: Kcal: 200; Fat 16.9g, Net Carbs 3.7g, Protein 9.4g

Ingredients

16 ounces cheddar cheese with jalapeño peppers
¾ cup grana padano cheese, grated
2 tbsp almond flour
1 tbsp flax meal
1 tsp baking powder
Salt and red pepper flakes, to taste
⅓ tsp cumin powder
½ tsp dried oregano
⅓ tsp dried rosemary
2 eggs
2 tbsp olive oil

Dipping sauce

1 cup cream cheese
⅓ cup natural yogurt
¾ cup jarred fire-roasted red peppers, chopped
1 tbsp mustard
1 chili pepper, deveined and minced
2 garlic cloves, chopped
Salt and black pepper to taste

Directions

Chop cheddar cheese crosswise into sticks. In a bowl, mix the dry ingredients. In a separate bowl, whisk the eggs. Dip each cheese stick into the eggs, and then roll in the dry mixture.
Set cheese sticks on a wax paper-lined baking sheet; freeze for 30 minutes. In a skillet over medium heat warm oil and fry cheese sticks for 5 minutes until the coating is golden brown and crisp. Set on paper towels to drain excess oil. Mix all ingredients for the dipping sauce, until smooth.

Mexican-Style Frittata

Ready in about: 25 minutes | Serves: 6
Per serving: Kcal: 225; Fat 17g, Net Carbs 5.1g, Protein 13.2g

Ingredients

10 eggs
Salt and black pepper to taste
⅓ cup chive & onion cream cheese
1 tbsp butter
1 onion, chopped
1 tsp garlic paste
2 red bell peppers, chopped
½ green bell pepper, chopped
1 tsp chipotle paste
1 ½ cups kale
½ cup cotija cheese, shredded

Directions

Set oven to 370ºF. Mix the eggs with onion cream cheese, black pepper, and salt.
Warm butter in a skillet over medium heat. Sauté onion until soft. Add in chipotle paste, bell peppers, and garlic paste, and cook for 4 minutes. Place in kale and cook for 2 minutes. Add in the egg/cheese mixture. Spread the mixture evenly over the skillet and set to the oven.
Bake for 8 minutes or until the frittata's top becomes golden brown but still slightly wobbly in the middle. Apply a topping of crumbled cotija cheese and bake for 3 more minutes or until the cheese melts completely. Slice into 6 wedges and serve while still warm.

Monterey Jack Cheese Soup

Ready in about: 20 minutes | Serves: 4
Per serving: Kcal 296; Fat 14.1g, Net Carbs 7.4g,
Protein 14.2g

Ingredients

2 tbsp butter
½ cup leeks, chopped
1 celery stalk, chopped
1 serrano pepper, finely chopped
1 tsp garlic puree
1 ½ tbsp flax seed meal
2 cups water
1 ½ cups coconut milk
6 ounces Monterey Jack cheese, shredded
Salt and black pepper, to taste
Fresh parsley, chopped to garnish

Directions

Set a pot over medium heat and melt butter. Add in serrano pepper, celery and leeks and sauté until soft. Place in coconut milk, garlic puree, water, and flax seed meal. Bring to a boil and reduce the heat. Allow simmering for 10 minutes or until cooked through.

Fold in the shredded cheese, kill the heat and stir to ensure the cheese is completely melted and you have a homogenous mixture. Add black pepper and salt to taste. Divide among serving bowls, decorate with parsley and serve warm.

Chorizo Scotch Eggs

Ready in about: 35 minutes | Serves: 8
Per serving: Kcal 247; Fat 11.4g, Net Carbs 0.6g,
Protein 33.7g

Ingredients

8 eggs
2 eggs, beaten
1 cup pork rinds, crushed
1 ½ pounds chorizo sausages, skinless
½ cup grana padano cheese, grated
1 garlic clove, minced
½ tsp onion powder
½ tsp chili pepper
1 tsp fresh parsley, chopped
Salt and black pepper to taste

Directions

Cook the 8 eggs in boiling salted water over medium heat for 10 minutes. Rinse under cold, running water and remove the shell; reserve. Preheat oven to 370ºF. In a mixing dish, mix the other ingredients, except for the beaten eggs and pork rinds. Take a handful of the mixture and wrap around each of the eggs. With fingers, mold the mixture until sealed to form balls. Dip the balls in the beaten eggs, coat with rinds and place in a greased baking dish. Bake for 25 minutes, until golden brown and crisp. Allow to cool before serving.

Ham & Egg Salad

Ready in about: 20 minutes | Serves: 4
Per serving: Kcal: 284; Fat 21.3g, Net Carbs 6.8g,
Protein 16.7g

Ingredients

8 eggs
⅓ cup mayonnaise
1 tbsp minced onion
½ tsp mustard
1 ½ tsp lime juice
Salt and black pepper, to taste
10 lettuce leaves
½ cup ham crumbs

Directions

In a pot, lay the eggs in a single layer; cover with salted water. Boil over high heat for 10 minutes. Remove and run under cold water. Then peel and chop the eggs.

Remove to a mixing bowl together with the mayonnaise, mustard, black pepper, lime juice, onion, and salt. Lay on a bed of lettuce leaves and ham crumbs to serve.

Mediterranean Cheese Balls

Ready in about: 5 minutes | Serves: 6
Per serving: Kcal 217; Fat: 18.7g, Net Carbs: 2.1g,
Protein: 10g

Ingredients

4 ounces prosciutto, chopped
4 ounces goat cheese, crumbled
¼ cup aioli
½ cup black olives, pitted and chopped
½ tsp red pepper flakes
2 tbsp fresh basil, finely chopped

Directions

In a mixing dish, mix aioli, prosciutto and goat cheese. Place in fresh basil, red pepper flakes and black olives. Form 10 balls from the mixture. Arrange on a serving platter and serve immediately.

Italian-Style Roasted Butternut Squash and Basil

Ready in about: 40 minutes | Serves: 8
Per serving: Kcal 155; Fat: 12.7g, Carbs 6.2g, Protein: 4.6g

Ingredients

1 small butternut squash, sliced
1 tbsp coconut oil, melted
¼ cup fresh basil, chopped
1 cup heavy cream
½ cup buttermilk
1 cup ricotta cheese
2 tsp powdered unflavored gelatin
Fresh rosemary, chopped
Celery salt to taste
¼ tsp onion flakes
½ tsp fennel seeds
½ tsp mixed peppercorns, crushed
½ tsp cayenne pepper

Directions

Sprinkle coconut oil over the squash slices. In the preheated to 360ºF oven, roast squash for 30

124

minutes. Set the squash in a blender and pulse to obtain a smooth and creamy mixture.

Het a pan on low heat, add in mixed with heavy cream basil and cook for 4 minutes. Place in the rest of the ingredients and cook for 5 more minutes until completely melted. Fold in pureed squash and stir to mix well. Ladle the mixture into 8 ramekins. Refrigerate overnight. Flip the ramekin onto serving plates.

Pork & Vegetable Tart

Ready in about: 45 minutes | Serves: 6
Per serving: Kcal 415; Fat: 26.3g, Net Carbs: 4.2g, Protein: 35g

Ingredients

2 pounds ground pork
1 onion, chopped
1 garlic clove, minced
1 bell pepper, chopped
Salt and black pepper to taste
2 zucchinis, sliced
2 tomatoes, sliced
¼ cup whipping cream
8 eggs
½ cup Monterey Jack cheese, grated

Directions

Set oven to 360ºF. Grease a baking dish with cooking spray.
In a bowl, mix onion, bell pepper, ground pork, garlic, pepper and salt. Layer the meat mixture on the bottom of the baking dish. Spread zucchini slices on top followed with tomato slices. Bake for 30 minutes. In a separate bowl, combine cheese, eggs and whipping cream. Top the tart with this creamy mixture and bake for 10 minutes, until the edges and top become brown.

Sopressata and Cheese Roast

Ready in about: 1 hour | Serves: 4
Per serving: Kcal 334; Fat: 23g, Net Carbs: 6.2g, Protein: 25.5g

Ingredients

8 eggs
Salt to taste
1 cup cheddar cheese, grated
½ cup goat cheese
1 bell pepper, chopped
1 poblano pepper, deveined and chopped
½ tsp dried dill weed
1 tsp mustard
4 slices soppressata, chopped
4 slices pancetta, chopped
6 cups hot water

Directions

Set oven to 360ºF and grease a casserole dish with cooking spray. Beat the eggs in a bowl, add cheddar, mustard, and salt and mix to incorporate everything. Place the mixture in the casserole.

Stir in the remaining ingredients. Set a roasting pan with hot water in the middle of the oven. Insert the casserole dish into the roasting pan.
Bake for around 1 hour. Let cool for some minutes before cutting into squares. Serve while warm!

Tuna & Monterey Jack Stuffed Avocado

Ready in about: 20 minutes | Serves: 4
Per serving: Kcal: 286; Fat 23.9g, Net Carbs 9g, Protein 11.2g

Ingredients

2 avocados, halved and pitted
4 ounces Monterey Jack cheese, grated
2 ounces canned tuna, flaked
2 tbsp chives, chopped
Salt and black pepper, to taste
½ cup curly endive, chopped

Directions

Set oven to 360ºF. Set avocado halves in an ovenproof dish. In a mixing bowl, mix Monterey Jack cheese, chives, black pepper, salt, and tuna. Stuff the cheese/tuna mixture in avocado halves. Bake for 15 minutes or until the top is golden brown. Serve with curly endive for garnish.

Bacon & Eggplant Boats

Ready in about: 35 minutes | Serves: 3
Per serving: Kcal 506; Fat 41g, Net Carbs 4.5g, Protein 27.5g

Ingredients

3 eggplants, cut into halves
1 tbsp deli mustard
2 bacon slices, cooked, crumbled
6 eggs
Salt, to taste
¼ tsp black pepper
¼ tsp dried parsley

Directions

Scoop flesh from eggplant halves to make shells; set the eggplant boats on a greased baking pan. Spread mustard on the bottom of every eggplant half. Split the bacon among eggplant boats.
Crack an egg in each half, sprinkle with parsley, black pepper, and salt. Set oven at 400ºF and bake for 30 minutes or until boats become tender.

Ham & Egg Mug Cups

Ready in about: 5 minutes | Serves: 2
Per serving: Kcal: 244; Fat 17.5g, Net Carbs 2.9g, Protein 19.2

Ingredients

4 eggs
4 tbsp coconut milk
¼ cup ham, cubed
½ tsp chili pepper
Salt and black pepper, to taste
2 tbsp chives, chopped

Directions

Mix all ingredients excluding chives. With a cooking spray, grease two microwave-safe cups. Divide the egg mixture into the cups. Microwave for 1 minute. Decorate with chives before serving.

Spicy Eggs with Turkey Ham
Ready in about: 15 minutes | Serves: 2
Per serving: Kcal 462; Fat: 40.6g, Net Carbs: 7.1g, Protein: 16.9g
Ingredients
2 tbsp olive oil
½ cup onion, chopped
1 tsp smashed garlic
1 tsp serrano pepper, deveined and minced
Salt and black pepper to taste
5 ounces turkey ham, chopped
4 eggs, whisked
1 thyme sprig, chopped
½ cup olives, pitted and sliced
Directions
Over medium heat, set a skillet and warm oil; add in onion and sauté for 4 minutes until tender. Stir in garlic, salt, ham, black pepper, and serrano pepper; cook for 5-6 more minutes. Add in eggs and sprinkle with thyme; cook for 5 minutes. Garnish with sliced olives before serving.

Crêpes with Lemon-Buttery Syrup
Ready in about: 25 minutes | Serves: 6
Per serving: Kcal 243, Fat: 19.6g, Net Carbs: 5.5g, Protein: 11g
Ingredients
Crêpes:
6 ounces mascarpone cheese, softened
6 eggs
1 ½ tbsp granulated swerve
¼ cup almond flour
1 tsp baking soda
1 tsp baking powder
Syrup:
¾ cup water
2 tbsp lemon juice
1 tbsp butter
¾ cup swerve, powdered
1 tbsp vanilla extract
½ tsp xanthan gum
Directions
With the use of an electric mixer, mix all crepes ingredients until well incorporated.
Use melted butter to grease a frying pan and set over medium heat; cook the crepes until the edges start to brown, about 2 minutes. Flip over and cook the other side for a further 2 minutes; repeat the process with the remaining batter. Put the crepes on a plate.
In the same pan, mix swerve, butter and water; simmer for 6 minutes as you stir. Transfer the mixture to a blender together with a ¼ teaspoon of xanthan gum and vanilla extract and mix well. Place in the remaining xanthan gum, lemon juice, and allow to sit until the syrup is thick.

Asian Tofu Egg Soup
Ready in about: 15 minutes | Serves: 3

Per serving: Kcal 153; Fat: 9.8g, Net Carbs: 2.7g, Protein: 15g
Ingredients
3 cups chicken stock
1 tbsp tamari sauce
1 tsp coconut oil, softened
2 eggs, beaten
½ tsp turmeric powder
1-inch piece ginger, grated
Salt and black ground, to taste
¼ tsp paprika
½ pound extra-firm tofu, cubed
A handful of fresh cilantro, chopped
Directions
Set a pan over medium heat, add in tamari sauce, stock, and coconut oil. Bring to a boil and reduce the heat; allow boiling for 10 minutes. Place in eggs as you whisk to incorporate completely.
Add in turmeric, salt, paprika, black pepper and ginger. Place in tofu and simmer for 1 to 2 minutes. Divide into soup bowls and serve sprinkled with fresh cilantro.

Greek Yogurt & Cheese Alfredo Sauce
Ready in about: 10 minutes | Serves: 12
Per serving: Kcal 154; Fat: 13g, Net Carbs: 3.3g, Protein: 6.2g
Ingredients
2 tbsp butter
6 ounces heavy cream
Salt and black pepper, to taste
2 cloves garlic, chopped
¾ cup sour cream
½ cup Gruyere cheese, grated
1 cup goat cheese
½ cup cooked bacon, chopped
1 cup Greek yogurt
Directions
Set a pan over medium heat and warm butter. Stir in heavy cream and cook for 2-3 minutes. Sprinkle with black pepper and salt; mix in the Greek yogurt and cook for 2 minutes. Stir in the remaining ingredients to mix well until smooth.

Caprese Stuffed Tomatoes
Ready in about: 35 minutes | Serves: 5
Per serving: Kcal 306; Fat: 27.5g, Net Carbs: 4.4g, Protein: 11.3g
Ingredients
5 tomatoes
5 slices fresh mozzarella cheese
¼ cup sour cream
1 egg, whisked
1 clove garlic, minced
4 tbsp fresh scallions, chopped
Salt and black pepper, to taste
2 tbsp butter, softened
Directions
Set oven to 360ºF. Lightly grease a rimmed baking sheet with cooking spray. Horizontally slice tomatoes

into halves and get rid of the hard cores; scoop out pulp and seeds.

In a bowl, mix egg, salt, butter, black pepper, garlic, sour cream, and scallions. Split the filling between tomatoes, cover each one with a mozzarella slice and bake in the preheated oven for 30 minutes. Place on a wire rack and allow to cool for 5 minutes; serve alongside fresh rocket leaves.

Vanilla-Coconut Cream Tart

Ready in about: 30 minutes + cooling time | Serves: 6
Per serving: Kcal 305, Fat: 30.6g, Net Carbs: 9.7g, Protein: 4.6g

Ingredients

½ cup butter
⅓ cup xylitol
¾ cup coconut flour
⅓ cup coconut shreds, unsweetened
2 ¼ cups heavy cream
3 egg yolks
⅓ cup almond flour
¾ cup water
½ tsp ground cinnamon
½ tsp star anise, ground
½ tsp vanilla extract
2 tbsp coconut flakes

Directions

Set a pan over medium heat and warm butter. Stir in xylitol and cook until fully dissolved.
Add in coconut shreds and coconut flour and cook for 2 more minutes. Scrape the crust mixture into the bottom of a baking dish. Refrigerate the mixture.
Preheat the pan over medium-low heat; place in 1 ¼ cups of heavy cream and warm. Fold in egg yolks and mix thoroughly. Mix in water and almond flour until thick. Place in cinnamon, vanilla extract, and anise star. Cook until thick.
Let cool for 10 minutes; sprinkle over the crust. Place in the refrigerator for some hours. Beat the remaining heavy cream until stiff peaks start to form. Spread the cream all over the cake. Top with coconut flakes to serve.

Raspberry & Rum Omelet

Ready in about: 10 minutes | Serves: 1
Per serving: Kcal 488, Fat: 42g, Net Carbs: 8g, Protein: 15.3g

Ingredients

2 eggs
2 tbsp heavy cream
½ tsp ground cloves
1 tbsp coconut oil
2 tbsp mascarpone cheese
6 fresh raspberries, sliced
1 tbsp powdered swerve
1 tbsp rum

Directions

Beat the eggs with ground cloves and heavy cream. Set pan over medium heat and warm oil. Place in the egg mixture; cook for 3 minutes. Set the omelet onto a plate; apply a topping of raspberries and mascarpone cheese. Roll it up and sprinkle with powdered swerve. Pour the warm rum over the omelet and ignite it. Let the flame die out and serve.

Cauli Mac and Cheese

Ready in about: 15 minutes | Serves: 4
Per serving: Kcal 357; Fat: 32.5g, Net Carbs: 10.9g, Protein: 8.4g

Ingredients

1 head cauliflower, cut into florets
2 tbsp ghee, melted
Salt and black pepper, to taste
½ cup crème fraiche
½ cup half-and-half
1 cup cream cheese
½ tsp turmeric powder
1 tsp garlic paste
½ tsp onion flakes

Directions

Set oven to 450ºF. Grease a baking sheet with cooking spray.
Shake cauliflower florets with melted ghee, salt, and black pepper. Arrange on the baking sheet and roast for 15 minutes. In a saucepan over medium heat, pour the remaining ingredients and heat through, stirring frequently. Reduce heat to low and simmer for 2-3 minutes until thickened. Coat the cauliflower florets in the cheese sauce and serve immediately in serving bowls.

Eggs in a Mug

Ready in about: 5 minutes | Serves: 2
Per serving: Kcal 197; Fat: 13.8g, Net Carbs: 2.7g, Protein: 15.7g

Ingredients

4 eggs
¼ cup coconut milk
¼ cup cheddar cheese, grated
1 garlic clove, minced
¼ tsp dried dill
¼ tsp turmeric powder
Sea salt and red pepper flakes, to taste

Directions

In a mixing bowl, mix the eggs, cheddar cheese, red pepper, garlic, coconut milk, turmeric powder and salt. Divide the mixture between 2 microwave-safe mugs. Place in the microwave for 40 seconds. Stir well and continue microwaving for 70 seconds. Sprinkle with dried dill and serve.

Spicy Cheese Chips

Ready in about: 18 minutes | Serves: 2
Per serving: Kcal: 100; Fat 8g, Net Carbs 0g, Protein 7g

Ingredients

3 cups cheddar cheese, grated
⅓ tsp salt
½ tsp garlic powder
½ tsp cayenne pepper
½ tsp dried rosemary
⅓ tsp chili powder

Directions

Set oven to 420ºF. Line a parchment paper on a baking sheet.
Mix grated cheddar cheese with spices. Create 2 tablespoons of cheese mixture into small mounds on the baking sheet. Bake for about 15 minutes; allow to cool to harden the chips.

Blue Cheese Stuffed Peppers

Ready in about: 35 minutes | Serves: 4
Per serving: Kcal 359; Fat: 29.7g, Net Carbs: 6.7g, Protein: 17.7g

Ingredients

4 bell peppers, tops sliced off and deseeded
6 ounces cottage cheese
6 ounces blue cheese, crumbled
½ cup pork rinds, crushed
2 cloves garlic, smashed
1 ½ cups pureed tomatoes
1 tsp dried basil
Salt and black pepper, to taste
½ tsp chili pepper
½ tsp oregano

Directions

Preheat oven to 360ºF and grease a casserole dish with cooking spray and pour in some water.
In a bowl, mix garlic, cottage cheese, pork rinds, blue cheese, tomatoes, oregano, salt, cayenne pepper, black pepper, and basil. Stuff the peppers and remove to the casserole dish. Bake for 30 minutes until the peppers are tender. Serve with mixed salad on the side.

Chili Egg Pickles

Ready in about: 20 minutes | Serves: 5
Per serving: Kcal: 145; Fat 9g, Net Carbs 2.8g, Protein 11.4g

Ingredients

10 eggs
½ cup onions, sliced
3 cardamom pods
1 tbsp chili powder
1 tsp yellow seeds
2 clove garlic, sliced
1 cup vinegar
1 ¼ cups water
1 tbsp salt

Directions

Boil eggs in salted water until hard-cooked, about 10 minutes; rinse under cold, running water; peel and discard the shells. Place the peeled eggs onto a large jar. Set a pan over medium heat. Stir in all remaining ingredients; bring to a rapid boil. Reduce heat to low; allow to simmer for 6 minutes. Spoon this mixture into the jar. Refrigerate for 2 to 3 weeks.

Gingery Tuna Mousse

Ready in about: 20 minutes + chilling time | Serves: 5
Per serving: Kcal 100; Fat: 5.8g, Net Carbs: 4.1g, Protein: 8g

Ingredients

1 ½ tsp gelatin, powdered
3 tbsp water
2 ounces ricotta cheese
3 tbsp mayonnaise
1 tsp mustard
3 ounces canned tuna, flaked
¼ cup onions, chopped
1 garlic clove, minced
½ tsp salt
¼ tsp black pepper
⅓ tsp ginger, grated

Directions

Mix gelatin in water; let sit for 10 minutes. Set a pan over medium heat and warm ricotta cheese; place in gelatin and mix to blend well; let the mixture cool. Place in the other ingredients and stir.
Split the mixture among 5 mousse molds and refrigerate overnight. Serve by inverting the molds over a serving platter.

Cheese & Pumpkin Chicken Meatballs

Ready in about: 35 minutes | Serves: 5
Per serving: Kcal 378; Fat: 24.5g, Net Carbs: 4.7g, Protein: 36g

Ingredients

1 egg, beaten
1 ½ pounds ground chicken
½ cup pumpkin, grated
2 garlic cloves, minced
1 onion, chopped
1 tbsp Italian mixed herbs
Salt and black pepper, to taste
2 tbsp olive oil
1 cup cheddar cheese, shredded

Directions

Preheat oven to 360ºF. Combine all ingredients excluding cheese. Form meatballs from the mixture; set them on a parchment-lined baking sheet. Bake for 25 minutes, flipping once.
Spread cheese over the balls and bake for 7 more minutes or until all cheese melts.

Chicken Meatloaf Cups with Pancetta

Ready in about: 30 minutes | Serves: 6
Per serving: Kcal 276, Fat: 18.3g, Net Carbs: 1.2g, Protein: 29.2g

Ingredients

2 tbsp onion, chopped
1 tsp garlic, minced
1 pound ground chicken
2 ounces cooked pancetta, chopped
1 egg, beaten
1 tsp mustard
Salt and black pepper, to taste
½ tsp crushed red pepper flakes
1 tsp dried basil
½ tsp dried oregano
4 ounces cheddar cheese, cubed

Directions

In a bowl, mix mustard, onion, ground chicken, egg, pancetta, and garlic. Season with oregano, red pepper, black pepper, basil and salt.
Split the mixture into greased muffin cups. Lower one cube of cheddar cheese into each meatloaf cup. Close the top to cover the cheese. Bake in the oven at 345ºF for 20 minutes, or until the meatloaf cups become golden brown. Let cool for 10 minutes before transferring from the muffin pan.

Ham and Emmental Eggs

Ready in about: 20 minutes | Serves: 5
Per serving: Kcal 444; Fat: 35.3g, Net Carbs: 2.7g, Protein: 29.8g

Ingredients

1 tbsp olive oil
4 slices ham, chopped
½ cup chives, chopped
½ cup broccoli, chopped
1 clove garlic, minced
1 tsp fines herbes
¼ cup vegetable broth
5 eggs
1 ½ cups emmental cheese, shredded

Directions

In a frying pan, warm oil. Add in ham and cook for 4 minutes, until brown and crispy; set aside.
Using the same pan, cook chives. Place in the garlic and broccoli and cook until soft as you stir occasionally. Stir in broth and fines herbes and cook for 6 more minutes.
Make 5 holes in the mixture until you are able to see the bottom of your pan. Crack an egg into each hole. Spread cheese over the top and cook for 6 more minutes. Scatter the reserved ham over to serve.

Chorizo and Cheese Gofre

Ready in about: 20 minutes | Serves: 3
Per serving: Kcal 453, Fat: 37g, Net Carbs: 4.5g, Protein: 25.6g

Ingredients

6 eggs, separate egg whites and egg yolks
½ tsp baking powder
6 tbsp almond flour
4 tbsp butter, melted
¼ tsp salt
½ tsp dried rosemary
3 tbsp tomato puree
3 ounces smoked chorizo, chopped
3 ounces cheddar cheese, shredded

Directions

In a mixing bowl, mix egg yolks, almond flour, rosemary, butter, baking powder, and salt. Beat the egg whites until pale and combine with the egg yolk mixture.
Grease waffle iron and set over medium heat, add in ¼ cup of the batter and cook for 3 minutes until golden. Repeat with the remaining batter.
Place one waffle back to the waffle iron; sprinkle 1 tbsp of tomato puree to the waffle; apply a topping of 1 ounce of cheese and 1 ounce of chorizo. Cover with another waffle; cook until all the cheese melts.
Do the same with all remaining ingredients.

Cheese, Ham and Egg Muffins

Ready in about: 20 minutes | Serves: 6
Per serving: Kcal: 268; Fat 18.3g, Net Carbs 0.7g, Protein 26.2g

Ingredients

24 slices smoked ham
6 eggs, beaten
Salt and black pepper, to taste
¼ cup fresh parsley, chopped
¼ cup ricotta cheese
¼ cup Brie, chopped

Directions

Set oven to 390ºF. Line 2 slices of smoked ham into each greased muffin cup, to circle each mold.
In a mixing bowl, mix the rest of the ingredients. Fill ¾ of the ham lined muffin cup with the egg/cheese mixture. Bake for 15 minutes. Serve warm!

Baked Chicken Legs with Cheesy Spread

Ready in about: 45 minutes | Serves: 4
Per serving: Kcal 119; Fat: 10.5g, Net Carbs: 1.1g, Protein: 5.1g

Ingredients

4 chicken legs
¼ cup goat cheese
2 tbsp sour cream
1 tbsp butter, softened
1 onion, chopped
Sea salt and black pepper, to taste

Directions

Preheat oven to 360ºF and season the legs with salt and black pepper. Roast in a greased baking dish for 25-30 minutes until crispy and browned. In a mixing bowl, mix the rest of the ingredients to form the spread. Scatter the spread over the chicken and serve with green salad.

Quatro Formaggio Pizza

Ready in about: 15 minutes | Serves: 4
Per serving: Kcal 266, Fat: 23.6g, Net Carbs: 6.6g, Protein: 9g

Ingredients

1 tbsp olive oil
½ cup cheddar cheese, shredded
1 ¼ cups mozzarella cheese, shredded
½ cup mascarpone cheese
½ cup blue cheese
2 tbsp sour cream
2 garlic cloves, chopped
1 red bell pepper, sliced
1 green bell pepper, sliced
10 cherry tomatoes, halved
1 tsp oregano
Salt and black pepper, to taste

Directions

In a bowl, mix the cheeses. Set a pan over medium heat and warm olive oil. Spread the cheese mixture on the pan and cook for 5 minutes until cooked through. Scatter garlic and sour cream over the crust. Add in tomatoes and bell peppers; cook for 2 minutes. Sprinkle with pepper, salt and oregano and serve.

Bacon Balls with Brie Cheese

Ready in about: 15 minutes | Serves: 5
Per serving: Kcal 206; Fat: 16.5g, Net Carbs: 0.6g, Protein: 13.4g

Ingredients

3 ounces bacon
6 ounces brie cheese
1 chili pepper, seeded and chopped
¼ tsp parsley flakes
½ tsp paprika

Directions

Set a pan over medium heat and fry the bacon until crispy; then crush it. Place the other ingredients in a bowl and mix to combine with the bacon grease. Refrigerate the mixture for 20 minutes. Remove and form balls from the mixture. Set the bacon in a plate and roll the balls around to coat.

Creamy Cheddar Deviled Eggs

Ready in about: 20 minutes | Serves: 5
Per serving: Kcal 177; Fat: 12.7g, Net Carbs: 4.6g, Protein: 11.4g

Ingredients

10 eggs
¼ cup mayonnaise
1 tbsp tomato paste
2 tbsp celery, chopped
2 tbsp carrot, chopped
2 tbsp chives, minced
2 tbsp cheddar cheese, grated
Salt and black pepper, to taste

Directions

Place the eggs in a pot and fill with water by about 1 inch. Bring the eggs to a boil over high heat, then reduce the heat to medium and simmer for 10 minutes.

Remove and rinse under running water until cooled. Peel and discard the shell. Slice each egg in half lengthwise and get rid of the yolks. Mix the yolks with the rest of the ingredients. Split the mixture amongst the egg whites and set deviled eggs on a plate to serve.

Jamon & Queso Balls

Ready in about: 15 minutes | Serves: 8
Per serving: Kcal: 168; Fat 13g, Net Carbs 2.5g, Protein 10.3g

Ingredients

1 egg
6 slices jamon serrano, chopped
6 ounces cotija cheese
6 ounces Manchego cheese
Salt and black pepper, to taste
¼ cup almond flour
1 tsp baking powder
1 tsp garlic powder

Directions

Preheat oven to 420 ºF.

Whisk the egg; place in the remaining ingredients and mix well. Split the mixture into 16 balls; set the balls on a baking sheet lined with parchment paper. Bake for 13 minutes or until they turn golden brown and become crispy.

Cajun Crabmeat Frittata

Ready in about: 25 minutes | Serves: 3
Per serving: Kcal 265; Fat: 15.8g, Net Carbs: 7.1g, Protein: 22.9g

Ingredients

1 tbsp olive oil
1 onion, chopped
4 ounces crabmeat, chopped
1 tsp cajun seasoning
6 large eggs, slightly beaten
½ cup Greek yogurt

Directions

Preheat oven to 350ºF. Set a large skillet over medium heat and warm the oil. Add in onion and sauté until soft, about 3 minutes. Stir in crabmeat and cook for 2 more minutes. Season with cajun seasoning. Evenly distribute the ingredients at the bottom of the skillet.

Whisk the eggs with yogurt. Transfer to the skillet. Set the skillet in the oven and bake for about 18 minutes or until eggs are cooked through. Slice into wedges and serve warm.

Crabmeat & Cheese Stuffed Avocado

Ready in about: 25 minutes | Serves: 4
Per serving: Kcal 264, Fat: 24.4g, Net Carbs: 11g, Protein: 3.7g

Ingredients

1 tsp olive oil
1 cup crabmeat
2 avocados, halved and pitted
3 ounces cream cheese
¼ cup almonds, chopped
1 tsp smoked paprika

Directions

Preheat oven to 425ºF and grease a baking pan with cooking spray.
In a bowl, mix crabmeat with cream cheese. To the avocado halves, place in almonds and crabmeat/cheese mixture and bake for 18 minutes. Decorate with smoked paprika and serve.

Juicy Beef Cheeseburgers

Ready in about: 20 minutes | Serves: 6
Per serving: Kcal 252; Fat: 15.5g, Net Carbs: 1.2g, Protein: 26g

Ingredients

1 pound ground beef
½ cup green onions, chopped
2 garlic cloves, finely chopped
¼ tsp black pepper
Salt and cayenne pepper, to taste
2 oz mascarpone cheese
3 oz pecorino romano cheese, grated
2 tbsp olive oil

Directions

In a mixing bowl, mix ground beef, garlic, cayenne pepper, black pepper, green onions, and salt. Shape into 6 balls; then flatten to make burgers.
In a separate bowl, mix mascarpone with grated pecorino romano cheeses. Split the cheese mixture among prepared patties. Wrap the meat mixture around the cheese mixture to ensure that the filling is sealed inside. Warm oil in a skillet over medium heat. Cook the burgers for 5 minutes each side.

Cilantro & Chili Omelet

Ready in about: 15 minutes | Serves: 2
Per serving: Kcal 319; Fat: 25g, Net Carbs: 10g, Protein: 14.9g

Ingredients

2 tsp butter
2 spring onions, chopped
2 spring garlic, chopped
4 eggs
1 cup sour cream, divided
2 tomatoes, sliced
1 green chili pepper, minced
2 tbsp fresh cilantro, chopped
Salt and black pepper, to taste

Directions

Set a pan over high heat and warm the butter. Sauté garlic and onions until tender and translucent.
Whisk the eggs with sour cream. Pour into the pan and use a spatula to smooth the surface; cook until eggs become puffy and brown to bottom. Add cilantro, chili pepper and tomatoes to one side of the omelet. Season with black pepper and salt. Fold the omelet in half and slice into wedges.

Zucchini with Blue Cheese and Walnuts

Ready in about: 15 minutes + chilling time | Serves: 6
Per serving: Kcal 489; Fat: 47.4g, Net Carbs: 6.9g, Protein: 12.7g

Ingredients

2 tbsp olive oil
6 zucchinis, sliced
1 ⅓ cups heavy cream
1 cup sour cream
8 ounces blue cheese
1 tsp Italian seasoning
¼ cup walnut halves

Directions

Set a grill pan over medium heat. Season zucchinis with Italian seasoning and drizzle with olive oil. Grill the zucchini until lightly charred. Remove to a serving platter.
In a dry pan over medium heat, toast the walnuts for 2-3 minutes and set aside. Add the heavy cream, blue cheese, and sour cream to the pan and mix until everything is well combined. Let cool for a few minutes and scatter over the grilled zucchini. Top with walnuts to serve.

Garlick & Cheese Turkey Slices

Ready in about: 20 minutes | Serves: 4
Per serving: Kcal 416; Fat: 26g, Net Carbs: 3.2g, Protein: 40.7g

Ingredients

2 tbsp olive oil
1 pound turkey breasts, sliced
2 garlic cloves, minced
½ cup heavy cream
⅓ cup chicken broth
2 tbsp tomato paste
1 cup cheddar cheese, shredded

Directions

Set a pan over medium heat and warm the oil; add in garlic and turkey and fry for 4 minutes; set aside. Stir in the broth, tomato paste, and heavy cream; cook until thickened.
Return the turkey to the pan; spread shredded cheddar cheese over. Let sit for 5 minutes covered or until the cheese melts. Serve instantly.

Prosciutto & Cheese Egg Cups
Ready in about: 30 minutes | Serves: 9
Per serving: Kcal 294, Fat: 21.4g, Net Carbs: 3.5g,
Protein: 21g
Ingredients
9 slices prosciutto
9 eggs
4 green onions, chopped
½ cup cheddar cheese, shredded
¼ tsp garlic powder
½ tsp dried dill weed
Sea salt and black pepper, to taste
Directions
Preheat oven to 390ºF and grease a 9-cup muffin pan
with oil. Line one slice of prosciutto on each cup. In a
mixing bowl, combine the remaining ingredients.
Split the egg mixture among muffin cups. Bake for 20
minutes. Leave to cool before serving.

Spanish Salsa Aioli
Ready in about: 10 minutes | Serves: 8
Per serving: Kcal 116; Fat: 13.2g, Net Carbs: 0.2g,
Protein: 0.4g
Ingredients
1 tbsp lemon juice
1 egg yolk, at room temperature
1 clove garlic, crushed
½ tsp salt
½ cup olive oil
¼ tsp black pepper
¼ cup fresh parsley, chopped
Directions
Using a blender, place in salt, lemon juice, garlic, and
egg yolk; pulse well to get a smooth and creamy
mixture. Set blender to slow speed.
Slowly sprinkle in olive oil and combine to ensure the
oil incorporates well. Stir in parsley and black pepper.
Refrigerate the mixture until ready.

Three-Cheese Fondue with Walnuts and Parsley
Ready in about: 15 minutes | Serves: 10
Per serving: Kcal 148; Fat: 10.2g, Net Carbs: 1.5g,
Protein: 9.3g
Ingredients
½ pound brie cheese, chopped
⅓ pound Swiss cheese, shredded
½ cup emmental cheese, grated
1 tbsp xanthan gum
½ tsp garlic powder
1 tsp onion powder
¾ cup white wine
½ tbsp lemon juice
Black pepper, to taste
1 cup walnuts, chopped
Directions
Set broiler to preheat. In a skillet, thoroughly mix
onion powder, brie, emmental, Swiss cheese, garlic
powder, and xanthan gum. Pour in lemon juice and
wine and sprinkle with black pepper.
Set the skillet under the broiler for 6 to 7 minutes,
until the cheese browns. Garnish with walnuts.

Berry Pancakes with Coconut Topping
Ready in about: 20 minutes | Serves: 4
Per serving: Kcal 237, Fat: 16.3g, Net Carbs: 8.5g,
Protein: 14.5g
Ingredients For the Batter:
5 eggs
6 ounces cream cheese, room temperature
1 tsp baking powder
3 tbsp coconut oil
A pinch of salt
Coconut topping:
1 cup fresh mixed berries
¼ tsp freshly grated nutmeg
2 tbsp swerve
½ cup natural coconut yogurt
Directions
Use an electric mixer to beat the eggs, cream cheese,
baking powder, and salt. Set a frying pan over
medium heat and brush lightly with oil. Ladle a small
amount of the batter into the pan and cook for 3
minutes for each side until golden; remove to a plate.
Repeat for the remaining pancakes.
Serve the pancakes in plates and scatter over fresh
berries. Sprinkle with swerve and ground nutmeg,
and finish with a dollop of coconut yogurt.

Carrot & Cheese Mousse
Ready in about: 15 minutes + cooling time | Serves: 6
Per serving: Kcal 368, Fat: 33.7g, Net Carbs: 5.6g,
Protein: 13.8g
Ingredients
1 ½ cups half & half
½ cup cream cheese
½ cup erythritol
3 eggs
1 ¼ cups canned carrots
½ tsp ground cloves
½ tsp ground cinnamon
¼ tsp grated nutmeg
A pinch of salt
Directions
Heat a pan over medium heat, mix erythritol, cream
cheese, and half & half, and warm, stirring frequently.
Remove from the heat. Beat the eggs; slowly place in
½ of the hot cream mixture to the beaten eggs. Pour
the mixture back to the pan. Cook for 3 minutes, until
thick. Kill the heat; add in carrots, cinnamon, salt,
nutmeg, and cloves. Blend with a blender. Let cool
before serving.

Italian Cakes with Gorgonzola and Salami

Ready in about: 25 minutes | Serves: 5
Per serving: Kcal 240, Fat: 15.3g, Net Carbs: 10g, Protein: 16.1g

Ingredients

3 slices salami
4 eggs, beaten
½ cup coconut flour
1 tsp baking powder
1 cup gorgonzola cheese, diced
A pinch of salt
A pinch of grated nutmeg

Directions

Set a frying pan over medium heat. Add in salami and cook as you turn with tongs until browned; use paper towels to drain the salami. Chop the salami and stir with the other ingredients to mix.
Grease cake molds. Fill them with batter (¾ full). Set oven to 390ºF and bake for 15 minutes.

One-Pot Cheesy Cauliflower & Bacon

Ready in about: 15 minutes | Serves: 4
Per serving: Kcal 323, Fat: 24g, Net Carbs: 7.4g, Protein: 18.8g

Ingredients

2 tbsp butter
½ pound bacon, cut into strips
1 head cauliflower, broken into florets
¼ cup sour cream
¾ cup heavy whipping cream
1 tsp smashed garlic
2 tbsp apple cider vinegar
½ cup queso fresco, crumbled

Directions

Set a frying pan over medium heat and melt the butter; brown the bacon for 3 minutes. Set aside. Add in cauliflower and cook until tender, about 4-5 minutes.
Add in the whipping and sour cream, then the vinegar and garlic; cook until warmed fully. Take the reserved bacon back to the pan. Fold in queso fresco and cook for 2 minutes, or until cheese melts.

Chorizo Egg Balls

Ready in about: 10 minutes + cooling time | Serves: 6
Per serving: Kcal 174, Fat: 15.2g, Net Carbs: 4.3g, Protein: 5.9g

Ingredients

2 eggs
½ cup butter, softened
8 black olives, pitted and chopped
3 tbsp mayonnaise
Salt and crushed red pepper flakes, to taste
1 pound cooked chorizo, chopped
2 tbsp chia seeds

Directions

In a food processor, place the eggs, olives, pepper flakes, mayo, butter, and salt and blitz until everything is incorporated. Stir in the chorizo. Refrigerate for 30 minutes.
Form balls from the mixture. Set the chia seeds on a serving bowl; roll the balls through to coat. Place in an airtight container and place in the refrigerator for 4 days.

Ginger & Walnut Porridge

Ready in about: 25 minutes | Serves: 2
Per serving: Kcal 430, Fat: 41.1g, Net Carbs: 9.8g, Protein: 11.4g

Ingredients

3 eggs
4 tbsp swerve
½ cup heavy cream
1 ½ tbsp coconut oil
½ tsp ginger paste
¼ tsp turmeric powder
¼ cup walnuts, chopped

Directions

In a bowl, mix swerve, eggs and heavy cream. Set a pot over medium heat and warm coconut oil. Add in egg/cream mixture and cook until cooked through. Kill the heat and place in turmeric and ginger paste. Split the porridge into bowls, top with chopped walnuts and serve.

Chili Chicken Breasts Wrapped in Bacon

Ready in about: 35 minutes | Serves: 6
Per serving: Kcal 275, Fat: 9.5g, Net Carbs: 1.3g, Protein: 44.5g

Ingredients

6 chicken breasts, flatten
1 tbsp olive oil
2 tbsp fresh parsley, chopped
3 garlic cloves, chopped
1 chili pepper, chopped
1 tsp tarragon
Salt and black pepper, to taste
1 tsp hot paprika
6 slices bacon

Directions

Preheat oven to 390ºF. Mix garlic, tarragon, hot paprika, salt, chili pepper, and black pepper; rub onto chicken and roll fillets in the bacon slices.
Arrange on a greased with the olive oil baking dish and bake for 30 minutes. Plate the chicken and serve sprinkled with fresh parsley.

Pureed Broccoli with Roquefort Cheese

Ready in about: 15 minutes | Serves: 4
Per serving: Kcal 230, Fat: 17.7g, Net Carbs: 7.2g,
Protein: 11.9g

Ingredients

1 ½ pounds broccoli, broken into florets
2 tbsp olive oil, divided
1 tsp crushed garlic
1 rosemary sprig, chopped
1 thyme sprig, chopped
2 cups Roquefort cheese, crumbled
Black pepper to taste

Directions

Place salted water in a deep pan over medium heat. Add in broccoli and boil for 8 minutes. Drain and remove the cooked florets to a casserole dish.

In a food processor, pulse ½ of the broccoli. Place in 1 tbsp oil and 1 cup of the cooking liquid. Repeat with the remaining water, broccoli, and 1 tbsp oil. Stir in the remaining ingredients, and serve.

Mini Egg Muffins

Ready in about: 40 minutes | Serves: 5
Per serving: Kcal 261; Fat: 16g, Net Carbs: 7.6g,
Protein: 21.1g

Ingredients

1 tbsp olive oil
1 onion, chopped
1 bell pepper, chopped
6 slices bacon, chopped
8 eggs, whisked
1 cup gruyere cheese, shredded
Salt and black pepper, to taste
¼ tsp rosemary
1 tbsp fresh parsley, chopped

Directions

Set oven to 390ºF. Place cupcake liners to your muffin pan. In a skillet over medium heat, warm the oil and sauté the onion and bell pepper for 4-5 minutes, as you stir constantly until tender.

Stir in bacon and cook for 3 more minutes. Add in the rest of the ingredients and mix well. Set the mixture to the lined muffin pan and bake for 23 minutes; let muffins cool, before serving.

Cheesy Bites with Turnip Chips

Ready in about: 25 minutes | Serves: 8
Per serving: Kcal 177; Fat: 12.9g, Net Carbs: 6.8g,
Protein: 8.8g,

Ingredients

1 cup Monterey Jack cheese, shredded
½ cup natural yogurt
1 cup pecorino cheese, grated
2 tbsp tomato puree
½ tsp dried rosemary leaves, crushed
1 tsp dried thyme leaves, crushed
Salt and black pepper, to taste
1 pound turnips, sliced
2 tbsp olive oil

Directions

In a mixing bowl, mix cheese, tomato puree, black pepper, salt, rosemary, yogurt, and thyme. Place in foil liners-candy cups and refrigerate until ready to serve.

Set oven to 430ºF. Coat turnips with salt, black pepper and oil. Arrange in a single layer on a cookie sheet. Bake for 20 minutes, shaking once or twice. Dip turnip chips in cheese cups.

Goat Cheese Muffins with Ajillo Mushrooms

Ready in about: 45 minutes | Serves: 6
Per serving: Kcal 263, Fat: 22.4g, Net Carbs: 6.1g,
Protein: 10g

Ingredients

1 ½ cups heavy cream
5 ounces goat cheese, crumbled
3 eggs
Salt and black pepper, to taste
1 tbsp butter, softened
2 cups mushrooms, chopped
2 garlic cloves, minced

Directions

Preheat oven to 320ºF. Insert 6 ramekins into a large pan. Add in boiling water up to 1-inch depth. In a pan, over medium heat, warm heavy cream. Reduce the heat and stir in goat cheese; cook until melted. Remove from the heat.

Beat the eggs in a bowl and gradually add the cream mixture. Sprinkle with pepper and salt. Ladle the mixture into ramekins. Bake for 40 minutes.

Melt butter in a pan over medium heat. Add garlic and mushrooms, season with salt and pepper and sauté for 5 minutes until tender. Spread the ajillo mushrooms on top of each cooled muffin to serve.

Grilled Halloumi Cheese with Eggs

Ready in about: 20 minutes | Serves: 4
Per serving: Kcal 542; Fat: 46.4g, Net Carbs: 11.2g,
Protein: 23.7g

Ingredients

4 slices halloumi cheese
2 tbsp olive oil
1 tsp dried Greek seasoning blend
6 eggs, beaten
½ tsp sea salt
¼ tsp crushed red pepper flakes
1 ½ cups avocado, pitted and sliced
1 cup grape tomatoes, halved
4 tbsp pecans, chopped

Directions

Preheat your grill to medium. Set the halloumi in the center of a piece of heavy-duty foil. Sprinkle oil over the halloumi and apply Greek seasoning blend. Close the foil to create a packet. Grill for about 15 minutes; then slice into four pieces.

In a frying pan, warm the olive oil and cook the eggs. Stir well to create large and soft curds. Season with salt and red pepper flakes. Put the eggs and grilled cheese on a serving bowl. Serve alongside tomatoes and avocado, decorated with chopped pecans.

Herbed Keto Bread

Ready in about: 40 minutes | Serves: 6
Per serving: Kcal 115, Fat: 10.2g, Net Carbs: 1g, Protein: 3.9g

Ingredients

5 eggs
½ tsp cream of tartar
2 cups almond flour
3 tablespoons butter, melted
3 tsp baking powder
1 tsp salt
1 tsp dried rosemary
½ tsp dried oregano
1 tbsp sunflower seeds
2 tbsp sesame seeds

Directions

Preheat oven to 360ºF and grease a loaf pan with cooking spray. Combine the eggs with cream of tartar until the formation of stiff peaks happens. In a food processor, place in the baking powder, flour, salt, and butter and blitz to incorporate fully.

Stir in the egg mixture. Ladle the batter into the prepared loaf pan. Spread the loaf with sesame seeds, dried rosemary, sunflower seeds, and oregano and bake for 35 minutes. Serve with butter.

DESERTS & DRINKS

Chocolate Marshmallows

Ready in about: 30 minutes | Serves: 4
Per serving: Kcal 55, Fat 2.2g, Net Carbs 5.1g, Protein 0.5g

Ingredients

2 tbsp unsweetened cocoa powder
½ tsp vanilla extract
½ cup swerve
1 tbsp xanthan gum mixed in 1 tbsp water
A pinch Salt
6 tbsp cool water
2 ½ tsp gelatin powder

Dusting:

1 tbsp unsweetened cocoa powder
1 tbsp swerve confectioner's sugar

Directions

Line the loaf pan with parchment paper and grease with cooking spray; set aside. In a saucepan, mix the swerve, 2 tbsp of water, xanthan gum mixture, and salt. Place the pan over medium heat and bring to a boil. Insert the thermometer and let the ingredients simmer to 240ºF, for 7 minutes.

In a small bowl, add 2 tbsp of water and sprinkle the gelatin on top. Let sit there without stirring to dissolve for 5 minutes. While the gelatin dissolves, pour the remaining water in a small bowl and heat in the microwave for 30 seconds. Stir in cocoa powder and mix it into the gelatin.

When the sugar solution has hit the right temperature, gradually pour it directly into the gelatin mixture while continuously whisking. Beat for 10 minutes to get a light and fluffy consistency.

Next, stir in the vanilla and pour the blend into the loaf pan. Let the marshmallows set for 3 hours and then use an oiled knife to cut it into cubes; place them on a plate. Mix the remaining cocoa powder and confectioner's sugar together. Sift it over the marshmallows.

Dark Chocolate Mousse with Stewed Plums

Ready in about: 45 minutes + cooling time | Serves: 6
Per serving: Kcal 288, Fat 23g, Net Carbs 6.9g, Protein 9.5g

Ingredients

12 oz unsweetened chocolate
8 eggs, separated into yolks and whites
2 tbsp salt
¾ cup swerve sugar
½ cup olive oil
3 tbsp brewed coffee

Stewed plums:

4 plums, pitted and halved
½ stick cinnamon
½ cup swerve
½ cup water
½ lemon, juiced

Directions

Put the chocolate in a bowl and melt in the microwave for 1 ½ minutes. In a separate bowl, whisk the yolks with half of the swerve until a pale yellow has formed, then, beat in the salt, olive oil, and coffee. Mix in the melted chocolate until smooth.

In a third bowl, whisk the whites with a hand mixer until a soft peak has formed. Sprinkle the remaining swerve over and gently fold in with a spatula. Fetch a tablespoon full of the chocolate mixture and fold in to combine. Pour in the remaining chocolate mixture and whisk to mix.

Pour the mousse into 6 ramekins, cover with plastic wrap, and refrigerate overnight. The next morning, pour water, swerve, cinnamon, and lemon juice in a saucepan and bring to a simmer for 3 minutes, occasionally stirring to ensure the swerve has dissolved and a syrup has formed.

Add the plums and poach in the sweetened water for 18 minutes until soft. Turn the heat off and discard the cinnamon stick. Spoon a plum each with syrup on the chocolate mousse and serve.

Granny Smith Apple Tart

Ready in about: 65 minutes | Serves: 8
Per serving: Kcal 302, Fat: 26g, Net Carbs: 6.7g, Protein: 7g

Ingredients

6 tbsp butter
2 cups almond flour
1 tsp cinnamon
⅓ cup sweetener

Filling:

2 cups sliced Granny Smith
¼ cup butter
¼ cup sweetener
½ tsp cinnamon
½ tsp lemon juice

Topping:

¼ tsp cinnamon
2 tbsp sweetener

Directions

Preheat oven to 370ºF and combine all crust ingredients in a bowl. Press this mixture into the bottom of a greased pan. Bake for 5 minutes.

Meanwhile, combine the apples and lemon juice in a bowl and let them sit until the crust is ready. Arrange them on top of the crust. Combine the rest of the filling ingredients, and brush this mixture over the apples. Bake for about 30 minutes.

Press the apples down with a spatula, return to oven, and bake for 20 more minutes. Combine the cinnamon and sweetener, in a bowl, and sprinkle over the tart.

Note: Granny Smith apples have just 9.5g of net carbs per 100g. Still high for you? Substitute with Chayote squash, which has the same texture and rich nutrients, and just around 4g of net carbs.

Coconut Cheesecake

Ready in about: 30 minutes + freezing time | Serves: 12

Per serving: Kcal 256, Fat: 25g, Net Carbs: 3g, Protein: 5g

Ingredients

Crust:

2 egg whites
¼ cup erythritol
3 cups desiccated coconut
1 tsp coconut oil
¼ cup melted butter

Filling:

3 tbsp lemon juice
6 ounces raspberries
2 cups erythritol
1 cup whipped cream
Zest of 1 lemon
24 ounces cream cheese

Directions

Grease bottom and sides of a springform pan with coconut oil. Line with parchment paper. Preheat oven to 350ºF and mix all crust ingredients. Pour the crust into the pan. Bake for about 25 minutes; let cool.

Meanwhile, beat the cream cheese with an electric mixer until soft. Add the lemon juice, zest, and erythritol. Fold the whipped cream into the cheese cream mixture. Fold in the raspberries gently. Spoon the filling into the baked and cooled crust. Place in the fridge for 4 hours.

Raspberry Nut Truffles

Ready in about: 6 minutes + cooling time | Serves: 4
Per serving: Kcal 251, Fat 18.3g, Net Carbs 3.5g, Protein 12g

Ingredients

2 cups raw cashews
2 tbsp flax seed
1 ½ cups sugar-free raspberry preserves
3 tbsp swerve
10 oz unsweetened chocolate chips
3 tbsp olive oil

Directions

Line a baking sheet with parchment paper and set aside. Grind the cashews and flax seeds in a blender for 45 seconds until smoothly crushed; add the raspberry and 2 tbsp of swerve.

Process further for 1 minute until well combined. Form 1-inch balls of the mixture, place on the baking sheet, and freeze for 1 hour or until firmed up.

Melt the chocolate chips, oil, and 1tbsp of swerve in a microwave for 1 ½ minutes. Toss the truffles to coat in the chocolate mixture, put on the baking sheet, and freeze further for at least 2 hours.

Passion Fruit Cheesecake Slices

Ready in about: 15 minutes + cooling time | Serves: 8
Per serving: Kcal 287, Fat 18g, Net Carbs 6.1g, Protein 4.4g

Ingredients

1 cup crushed almond biscuits
½ cup melted butter

Filling:

1 ½ cups cream cheese
¾ cup swerve sugar
1 ½ whipping cream
1 tsp vanilla bean paste
4-6 tbsp cold water
1 tbsp gelatin powder

Passionfruit jelly:

1 cup passion fruit pulp
¼ cup swerve confectioner's sugar
1 tsp gelatin powder
¼ cup water, room temperature

Directions

Mix the crushed biscuits and butter in a bowl, spoon into a spring-form pan, and use the back of the spoon to level at the bottom. Set aside in the fridge. Put the cream cheese, swerve sugar, and vanilla paste into a bowl, and use the hand mixer to whisk until smooth; set aside.

In a bowl, add 2 tbsp of cold water and sprinkle 1 tbsp of gelatin powder. Let dissolve for 5 minutes. Pour the gelatin liquid along with the whipping cream in the cheese mixture and fold gently.

Remove the spring-form pan from the refrigerator and pour over the mixture. Return to the fridge.

For the passionfruit jelly: add 2 tbsp of cold water and sprinkle 1 tsp of gelatin powder. Let dissolve for 5 minutes. Pour confectioner's sugar and ¼ cup of water into it. Mix and stir in passion fruit pulp.

Remove the cake again and pour the jelly over it. Swirl the pan to make the jelly level up. Place the pan back into the fridge to cool for 2 hours. When completely set, remove and unlock the spring-pan. Lift the pan from the cake and slice the dessert.

Blueberry Tart with Lavender

Ready in about: 35 minutes + cooling time | Serves: 6
Per serving: Kcal 198, Fat 16.4g, Net Carbs 10.7g, Protein 3.3g

Ingredients

1 large low carb pie crust
1 ½ cups heavy cream
2 tbsp swerve
1 tbsp culinary lavender
1 tsp vanilla extract
2 cups fresh blueberries
Erythritol for topping

Directions

Preheat oven to 400ºF. Place the pie crust with its pan on a baking tray and bake in the oven for 30 minutes, until golden brown; remove and let cool.

Mix the heavy cream and lavender in a saucepan. Set the pan over medium heat and bring the mixture to a boil; turn the heat off and let cool. Strain the cream through a colander into a bowl to remove the lavender pieces. Mix swerve and vanilla into the cream, and pour into the cooled crust.

Scatter the blueberries on and refrigerate the pie for 45 minutes. Remove and top with erythritol.

Vanilla Flan with Mint

Ready in about: 60 minutes + cooling time | Serves: 4
Per serving: Kcal 269, Fat: 26g, Net Carbs: 1.7g, Protein: 7.6g

Ingredients
⅓ cup erythritol, for caramel
2 cups almond milk
4 eggs
1 tbsp vanilla extract
1 tbsp lemon zest
½ cup erythritol, for custard
2 cup heavy whipping cream
Mint leaves, to serve

Directions
Heat erythritol for the caramel in a deep pan. Add 2-3 tablespoons of water, and bring to a boil. Reduce the heat and cook until the caramel turns golden brown. Divide between 4-6 metal tins. Set aside to cool.
In a bowl, mix eggs, remaining erythritol, lemon zest, and vanilla. Add almond milk and beat until well combined. Pour the custard into each caramel-lined ramekin and place in a deep baking tin.
Fill over the way with the remaining hot water. Bake at 345ºF for 45-50 minutes. Take out the ramekins and let cool for at least 4 hours in the fridge. Run a knife slowly around the edges to invert onto a dish. Serve with dollops of whipped cream, scattered with mint leaves.

Chocolate Cakes

Ready in about: 25 minutes | Serves: 6
Per serving: Kcal 218, Fat: 20g, Net Carbs: 10g, Protein: 4.8g

Ingredients
½ cup almond flour
¼ cup xylitol
1 tsp baking powder
½ tsp baking soda
1 tsp cinnamon, ground
A pinch of salt
A pinch of ground cloves
½ cup butter, melted
½ cup buttermilk
1 egg
1 tsp pure almond extract
For the Frosting:
1 cup heavy cream
1 cup dark chocolate, flaked

Directions
Preheat oven to 360ºF. Use a cooking spray to grease a donut pan.
In a bowl, mix the cloves, almond flour, baking powder, salt, baking soda, xylitol, and cinnamon. In a separate bowl, combine the almond extract, butter, egg, and buttermilk. Mix the wet mixture into the dry mixture. Evenly ladle the batter into the donut pan. Bake for 17 minutes.

Set a pan over medium heat and warm heavy cream; simmer for 2 minutes. Fold in the chocolate flakes; combine until all the chocolate melts; let cool. Spread the top of the cakes with the frosting.

Lemon Cheesecake Mousse

Ready in about: 5 minutes + cooling time | Serves: 4
Per serving: Kcal 223, Fat 18g, Net Carbs 3g, Protein 12g

Ingredients
24 oz cream cheese, softened
2 cups swerve confectioner's sugar
2 lemons, juiced and zested
Pink salt to taste
1 cup whipped cream + extra for garnish

Directions
Whip the cream cheese in a bowl with a hand mixer until light and fluffy. Mix in the swerve sugar, lemon juice, and salt. Fold in the whipped cream to evenly combine.
Spoon the mousse into serving cups and refrigerate to thicken for 1 hour. Swirl with extra whipped cream and garnish lightly with lemon zest. Serve immediately.

Ice Cream Bars Covered with Chocolate

Ready in about: 20 minutes + freezing time | Serves: 15
Per serving: Kcal 345 Fat: 32g, Net Carbs: 5g, Protein: 4g

Ingredients
Ice cream:
1 cup heavy whipping cream
1 tsp vanilla extract
¾ tsp xanthan gum
½ cup peanut butter
1 cup half and half
1 ½ cups almond milk
⅓ tsp stevia powder
1 tbsp vegetable glycerin
3 tbsp xylitol
Chocolate:
¾ cup coconut oil
¼ cup cocoa butter pieces, chopped
2 ounces unsweetened chocolate
3 ½ tsp THM super sweet blend

Directions
Blend all ice cream ingredients until smooth. Place in an ice cream maker and follow the instructions. Spread the ice cream into a lined pan, and freezer for about 4 hours.
Combine all chocolate ingredients in a microwave-safe bowl and heat until melted. Allow cooling. Remove the ice cream from the freezer and slice into bars. Dip them into the cooled chocolate mixture and return to the freezer for about 10 minutes before serving.

Green Tea Brownies with Macadamia Nuts

Ready in about: 28 minutes | Serves: 4
Per serving: Kcal 248, Fat 23.1g, Net Carbs 2.2g, Protein 5.2g

Ingredients

1 tbsp green tea powder
¼ cup unsalted butter, melted
4 tbsp swerve confectioner's sugar
A pinch of salt
¼ cup coconut flour
½ tsp baking powder
1 egg
¼ cup chopped macadamia nuts

Directions

Preheat oven to 350ºF and line a square baking dish with parchment paper. Pour the melted butter into a bowl, add sugar and salt, and whisk to combine. Crack the egg into the bowl.
Beat the mixture until the egg has incorporated. Pour coconut flour, green tea, and baking powder into a fine-mesh sieve and sift them into the egg bowl; stir. Add the nuts, stir again, and pour the mixture into the lined baking dish. Bake for 18 minutes, remove and slice into brownie cubes.

Eggless Strawberry Mousse

Ready in about: 6 minutes + cooling time | Serves: 6
Per serving: Kcal 290, Fat 24g, Net Carbs 5g, Protein 5g

Ingredients

2 cups chilled heavy cream
2 cups fresh strawberries, hulled
5 tbsp erythritol
2 tbsp lemon juice
¼ tsp strawberry extract
2 tbsp sugar-free strawberry preserves

Directions

Beat the heavy cream, in a bowl, with a hand mixer at high speed until a stiff peak forms, for about 1 minute; refrigerate immediately. Puree the strawberries in a blender and pour into a saucepan.
Add erythritol and lemon juice, and cook on low heat for 3 minutes while stirring continuously. Stir in the strawberry extract evenly, turn off the heat and allow cooling. Fold in the whipped cream until evenly incorporated, and spoon into six ramekins. Refrigerate for 4 hours to solidify.
Garnish with strawberry preserves and serve immediately.

Chocolate Chip Cookies

Ready in about: 20 minutes | Serves: 4
Per serving: Kcal 317, Fat 27g, Net Carbs 8.9g, Protein 6.3g

Ingredients

1 cup butter, softened
2 cups swerve brown sugar
3 eggs
2 cups almond flour

2 cups unsweetened chocolate chips

Directions

Preheat oven to 350ºF and line a baking sheet with parchment paper.
Whisk the butter and sugar with a hand mixer for 3 minutes or until light and fluffy. Add the eggs one at a time, and scrape the sides as you whisk. Mix in almond flour at low speed until well combined.
Fold in the chocolate chips. Scoop 3 tablespoons each on the baking sheet creating spaces between each mound and bake for 15 minutes to swell and harden. Remove, cool and serve.

Coconut Bars

Ready in about: 40 minutes + freezing time | Serves: 4
Per serving: Kcal 215, Fat: 22g, Net Carbs: 1.4g, Protein: 2g

Ingredients

3 ½ ounces ghee
10 saffron threads
1 ⅓ cups coconut milk
1 ¾ cups shredded coconut
4 tbsp sweetener
1 tsp cardamom powder

Directions

Combine the shredded coconut with 1 cup of the coconut milk. In another bowl, mix together the remaining coconut milk with the sweetener and saffron. Let sit for 30 minutes.
Heat the ghee in a wok. Add the coconut mixtures and cook for 5 minutes on low heat, mixing continuously. Stir in the cardamom and cook for another 5 minutes. Spread the mixture onto a small container and freeze for 2 hours. Cut into bars and enjoy!

Berry Tart

Ready in about: 45 minutes | Serves: 4
Per serving: Kcal 305, Fat: 26.5g, Net Carbs: 4.9g, Protein: 15g

Ingredients

4 eggs
2 tsp coconut oil
2 cups berries
1 cup coconut milk
1 cup almond flour
¼ cup sweetener
½ tsp vanilla powder
1 tbsp powdered sweetener
A pinch of salt

Directions

Preheat oven to 350ºF. Place all ingredients except coconut oil, berries, and powdered sweetener, in a blender; blend until smooth. Gently fold in the berries. Grease a baking dish with the oil. Pour the mixture into the prepared pan and bake for 35 minutes. Sprinkle with powdered sugar to serve.

Lychee and Coconut Lassi

Ready in about: 28 minutes + cooling time | Serves: 4
Per serving: Kcal 285, Fat 26.1g, Net Carbs 1.5g, Protein 5.3g

Ingredients

2 cups lychee pulp, seeded
2 ½ cups coconut milk
4 tsp swerve
2 limes, zested and juiced
1 ½ cups plain yogurt
1 lemongrass, white part only, crushed
Toasted coconut shavings for garnish

Directions

In a saucepan, add the lychee pulp, coconut milk, swerve, lemongrass, and lime zest. Stir and bring to boil on medium heat for 2 minutes, stirring continually. Then reduce the heat, and simmer for 1 minute. Turn the heat off and let the mixture sit for 15 minutes.

Remove the lemongrass and pour the mixture into a smoothie maker or a blender, add the yogurt and lime juice, and process the ingredients until smooth, for about 60 seconds. Pour into a jug and refrigerate for 2 hours until cold; stir. Serve garnished with coconut shavings.

Blackcurrant Iced Tea

Ready in about: 8 minutes | Serves: 4
Per serving: Kcal 22, Fat 0g, Net Carbs 5g, Protein 0g

Ingredients

6 unflavored tea bags
2 cups water
½ cup sugar-free blackcurrant extract
Swerve to taste
Ice cubes for serving
Lemon slices to garnish, cut on the side

Directions

Pour the ice cubes in a pitcher and place it in the fridge.

Bring the water to boil in a saucepan over medium heat for 3 minutes and turn the heat off. Stir in the sugar to dissolve and steep the tea bags in the water for 2 minutes.

Remove the bags after and let the tea cool down. Stir in the blackcurrant extract until well incorporated, remove the pitcher from the fridge, and pour the mixture over the ice cubes.

Let sit for 3 minutes to cool and after, pour the mixture into tall glasses. Add some more ice cubes, place the lemon slices on the rim of the glasses, and serve the tea cold.

White Chocolate Cheesecake Bites

Ready in about: 4 minutes + cooling time | Serves: 12
Per serving: Kcal 241, Fat 22g, Net Carbs 3.1g, Protein 5g

Ingredients

10 oz unsweetened white chocolate chips
½ half and half
20 oz cream cheese, softened
½ cup swerve
1 tsp vanilla extract

Directions

In a saucepan, melt the chocolate with half and a half on low heat for 1 minute. Turn the heat off.

In a bowl, whisk the cream cheese, swerve, and vanilla extract with a hand mixer until smooth. Stir into the chocolate mixture. Spoon into silicone muffin tins and freeze for 4 hours until firm.

Vanilla Chocolate Mousse

Ready in about: 30 minutes | Serves: 4
Per serving: Kcal 370, Fat: 25g, Net Carbs: 3.7g, Protein: 7.6g

Ingredients

3 eggs
1 cup dark chocolate chips
1 cup heavy cream
1 cup fresh strawberries, sliced
1 vanilla extract
1 tbsp swerve

Directions

Melt the chocolate in a bowl, in your microwave for a minute on high, and let it cool for 10 minutes.

Meanwhile, in a medium-sized mixing bowl, whip the cream until very soft. Add the eggs, vanilla extract, and swerve; whisk to combine. Fold in the cooled chocolate. Divide the mousse between four glasses, top with the strawberry slices and chill in the fridge for at least 30 minutes before serving.

Blueberry Ice Pops

Ready in about: 5 minutes + cooling time | Serves: 6
Per serving: Kcal 48, Fat 1.2g, Net Carbs 7.9g, Protein 2.3g

Ingredients

3 cups blueberries
½ tbsp lemon juice
¼ cup swerve
¼ cup water

Directions

Pour the blueberries, lemon juice, swerve, and water in a blender, and puree on high speed for 2 minutes until smooth. Strain through a sieve into a bowl, discard the solids.

Mix in more water if too thick. Divide the mixture into ice pop molds, insert stick cover, and freeze for 4 hours to 1 week. When ready to serve, dip in warm water and remove the pops.

Strawberry Vanilla Shake

Ready in about: 2 minutes | Serves: 4
Per serving: Kcal 285, Fat 22.6g, Net Carbs 3.1g,
Protein 16g

Ingredients

2 cups strawberries, stemmed and halved
12 strawberries to garnish
½ cup cold unsweetened almond milk
2/3 tsp vanilla extract
½ cup heavy whipping cream
2 tbsp swerve

Directions

Process the strawberries, milk, vanilla extract, whipping cream, and swerve in a large blender for 2 minutes; work in two batches if needed . The shake should be frosty.
Pour into glasses, stick in straws, garnish with strawberry halves, and serve.

Cranberry White Chocolate Barks

Ready in about: 5 minutes + cooling time | Serves: 6
Per serving: Kcal 225, Fat 21g, Net Carbs 3g, Protein 6g

Ingredients

10 oz unsweetened white chocolate, chopped
½ cup erythritol
⅓ cup dried cranberries, chopped
⅓ cup toasted walnuts, chopped
¼ tsp pink salt

Directions

Line a baking sheet with parchment paper. Pour chocolate and erythritol in a bowl, and melt in the microwave for 25 seconds, stirring three times until fully melted. Stir in the cranberries, walnuts, and salt, reserving a few cranberries and walnuts for garnishing.
Pour the mixture on the baking sheet and spread out. Sprinkle with remaining cranberries and walnuts. Refrigerate for 2 hours to set. Break into bite-size pieces to serve.

Vanilla Ice Cream

Ready in about: 5 minutes + cooling time | Serves: 4
Per serving: Kcal 290, Fat 23g, Net Carbs 6g, Protein 13g

Ingredients

½ cup smooth peanut butter
½ cup swerve
3 cups half and half
1 tsp vanilla extract
2 pinches salt

Directions

Beat peanut butter and swerve in a bowl with a hand mixer until smooth. Gradually whisk in half and half until thoroughly combined. Mix in vanilla and salt. Pour mixture into a loaf pan and freeze for 45 minutes until firmed up. Scoop into glasses when ready to eat and serve.

Chia and Blackberry Pudding

Ready in about: 10 minutes | Serves: 2
Per serving: Kcal 169, Fat: 10g, Net Carbs: 4.7g,
Protein: 7.5g

Ingredients

1 cup full-fat natural yogurt
2 tsp swerve
2 tbsp chia seeds
1 cup fresh blackberries
1 tbsp lemon zest
Mint leaves, to serve

Directions

Mix together the yogurt and the swerve. Stir in the chia seeds. Reserve 4 blackberries for garnish and mash the remaining ones with a fork until pureed. Stir in the yogurt mixture
Chill in the fridge for 30 minutes. When cooled, divide the mixture between 2 glasses. Top each with a couple of blackberries, mint leaves, lemon zest and serve.

Mint Chocolate Protein Shake

Ready in about: 4 minutes | Serves: 4
Per serving: Kcal 191, Fat 14.5g, Net Carbs 4g,
Protein 15g

Ingredients

3 cups flax milk, chilled
3 tsp unsweetened cocoa powder
1 avocado, pitted, peeled, sliced
1 cup coconut milk, chilled
3 mint leaves + extra to garnish
3 tbsp erythritol
1 tbsp low carb Protein powder
Whipping cream for topping

Directions

Combine the milk, cocoa powder, avocado, coconut milk, mint leaves, erythritol, and protein powder into a blender, and blend for 1 minute until smooth.
Pour into serving glasses, lightly add some whipping cream on top, and garnish with mint leaves.

Almond Butter Fat Bombs

Ready in about: 3 minutes + cooling time | Serves: 4
Per serving: Kcal 193, Fat 18.3g, Net Carbs 2g,
Protein 4g

Ingredients

½ cup almond butter
½ cup coconut oil
4 tbsp unsweetened cocoa powder
½ cup erythritol

Directions

Melt butter and coconut oil in the microwave for 45 seconds, stirring twice until properly melted and mixed. Mix in cocoa powder and erythritol until completely combined. Pour into muffin moulds and refrigerate for 3 hours to harden.

Almond Milk Hot Chocolate

Ready in about: 7 minutes | Serves: 4
Per serving: Kcal 225, Fat 21.5g, Net Carbs 0.6g, Protein 4.5g

Ingredients

3 cups almond milk
4 tbsp unsweetened cocoa powder
2 tbsp swerve
3 tbsp almond butter
Finely chopped almonds to garnish

Directions

In a saucepan, add the almond milk, cocoa powder, and swerve. Stir the mixture until the sugar dissolves. Set the pan over low to heat through for 5 minutes, without boiling.
Swirl the mix occasionally. Turn the heat off and stir in the almond butter to be incorporated. Pour the hot chocolate into mugs and sprinkle with chopped almonds. Serve hot.

Berry Merry

Ready in about: 6 minutes | Serves: 4
Per serving: Kcal 83, Fat 3g, Net Carbs 8g, Protein 2.7g

Ingredients

1 ½ cups blackberries
1 cup strawberries + extra for garnishing
1 cup blueberries
2 small beets, peeled and chopped
2/3 cup ice cubes
1 lime, juiced

Directions

For the extra strawberries for garnishing, make a single deep cut on their sides; set aside.
Add the blackberries, strawberries, blueberries, beet, and ice into the smoothie maker and blend the ingredients at high speed until smooth and frothy, for about 60 seconds.
Add the lime juice, and puree further for 30 seconds. Pour the drink into tall smoothie glasses, fix the reserved strawberries on each glass rim, stick a straw in, and serve the drink immediately.

Coffee Fat Bombs

Ready in about: 3 minutes + cooling time | Serves: 6
Per serving: Kcal 145, Fat 14g, Net Carbs 2g, Protein 4g

Ingredients

1 ½ cups mascarpone cheese
½ cup melted butter
3 tbsp unsweetened cocoa powder
¼ cup erythritol
6 tbsp brewed coffee, room temperature

Directions

Whisk the mascarpone cheese, butter, cocoa powder, erythritol, and coffee with a hand mixer until creamy and fluffy, for 1 minute. Fill into muffin tins and freeze for 3 hours until firm.

Strawberry and Basil Lemonade

Ready in about: 3 minutes | Serves: 4
Per serving: Kcal 66, Fat 0.1g, Net Carbs 5.8g, Protein 0.7g

Ingredients

4 cups water
12 strawberries, leaves removed
1 cup fresh lemon juice
⅓ cup fresh basil
¾ cup swerve
Crushed Ice
Halved strawberries to garnish
Basil leaves to garnish

Directions

Spoon some ice into 4 serving glasses and set aside. In a pitcher, add the water, strawberries, lemon juice, basil, and swerve. Insert the blender and process the ingredients for 30 seconds.
The mixture should be pink and the basil finely chopped. Adjust the taste and add the ice in the glasses. Drop 2 strawberry halves and some basil in each glass and serve immediately.

Mixed Berry Nuts Mascarpone Bowl

Ready in about: 8 minutes | Serves: 4
Per serving: Kcal 480, Fat 40g, Net Carbs 5g, Protein 20g

Ingredients

4 cups Greek yogurt
Liquid stevia to taste
1 ½ cups mascarpone cheese
1 ½ cups blueberries and raspberries
1 cup toasted pecans

Directions

Mix the yogurt, stevia, and mascarpone in a bowl until evenly combined. Divide the mixture into 4 bowls, share the berries and pecans on top of the cream. Serve the dessert immediately.

Mixed Berry Trifle

Ready in about: 3 minutes + cooling time | Serves: 4
Per serving: Kcal 321, Fat 28.5g, Net Carbs 8.3g, Protein 9.8g

Ingredients

½ cup walnuts, toasted
1 avocado, chopped
1 cup mascarpone cheese, softened
1 cup fresh blueberries
1 cup fresh raspberries
1 cup fresh blackberries

Directions

In four dessert glasses, share half of the mascarpone, half of the berries (mixed), half of the walnuts, and half of the avocado, and repeat the layering process for a second time to finish the ingredients. Cover the glasses with plastic wrap and refrigerate for 45 minutes until quite firm.

Walnut Cookies

Ready in about: 15 minutes | Serves: 12
Per serving: Kcal 101, Fat: 11g, Net Carbs: 0.6g,
Protein: 1.6g

1 egg
2 cups ground pecans
¼ cup sweetener
½ tsp baking soda
1 tbsp butter
20 walnuts halves

Preheat oven to 350ºF. Mix the ingredients, except the walnuts, until combined. Make 20 balls out of the mixture and press them with your thumb onto a lined cookie sheet. Top each cookie with a walnut half. Bake for about 12 minutes.

Raspberry Sorbet

Ready in about: 10 minutes + cooling time | Serves: 1
Per serving: Kcal 173, Fat: 10g, Net Carbs: 3.7g,
Protein: 4g

¼ tsp vanilla extract
1 packet gelatine, without sugar
1 tbsp heavy whipping cream
⅓ cup boiling water
2 tbsp mashed raspberries
1 ½ cups crushed Ice
⅓ cup cold water

Combine the gelatin and boiling water, until completely dissolved; then transfer to a blender. Add the remaining ingredients. Blend until smooth and freeze for at least 2 hours.

Cinnamon and Turmeric Latte

Ready in about: 7 minutes | Serves: 4
Per serving: Kcal 132, Fat 12g, Net Carbs 0.3g,
Protein 3.9g

3 cups almond milk
⅓ tsp cinnamon powder
1 cup brewed coffee
½ tsp turmeric powder
1 ½ tsp erythritol
Cinnamon sticks to garnish

In the blender, add the almond milk, cinnamon powder, coffee, turmeric, and erythritol. Blend the ingredients at medium speed for 45 seconds and pour the mixture into a saucepan.
Set the pan over low heat and heat through for 5 minutes; do not boil. Keep swirling the pan to prevent from boiling. Turn the heat off, and serve in latte cups, with a cinnamon stick in each one.

Cinnamon Cookies

Ready in about: 25 minutes | Serves: 4
Per serving: Kcal 134, Fat: 13g, Net Carbs: 1.5g,
Protein: 3g

Cookies:
2 cups almond flour
½ tsp baking soda
¾ cup sweetener
½ cup butter, softened
A pinch of salt
Coating:
2 tbsp erythritol sweetener
1 tsp cinnamon

Preheat oven to 350ºF. Combine all cookie ingredients in a bowl. Make 16 balls out of the mixture and flatten them with hands. Combine the cinnamon and erythritol. Dip the cookies in the cinnamon mixture and arrange them on a lined cookie sheet. Cook for 15 minutes, until crispy.

Creamy Coconut Kiwi Drink

Ready in about: 3 minutes | Serves: 4
Per serving: Kcal 351, Fat 28g, Net Carbs 9.7g,
Protein 16g

5 kiwis, pulp scooped
2 tbsp erythritol
2 cups unsweetened coconut milk
2 cups coconut cream
7 ice cubes
Mint leaves to garnish

In a blender, process the kiwis, erythritol, milk, cream, and ice cubes until smooth, about 3 minutes. Pour into four serving glasses, garnish with mint leaves, and serve.

Coconut Fat Bombs

Ready in about: 2 minutes +cooling time | Serves: 4
Per serving: Kcal 214, Fat 19g, Net Carbs 2g, Protein 4g

2/3 cup coconut oil, melted
1 (14 oz) can coconut milk
18 drops stevia liquid
1 cup unsweetened coconut flakes

Mix the coconut oil with the milk and stevia to combine. Stir in the coconut flakes until well distributed. Pour into silicone muffin molds and freeze for 1 hour to harden.

Vanilla Bean Frappuccino

Ready in about: 6 minutes | Serves: 4
Per serving: Kcal 193, Fat 14g, Net Carbs 6g, Protein 15g

Ingredients

3 cups unsweetened vanilla almond milk, chilled
2 tsp swerve
1 ½ cups heavy cream, cold
1 vanilla bean
¼ tsp xanthan gum
Unsweetened chocolate shavings to garnish

Directions

Combine the almond milk, swerve, heavy cream, vanilla bean, and xanthan gum in the blender, and process on high speed for 1 minute until smooth. Pour into tall shake glasses, sprinkle with chocolate shavings, and serve immediately.

Chocolate Bark with Almonds

Ready in about: 5 minutes + cooling time | Serves: 12
Per serving: Kcal 161, Fat: 15.3g, Net Carbs: 1.9g, Protein: 1.9g

Ingredients

½ cup toasted almonds, chopped
½ cup butter
10 drops stevia
¼ tsp salt
½ cup unsweetened coconut flakes
4 ounces dark chocolate

Directions

Melt together the butter and chocolate, in the microwave, for 90 seconds. Remove and stir in stevia. Line a cookie sheet with waxed paper and spread the chocolate evenly. Scatter the almonds on top, coconut flakes, and sprinkle with salt. Refrigerate for one hour.

Dark Chocolate Mochaccino Ice Bombs

Ready in about: 5 minutes + cooling time | Serves: 4
Per serving: Kcal 127, Fat: 13g, Net Carbs: 1.4g, Protein: 1.9g

Ingredients

½ pound cream cheese
4 tbsp powdered sweetener
2 ounces strong coffee
2 tbsp cocoa powder, unsweetened
1 ounce cocoa butter, melted
2 ½ ounces dark chocolate, melted

Directions

Combine cream cheese, sweetener, coffee, and cocoa powder, in a food processor. Roll 2 tbsp of the mixture and place on a lined tray.
Mix the melted cocoa butter and chocolate, and coat the bombs with it. Freeze for 2 hours.

Raspberry Flax Seed Dessert

Ready in about: 5 minutes | Serves: 4
Per serving: Kcal 390, Fat 33.5g, Net Carbs 3g, Protein 13g

Ingredients

2 cups raspberries, reserve a few for topping
3 cups unsweetened vanilla almond milk
1 cup heavy cream
½ cup chia seeds
½ cup flaxseeds, ground
4 tsp liquid stevia
Chopped mixed nuts for topping

Directions

In a medium bowl, crush the raspberries with a fork until pureed.
Pour in the almond milk, heavy cream, chia seeds, and liquid stevia. Mix and refrigerate the pudding overnight. Spoon the pudding into serving glasses, top with raspberries, mixed nuts, and serve

14-DAY MEAL PLAN TO LOSE UP TO 20 POUNDS

Drink 7 to 9 glasses of water daily

Day	Breakfast	Lunch	Dinner	Dessert/Snacks	Kkal
1	Morning Berry-Green Smoothie	Bacon Wrapped Chicken with Grilled Asparagus	Russian Beef Gratin	Passion Fruit Cheesecake Slices	1,672
2	Duo-Cheese Omelet with Pimienta & Basil	Peanut Butter Pork Stir-fry	Green Mackerel Salad	Berry Tart	1,784
3	Egg Tofu Scramble with Kale & Mushrooms	Parmesan Wings with Yogurt Sauce	Spicy Sea Bass with Hazelnuts	Peanut Butter Ice Cream	1,678
4	Dark Chocolate Smoothie	Chili Turkey Patties with Cucumber Salsa	Grilled Halloumi Cheese with Eggs	Chocolate Bark with Almonds (x2)	1,642
5	Spicy Egg Muffins with Bacon & Cheese	Zoodles with Avocado & Olives	Homemade Classic Beef Burgers	Peanut Butter Ice Cream	1,705
6	Avocado and Kale Eggs	Mexican Beef Chili	One Pot Chicken with Mushrooms	Vanilla Chocolate Mousse	1,628
7	Almond Waffles with Cinnamon	Cheesy Lettuce Rolls	Pumpkin & Meat Peanut Stew	Coconut Fat Bombs (x4)	1,642
8	Giant Egg Quiche	Warm Rump Steak Salad	Blue Cheese Stuffed Peppers	Raspberry Nut Truffles (x2)	1,610
9	Coconut Flour Bagels	Chicken Paella with Chorizo	Strawberry Salad with Spinach, Cheese & Almonds	Chocolate Chip Cookies (x1)	1,801
10	Bacon and Cheese Pesto Mug Cake	Monterrey Jack Cheese Soup	Bianca Pizza	Raspberry Nut Truffles	1,650
11	Chorizo and Mozzarella Omelet	Vegetable Burritos	Chicken Breasts with Cheddar & Pepperoni	Mixed Berry Nuts Mascarpone Bowl	1,691
12	Breakfast Buttered Eggs	Power Green Soup + Devilled Eggs with Sriracha Mayo	Spiced Pork Roast with Collard Greens	Strawberry Vanilla Shake	1,632
13	Morning Almond Shake	Creamy Stuffed Chicken with Parma Ham	Chipotle Pizza with Cotija & Cilantro	Chocolate Cakes (x2)	1,612
14	Chocolate Creps with Caramel Cream	Coconut, Green Beans, and Shrimp Curry Soup	Chicken in Creamy Spinach Sauce	Green Tea Brownies with Macadamia (x2)	1,541

Appendix : Recipes Index

Cheese, Ham and Egg Muffins 129
Cheesy Basil Omelet 123
Cheesy Bites with Turnip Chips 134
Cheesy Cauliflower Bake with Mayo Sauce 115
Cheesy Cauliflower Falafel 89
Cheesy Cauliflower Fritters 117
Cheesy Chicken Bake with Zucchini 42
Cheesy Chicken Fritters with Dill Dip 113
Cheesy Green Bean Crisps 116
Cheesy Lettuce Rolls 120
Cheesy Sausage Quiche 27
Cheesy Turkey and Broccoli Traybake 54
Cheesy Turkey Sausage Egg Muffins 32
Chia and Blackberry Pudding 141
Chicken & Squash Traybake 45
Chicken and Bacon Rolls 53
Chicken and Green Cabbage Casserole 50
Chicken and Zucchini Bake 47
Chicken Breasts with Cheddar & Pepperoni 51
Chicken Breasts with Spinach & Artichoke 53
Chicken Breasts with Walnut Crust 53
Chicken Cauliflower Bake 36
Chicken Creamy Soup 106
Chicken Drumsticks in Tomato Sauce 37
Chicken Garam Masala 40
Chicken Goujons with Tomato Sauce 42
Chicken Gumbo 49
Chicken in Creamy Mushroom Sauce 45
Chicken in Creamy Spinach Sauce 39
Chicken in Creamy Tomato Sauce 43
Chicken in White Wine Sauce 47
Chicken Meatloaf Cups with Pancetta 129
Chicken Paella with Chorizo 36
Chicken Skewers with Celery Fries 42
Chicken Stew with Sun-Dried Tomatoes 52
Chicken Stroganoff 44
Chicken Thighs with Broccoli & Green Onions 52
Chicken Wings with Thyme Chutney 38
Chicken with Anchovy Tapenade 44
Chicken with Asparagus & Root Vegetables 48
Chicken with Green Sauce 49
Chicken with Monterey Jack Cheese 48
Chicken with Parmesan Topping 52
Chicken, Broccoli & Cashew Stir-Fry 37
Chicken, Eggplant and Gruyere Gratin 50
Chili Chicken Breasts Wrapped in Bacon 133
Chili Egg Pickles 128
Chili Turkey Patties with Cucumber Salsa 38
Chipotle Pizza with Cotija & Cilantro 122
Chocolate Bark with Almonds 144
Chocolate Cakes 138
Chocolate Chip Cookies 139
Chocolate Crepes with Caramel Cream 26
Chocolate Marshmallows 136
Chocolate Protein Coconut Shake 30
Chocolate, Yogurt & Egg Muffins 19
Chorizo and Cheese Gofre 129
Chorizo and Mozzarella Omelet 29
Chorizo Egg Balls 133
Chorizo Scotch Eggs 124
Chuck Roast Beef 78
Cilantro & Chili Omelet 131

Cilantro Chicken Breasts with Mayo-Avocado Sauce 34
Cinnamon and Turmeric Latte 143
Cinnamon Cookies 143
Classic Italian Bolognese Sauce 71
Classic Tangy Ratatouille 93
Cobb Egg Salad in Lettuce Cups 106
Cobb Salad with Blue Cheese Dressing 110
Cocoa Nuts Goji Bars 119
Coconut & Walnut Chia Pudding 33
Coconut Bars 139
Coconut Cauliflower & Parsnip Soup 101
Coconut Cheesecake 137
Coconut Chicken Soup 51
Coconut Crab Patties 83
Coconut Curry Mussels 84
Coconut Fat Bombs 143
Coconut Flour Bagels 27
Coconut Ginger Macaroons 115
Coconut, Green Beans & Shrimp Curry Soup 104
Cod in Garlic Butter Sauce 85
Coffee Fat Bombs 142
Colorful Vegan Soup 95
Crabmeat & Cheese Stuffed Avocado 131
Cranberry White Chocolate Barks 141
Cream of Thyme Tomato Soup 103
Cream of Zucchini and Avocado 96
Creamy Almond and Turnip Soup 101
Creamy Cauliflower Soup with Bacon Chips 103
Creamy Cauliflower Soup with Chorizo Sausage 106
Creamy Cheddar Deviled Eggs 130
Creamy Coconut Kiwi Drink 143
Creamy Cucumber Avocado Soup 87
Creamy Hoki with Almond Bread Crust 81
Creamy Pork Chops 64
Creamy Stuffed Chicken with Parma Ham 37
Creamy Vegetable Stew 87
Cremini Mushroom Stroganoff 92
Crêpes with Lemon-Buttery Syrup 126
Crispy Bacon Salad with Mozzarella & Tomato 109
Crispy Chorizo with Cheesy Topping 116
Crispy-Topped Baked Vegetables 100
Crunchy Pork Rind and Zucchini Sticks 114

D

Dark Chocolate Mochaccino Ice Bombs 144
Dark Chocolate Mousse with Stewed Plums 136
Dark Chocolate Smoothie 23
Devilled Eggs with Sriracha Mayo 114
Dill Pickles with Tuna-Mayo Topping 119
Dilled Salmon in Creamy Sauce 85
Duck & Vegetable Casserole 57
Duo-Cheese Chicken Bake 115
Duo-Cheese Omelet with Pimenta and Basil 32

E

Easy Cauliflower Soup 100
Easy Chicken Chili 41
Easy Chicken Meatloaf 50
Easy Vanilla Granola 102
Easy Zucchini Beef Lasagna 68
Egg in a Cheesy Spinach Nests 24

Egg Omelet Roll with Cream Cheese & Salmon 30
Egg Tofu Scramble with Kale & Mushrooms 24
Eggless Strawberry Mousse 139
Eggplant & Tomato Braised Chicken Thighs 35
Eggs & Crabmeat with Creme Fraiche Salsa 31
Eggs in a Mug 127

F

Fall Roasted Vegetables 101
Five Greens Smoothie 23
Fontina Cheese and Chorizo Waffles 31
Fried Chicken Breasts 53
Fried Chicken with Coconut Sauce 46
Fried Tofu with Mushrooms 97

G

Garlic & Ginger Chicken with Peanut Sauce 37
Garlic and Basil Mashed Celeriac 120
Garlic Chicken Salad 109
Garlic Pork Chops with Mint Pesto 65
Garlick & Cheese Turkey Slices 131
Garlicky Bok Choy 99
Garlicky Cheddar Biscuits 117
Garlicky Pork with Bell Peppers 60
Giant Egg Quiche 25
Ginger & Walnut Porridge 133
Gingery Tuna Mousse 128
Goat Cheese Muffins with Ajillo Mushrooms 134
Granny Smith Apple Tart 136
Greek Chicken with Capers 44
Greek Pork with Olives 64
Greek Salad with Poppy Seed Dressing 96
Greek Yogurt & Cheese Alfredo Sauce 126
Greek-Style Zucchini Pasta 99
Green Mackerel Salad 108
Green Minestrone Soup 103
Green Salad with Bacon and Blue Cheese 109
Green Tea Brownies with Macadamia Nuts 139
Grilled Cheese the Keto Way 90
Grilled Chicken Wings 39
Grilled Halloumi Cheese with Eggs 134
Grilled Lamb on Lemony Sauce 80
Grilled Paprika Chicken with Steamed Broccoli 44
Grilled Pork Loin Chops with Barbecue Sauce 58
Grilled Shrimp with Chimichurri Sauce 83
Grilled Sirloin Steak with Sauce Diane 69
Grilled Steak Salad with Pickled Peppers 111

H

Habanero and Beef Balls 71
Habanero Chicken Wings 49
Ham & Egg Broccoli Bake 23
Ham & Egg Mug Cups 125
Ham & Egg Salad 124
Ham and Emmental Eggs 129
Ham and Vegetable Frittata 31
Hashed Zucchini & Bacon Breakfast 29
Herb Cheese Sticks 117
Herb Pork Chops with Raspberry Sauce 59
Herbed Keto Bread 135
Herby Beef & Veggie Stew 77
Herby Chicken Meatballs 45
Homemade Chicken Pizza Calzone 50
Homemade Classic Beef Burgers 73
Homemade Cold Gazpacho Soup 103

Homemade Pizza Crust 122
Hot Pork with Dill Pickles 65

I

Ice Cream Bars Covered with Chocolate 138
Italian Beef Ragout 69
Italian Cakes with Gorgonzola and Salami 133
Italian Sausage Stacks 23
Italian Sausage Stew 76
Italian-Style Chicken Wraps 118
Italian-Style Roasted Butternut Squash and Basil 124

J

Jalapeno Beef Pot Roasted 73
Jamaican Pork Oven Roast 65
Jamon & Queso Balls 130
Juicy Beef Cheeseburgers 131
Juicy Pork Medallions 65

k

Kale Cheese Waffles 102
Kale Frittata with Crispy Pancetta Salad 25
Keto Pizza Margherita 90
Kielbasa and Roquefort Waffles 33

L

Lamb Shashlyk 79
Lamb Stew with Veggies 80
Lemon & Rosemary Chicken in a Skillet 38
Lemon Cauliflower "Couscous" with Halloumi 88
Lemon Cheesecake Mousse 138
Lemon Chicken Bake 46
Lemon Chicken Wings 40
Lemon Garlic Shrimp 84
Lemon Pork Chops with Buttered Brussels
Sprouts 60
Lemon Threaded Chicken Skewers 36
Lemony Fried Artichokes 120
Lobster Salad with Mayo Dressing 107
Lychee and Coconut Lassi 140

M

Mascarpone & Vanilla Breakfast Cups 28
Mascarpone Snapped Amaretti Biscuits 113
Meatballs and Squash Pasta 20
Mediterranean Cheese Balls 124
Mediterranean Salad 106
Mexican Beef Chili 75
Mexican-Style Frittata 123
Mini Egg Muffins 134
Mint Chocolate Protein Shake 141
Mixed Berry Nuts Mascarpone Bowl 142
Mixed Berry Trifle 142
Mixed Roast Vegetables 116
Mocha Mug Cake 20
Monterey Jack Cheese Soup 124
Morning Almond Shake 30
Morning Berry-Green Smoothie 22
Morning Coconut Smoothie 98
Morning Granola 100
Mozzarella & Prosciutto Wraps 119
Mushroom & Cauliflower Bake 102
Mushroom & Cheese Lettuce Wraps 28
Mushroom & Jalapeño Stew 99
Mustard-Lemon Beef 72
Mustardy Pork Chops 64

Spicy Cheese Chips 128
Spicy Chicken Cucumber Bites 115
Spicy Chicken Kabobs 39
Spicy Devilled Eggs with Herbs 119
Spicy Egg Muffins with Bacon & Cheese 23
Spicy Eggs with Turkey Ham 126
Spicy Mesquite Pork Ribs 61
Spicy Sea Bass with Hazelnuts 81
Spicy Spinach Pinwheel Steaks 67
Spicy Tofu with Worcestershire Sauce 96
Spinach & Ricotta Stuffed Chicken Breasts 51
Spinach and Ricotta Gnocchi 121
Spinach Chicken Cheesy Bake 34
Spinach Frittata with Chorizo & Tomato Salad 20
Spinach Turnip Salad with Bacon 111
Spring Salad with Cheese Balls 110
Squid Salad with Mint, Cucumber & Chili Dressing 110
Sriracha Egg Salad with Mustard Dressing 110
Sriracha Tofu with Yogurt Sauce 90
Sticky Cranberry Chicken Wings 43
Strawberry and Basil Lemonade 142
Strawberry Salad with Spinach, Cheese & Almonds 109
Strawberry Vanilla Shake 141
Stuffed Avocados with Chicken 53
Stuffed Chicken Breasts with Cucumber Noodle Salad 41
Stuffed Cremini Mushrooms 92
Stuffed Mushrooms with Chicken 48
Stuffed Pork with Red Cabbage Salad 61
Stuffed Portobello Mushrooms 94
Sushi Shrimp Rolls 83
Sweet Chipotle Grilled Ribs 67
Sweet Garlic Chicken Skewers 35
Swiss Chard Pesto Scrambled Eggs 121
Swiss-Style Italian Sausage 65

T

Tasty Cauliflower Dip 100
Thai Beef with Shiitake Mushrooms 77
Three-Cheese Fondue with Walnuts and Parsley 132
Thyme & Wild Mushroom Soup 106
Thyme Chicken Thighs 41
Tilapia with Olives & Tomato Sauce 84
Tofu Sandwich with Cabbage Slaw 87
Tofu Sesame Skewers with Warm Kale Salad 89
Tofu Stir Fry with Asparagus 99
Tomato Stuffed Avocado 97
Traditional Greek Salad 108
Traditional Spinach and Feta Frittata 30
Trout and Fennel Parcels 81
Tuna & Monterey Jack Stuffed Avocado 125
Tuna Caprese Salad 107
Tuna Salad with Lettuce & Olives 107

Tuna Steaks with Shirataki Noodles 82
Turkey & Cheese Stuffed Mushrooms 54
Turkey & Leek Soup 56
Turkey & Mushroom Bake 57
Turkey Breast Salad 56
Turkey Burgers with Fried Brussels Sprouts 55
Turkey Enchilada Bowl 54
Turkey Fajitas 56
Turkey Pastrami & Mascarpone Cheese Pinwheels 117
Turkey Stew with Salsa Verde 56
Turkey, Coconut and Kale Chili 57

V

Vanilla Bean Frappuccino 144
Vanilla Chocolate Mousse 140
Vanilla Flan with Mint 138
Vanilla Ice Cream 141
Vanilla-Coconut Cream Tart 127
Veal Stew 79
Vegan Cheesy Chips with Tomatoes 96
Vegan Mushroom Pizza 91
Vegetable Burritos 92
Vegetable Greek Mousaka 86
Vegetable Tempeh Kabobs 86
Vegetable Tempura 93
Vegetarian Burgers 93
Venison Tenderloin with Cheese Stuffing 79

W

Walnut Cookies 143
Walnut Tofu Sauté 92
Walnuts with Tofu 101
Warm Baby Artichoke Salad 109
Warm Rump Steak Salad 69
White Chocolate Cheesecake Bites 140
White Wine Lamb Chops 80
Wild Mushroom and Asparagus Stew 92
Winter Veal and Sauerkraut 79

Y

Yummy Chicken Nuggets 45

Z

Zesty Frittata with Roasted Chilies 91
Zesty Ginger Pancakes with Lemon Sauce 26
Zesty Grilled Chicken 52
Zoodle, Bacon, Spinach, and Halloumi Gratin 63
Zoodles with Avocado & Olives 97
Zucchini Boats 99
Zucchini Boats with Beef and Pimiento Rojo 67
Zucchini Gratin with Feta Cheese 115
Zucchini Lasagna with Ricotta and Spinach 87
Zucchini Parmesan Chips with Greek Yogurt Dip 18
Zucchini Spaghetti with Turkey Bolognese Sauce 40
Zucchini with Blue Cheese and Walnuts 131

CPSIA information can be obtained
at www.ICGtesting.com
Printed in the USA
BVHW082211220321
603179BV00002B/157